Diabetes
An Answer to My Prayer
(JUST NOT THE ONE I WAS LOOKING FOR)

BY GERARD GARDNER

Diabetes: An Answer to My Prayer (Just Not The One I Was Looking For)
Publishing ❦ G. Gardner Publications
San Clemente, California/Virginia Beach, VA
Permission Requests ❦ inquiry@diabetesanswerbook.com
Web: www.diabetesanswerbook.com

Editor ❦ Mena Valiket
Assistant Editor ❦ Charmaine Rosenfield
Design & Layout ❦ Scott Mosher (www.theambientmind.com)

Copyright ©2015 by Gerard Gardner. All rights reserved.
ISBN-13: 978-1492358930 ❦ ISBN-10: 1492358932

This book or parts thereof may not be reproduced in any form, stored in a retrieval system or transmitted in any form by any means - electronic, mechanical, photocopy, recording or otherwise- without prior written permission of the publisher, except as provided by United States copyright law.

Limit of Liability / Disclaimer of Warranty: The Publisher and the Author make no representations or warranties with respect to the accuracy or completeness of the contents of this work and specifically disclaim all warranties, including without limitation warranties of fitness for a particular purpose. No warranty may be created or extended by the ideas, concepts, and / or opinions expressed herein. The advice and strategies contained herein may not be suitable for every situation. This work is sold with the understanding that the Publisher and /or Author are not engaged in rendering medical, legal, or other professional advice or services. If professional assistance is required, the services of a competent professional person should be sought. Neither the Publisher nor the Author shall be liable for damages arising herefrom. The fact that an individual, organization, or website is referred to in this work as a citation and / or potential source of further information does not mean that the Author or the Publisher endorses the information dispensed by the respective entities referenced above unless such an endorsement is expressly stated in the work. Furthermore, any opinions expressed by the Author in this work are purely the opinions of the Author and cannot be attributed to or be deemed to be held any individual or entity referenced within this work. Further, readers should be aware that websites listed in this work may have changed or disappeared between when this work was written and when it was read.

dedications

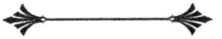

Charmaine and Mena.

Marguerite and Suzy, Alex, Andrew, Austin, and Renee.

Carmen, Jeannie, Claire, Jone, Anne Marie, Christina, and Antonio, Joanie B, Courtney, John C., Emmett (Dr. Em and his child bride Merle), Mick (Mickey Nine-toes), Beatrix, Michael, Dave M., Deidre, Deanna, James J., Sean M. and Eric W., Kathy and Bob (in memoriam of Bob).

There aren't proper words to adequately describe the impacts made on my life by these individuals. Some through even the tiniest of considerations, yet whether small or huge, consistent or just once or twice, the timing of their outreach and kindness made all the difference in the world to me.

First and foremost are my kids, who literally held my life in their hands and in their hearts. There were times when my outlook was so bleak that death in any form would have been a welcome relief; but what kept me alive was their love and my commitment to leaving them with a legacy that didn't include my giving up, ever. But had they not loved me or instead chose to reject me, I could never have found the strength to move ahead.

I have many thanks to give to my sisters who never abandoned me after all these years. Suzy and Marguerite gave me so much encouragement early on in this book, but a special thanks goes to Charmaine who became my second editor and did such an incredible job of guiding me while putting the right finishing touches on this book. She too gave me such incredible inspiration and helped me to stay on course so I could see it through.

And as I count these blessings in my life, right up there with my family is Mena, my editor. Thanks to her dedication and skillful insights, she helped me shape this into what it has become. Words can't express my thanks for her sacrifices to make this happen, something for which I'll be forever grateful.

Not least are Bob and Kathy, to whom I owe my life. Thank you.

To everyone else whose names are listed above, you are there because you helped me at those times when I needed a friend. You are the people who make the world a far better place because you are in it, and I thank you for that and for letting me be a part of your lives.

table of contents

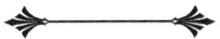

A PERSONAL JOURNEY

Introduction 1
Chapter 01 ❧ Out of Control..................................7
Chapter 02 ❧ The Early Years................................32
Chapter 03 ❧ California: Part 1 64
Chapter 04 ❧ California: Part 2 89
Chapter 05 ❧ The Corporate Ladder 112
Chapter 06 ❧ The Unhealthy Years...........................148
Chapter 07 ❧ The Road to Recovery..........................176
Chapter 08 ❧ How Diabetes Got Me on the Right Road 204

DIABETES

Chapter 09 ❧ What is Diabetes?.............................237
Chapter 10 ❧ Stress and Depression 262
Chapter 11 ❧ Myths, Misinformation, Medications, and Lawsuits:
             All About Diabetes 289
Chapter 12 ❧ Diabetes and the ACA:
             The Politics of Healthcare 308

BOOKENDS

Chapter 13 ❧ Introspection and the Next Steps 325
Bibliography 331

introduction

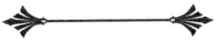

When I submitted my first draft so a friend of a friend could share his thoughts I wasn't too surprised at his initial assessment. He read the first few chapters then commented that he didn't really know what this book was going to deliver. He wasn't sure what to expect or what the average reader should expect. His comments were fair and appreciated, but he wasn't telling me anything I didn't know. In truth, I didn't know what to expect because I was chronicling events in my life that led me to a disease I really knew nothing about. I learned as I went but I had no idea how the story would end.

The more I learned, the more I wanted out of the circumstances I was dealing with, like my long term unemployment and a very ugly divorce, yet external forces were keeping me in a place where I couldn't see a way out. I really didn't know until the last chapter if I was going to survive it all. It wasn't just the disease I needed to survive, but would I be able to survive the dark clouds that kept surrounding me? I had already thought seriously about suicide; and once you think too deeply about taking your own life you've already accepted the ugly truth. When this happens, the threshold to actually doing it becomes much easier to cross.

"Enough!" he said. Now this was no ordinary friend of a friend. This person happened to be a world renowned expert on the disease, and from everything I'd seen and heard about him he's a champion of life itself.

"You need to give the reader a break," he said firmly, yet almost in exasperation. He was right of course, but the point he was missing was that I was the one who needed a break. And the source of his frustration, those parts of my life in print, was only a fraction of what really happened to me and continued to happen with very little relief.

At times it often boiled down to just two options, at least in my view: suicide or writing this book. Obviously I chose the latter, and it gave me a chance to look back at all that I had done then see what I still have left to do. Some of what I accomplished over the years was grand, some stupid, and some even exciting.

As I was completing this manuscript I had no place where I could provide a home for my youngest son and me to live together, for him at least fifty percent of the time since I have joint custody. That is what hit me the hardest, since I only got to spend time with him every other weekend if his schedule permitted. My son revealed to me that his mother forced him to skip holidays with me, ignoring the fact that he wanted to spend the time with me and also ignoring that I had a legal right to spend that time with him.

So yes, I wanted a break and more important than that, I wanted a life with my son and there's no question that the emotions I was battling to keep in check often took hold and at times clouded my perspectives. It's hard to feel light and free when it seems like everyone in the world around you is against you. Yet being able to find peace is a critical component to gaining the control needed to manage this deadly disease.

But it wasn't only a messy divorce that kept me in this ugly situation. I was unemployed and broke in a lousy economy and could barely find work to survive. After sending out more than six thousand resumes since finding out my contract position with the government was ending, I landed nine interviews and got two offers that I couldn't take because they were commission only and required upfront investments. I also got four contract positions that I did take but they started and ended within the same year. I lived below the poverty level and had few prospects. Fortunately and miraculously there were people around me who didn't lose faith in me. That proved to be a very bright spot in what could have been an even darker existence.

Eventually I got to see little breaks in the onslaught of disappointments in applying for hundreds of jobs that gave me a little relief. I went through months without knowing how the money was going to come in while dealing with the humiliation that came with it. Worse, because I had no steady income I had to go without health insurance for nearly three years and the stress of everything going on around me eventually undid all of the headway I had made toward getting healthy.

The breaks eventually got bigger until I began to see a clearer path where I could finally set goals for my financial and physical health. I even managed to finally start my real estate and insurance brokerage in the process, though over three years later than I had planned. I also have to credit the persistence and dedication of my editor who had my back while I was bouncing in and out of the turmoil.

But enough of me talking about me, now it's time to talk about my book. Just what is it really all about, and why does it matter? In short, it's a story about an average guy who started out healthy then took his life and health for granted and later ended up with a deadly disease. And it's about a disease that scared the hell out of me and finally made me sit up and take notice of the path I had taken, a path that was leading toward an untimely death. But when you look at the statistics, you'll see that I'm not alone.

In 2007 the National Diabetes Information Clearinghouse (NDIC) reported that 17 million Americans alone were diabetic and 39 million more were pre-diabetic. By 2010, that statistic changed to 25.6 million diabetics with 79 million Americans in pre-diabetic stages. And while talking to others who had this disease including some of my friends and colleagues, I found that they knew very little about it and how they got there.

This book is about knowing that simple changes in lifestyles and habits can help to reverse the path to this disease. It's also about how to be a survivor. If you were to look up the subject of diabetes, you'll find all sorts of information by experts and sufferers-turned experts, and the information is indeed very valuable. But the crux of it all boils down to some simple basics, at least for type 2 diabetes which is the most common and often brought about by poor lifestyle habits. The bottom line for those of us seeking information is this: Diabetes is bad and often deadly. In fact it is the seventh leading cause of death in the U.S., not to mention the other serious diseases connected to it. The best way to survive it and possibly send it into dormancy is to lose weight, eat right, and live healthy by getting plenty of rest and exercise.

I'm not diminishing the information or any of the authors in any way whatsoever, especially since the expert information you'll find in this book comes from many of those resources in a digest format. And while we're on the subject of experts, make no mistake here. I am no expert when it comes to this disease or anything else related to it. Not hardly, and that's why I chose to write this. This book is for those of you who might be just like me or my group of friends who were living their lives in what seemed like a normal existence and then one day learned they had this disease. What I found through this process saved my life, but whether or not it could help you save your life is up to you and the disease itself. There are no guarantees when it comes to any disease, but paying attention and doing the right things after getting diabetes can only help.

This book is also about overcoming the fear of having the disease and how you can use it to help you.

I've structured this project in a simple way. The first section of the book, chapters 1 through 8 cover my life to show how I went from being very healthy to how over time I started to develop some unhealthy patterns that led me to high blood pressure, heart problems, and finally to type 2 diabetes. Chapters 6 and 7 are the darkest chapters because they deal with the hardships I went through and calculated attacks by my ex-wife which caused me the most difficulties. To the average person, it might seem like I'm choosing to blame her for my ailments and while there is plenty of blame to go around there is a much bigger picture to be gained from those chapters. As you will see in later chapters, Stress and Depression are major factors in poor health, and Chapters 6 and 7 show the kind of stress that led me to and kept me afflicted with the deadly conditions I still have to live with each day.

The second section of the book, chapters 9 through 12 covers the disease itself, how I managed it, and where I went to learn about it. It also covers some of the misinformation that is out there and highlights the value of doing your homework when researching the consequences of diabetes.

Finally, Chapter 13 brings about some of the victories that I managed to achieve along the way. In some cases they might seem subtle but to me they're not. Stress, depression, and poor life choices brought me to a place where not only did I almost die more than once, I was actually welcoming death. The welcome mat I was laying out though got pulled back once I realized just what was really happening. Part of what I learned was how the disease could bring on things that frankly were worse than death, especially given my living situation. The rotten and very difficult circumstances I was dealing with put me in a life-laboratory to test how I could adapt to and survive those events while managing my multiple diseases often without having access to medications.

This was important for me because those same situations along with my inability and unwillingness to deal with them in the past are what led me to actually contract the disease. But now it's different, those circumstances force me to look at my health much more closely. I still have much to fix, but the strides I've made since knowing how this disease could impact me were tremendous because I have no other choices. This is where it shows how having the disease saved my life, because back when I had choices I never cared enough to try and help myself. But now I do.

I have a lot of work left to do but for now this part of the journey is over. The fact that I learned to care enough in order to fix myself is significant, and since I now have more successes than failures when dealing with the disease I have new hope.

As strange as this will seem, getting this disease really was an answer to my prayer. Back in my darkest moments, I prayed for a few very important things, and not least of which was to get healthy, fit, and lose a lot of weight. What I really had in mind when I prayed was winning the lottery so I'd have nothing to do all day but work out, of course for that to happen I'd actually have to start playing the lottery.

In retrospect, if the prayer was answered that way, it never would have changed the person that I was and I probably would have been worse off than before. Getting hit with diabetes and its consequences forced me to decide if I truly wanted to live or die, and how I was going to choose to live. It was scary at first, but now I know I never would have had the incentive to move ahead had I not been forced to make those choices. I hope and pray that you too will find some hope in what you're facing, or at the very least I hope you'll find some inspiration here and have a little fun and adventure in the process.

ONE

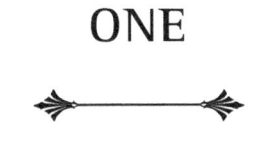

Out Of Control

*Two things define you. Your Patience when you have nothing,
And your Attitude when you have everything.*

- Author Unknown

It had only been ten months since I was seconds away from taking my own life when a colleague and I were talking; what started as a solicitation for opinion about my nearly-complete mystery novel manuscript digressed into the disaster that had become my life. Joel said, "Forget the mystery, the real story is what you just told me. That's what you ought to be writing."

So I began writing a story that was going to be about my life in review, but not long after I started it I learned that I had diabetes. Diabetes was a very unwelcome addition to the high blood pressure and heart disease that I already had and wasn't doing a good job at managing either of them. I decided to research the disease so I would know what I was up against and what I learned scared the hell out of me. I got scared for good reason.

Diabetes can be managed and doesn't mean you have to give up your life, or rather it doesn't mean that you have to give up the good parts. But here's the rub: If you choose not to manage it and avoid fixing what's wrong, it will become an ugly, devastating disease. Once I knew what I was up against, I realized I had some life changing choices to make, but in order to do that I took an inventory of how I got there in the first place.

I'm sure my story isn't unique. I lost a fortune to the fallout from the real estate and mortgage mess. It left millions of lives in ruins including mine and my family's. At the time, it was almost commonplace to turn on the news and hear about people who lost hope because of their financial losses, even committing suicide since they didn't know where else to turn. I almost became one of those news items.

Rags to Riches to Rags

Before I became a career mortgage banking executive, I struggled financially for the first three or four years while developing my expertise and client base in the mortgage industry. I'm traditional and conservative, and while my three kids were little I was happy that my wife wanted to stay home to take care of them. It gave them the security they needed and my wife cared for them well. It always bothered me when I saw parents take their kids in to daycare when the kids were sick but not sick enough to be turned away from daycare. Sometimes I would see little kids who were obviously feeling rotten and who just wanted to stay in bed and be cared for but had to go to daycare because their parents couldn't afford to take the time off to be with them. I didn't want that to happen to my kids. But there were trade-offs for mom staying at home. Things were really tough because my income was based upon commission with a small advance each month; there were days when we just didn't know how we would survive financially. As my expertise grew so did my income and our financial struggles became less intense.

I got a big break when Myrna, one of my fiercest competitors, had her boss Chuck recruit me so that I would be out of her territory and eliminated as her competition. I didn't mind because it was a great company. I welcomed the new challenge, and they offered a salary and benefits in addition to a great commission plan. Within six months I was Myrna's boss and in less than two years I was promoted to vice president with a six-figure salary plus bonus and commission. I worked at Home Savings of America, a Fortune 500 Savings and Loan so the promotion was significant, and of course I let it go to my head.

Even though the many years of struggling taught us to live modestly, we bought a very nice house with a payment that was triple our previous rent. Two months after buying it, I got the announcement that Home Savings had been acquired by Washington Mutual, a major competitor. Within eight months I was out of a job.

It wasn't all bad news though. As an officer with a golden parachute, I received a generous severance package when the sale of the company was completed. I remained cocky, and in fact was so cocky that I blew a great job offer over my arrogance and stupidity. That cockiness led to a downward spiral because I wasn't able to find work until nearly nine months later. When I did finally land a job with a mortgage division of an automobile company, the pay was so low that I had to pay most of our monthly expenses with what was left of my severance money. We reached a point of desperation that led us nearly to foreclosure.

Most of us have heard about pride coming before a fall, well I can tell you it is true. Once we started heading downward, my pride went right out the window and I was humbled in a way that I never had before in my entire working life. It also sent me into an emotional place where I kept taking it out on myself. I didn't eat right, stopped exercising and stayed up all hours of the night watching TV. I started praying and made a commitment that if I got a big salary I would pay our house off and we'd live within our means.

Incredibly, I got a call from a recruiter with whom I had worked before. A company that shot me down a year earlier was ready to hire me as a vice president. The company was a division of Chase Manhattan and was a Fortune 100 bank with income potential that was even better than when I was with Home Savings, so I was very interested to say the least.

Even though I had been so humble when asking for this good fortune to come my way, it wasn't long before I became cocky again. But this time I wasn't so stupid as to make the same mistakes that would keep me from being hired.

My income was higher than it had ever been, yet it didn't stop me from looking for ways to double it. I forgot the commitment I had made out loud should I find good fortune again. Instead of being smart with what I had, I focused on getting more. Recruited by another Fortune 100 bank for a position that paid triple what I was making at Chase, I soon focused on how quickly I could pass seven figures a year like some of my friends were already doing. The stress of the new job was intense and it started taking me down a very unhealthy path, but I wasn't paying attention and was more cocky and more arrogant than ever.

In order to get the new job I committed to relocating my family to a new and very expensive county, Orange County, California. Instead of buying a nice house that we could pay off in a few years, we bought a custom home in Coto de Caza which was the original setting for the Rich Housewives of Orange County reality series. The $100,000 down payment it only took six months to save would have been a nice down payment on a more modest home closer to the beach, but it was a small down on the home we did buy. Even though we could have afforded to keep our first home in Rancho, which was a great home that we could have paid off in a couple of years, I sold it anyway proving once again that I hadn't gotten any smarter.

It took a few years, but things really started going downhill and we waited too long to take steps to avoid the disaster that was heading our way. At the very least we could have sold the Coto house while the market was high. Although we put little money down in the beginning, the market value had increased giving us about $400,000 in net equity had we sold it at the right time. My income had dropped from about $600,000 a year to $200,000 and getting lower. If my wife would have had her real estate license as she promised, we could have pocketed up to about another $80,000 in commission on top of the equity. And had we been smarter, we would have sold and then waited for the market to cool down so we could pay cash for something more modest.

It would have been so smart if I would have paid off our Rancho home then sold the Coto house then when times got really tough we could have moved back to Rancho with about $450,000 in the bank and lived comfortably. But it takes brains, humility, and not much of an ego to have that much sense, none of which applied to me.

My three kids attended private Christian schools all their lives and were caught up in the wealth; and they, along with my wife became very spoiled. There wasn't a single need they had that I wouldn't accommodate. My wife sat around complaining all the time about how unhappy she was. I'd offer to send her and a friend or her sister on trips that she might enjoy like to Hawaii or New York but she never would do it. I'd buy her day spa pamperings and gave her unlimited spending out of our account. She had freedom to do whatever she wanted; no questions asked but always had reasons for not wanting to do anything. I'd book us great vacations and all she would do was complain about them. So I would ask her to book some for us but she never would.

My kids were a little easier to please, but they had their issues too. I bought them some really cool jet skis which we all had a blast on, but often when I'd buy them something they'd complain that somebody had something better. So the $600 guitar wasn't as good as the $1,000 guitar that an acquaintance had, and it didn't get taken care of as a result. Each kid had their own computer but I constantly had to fix or replace them because of the viruses they'd download. The private school they went to had a lot of snooty people in it, and frankly I was an arrogant bastard so I fit right in.

In order to keep making more and more money I traded comfort and common sense for daily doses of intense stress. Imagine if you will, making on average about $50,000 per month, with my biggest monthly check at just over $300,000, but going to bed each night wishing I would die in my sleep because the pressure at work and home was unbearable.

My weight ballooned and I had eight prescription medicines to take each day just to stay alive. I was taking drugs for cholesterol, high blood pressure, and heart disease. I was dealing with skin problems and was supposed to be taking drugs for depression, but I skipped that one.

I put a lot of money in the bank as part of the lessons I learned from our previous struggles, but I put more into spending and bad investments.

I lived in the present and became even more arrogant as a way to detract from my excessive weight. Financially, we were living a very good life but the rest of our household was a disaster on moral, physical, and spiritual planes. My wife and I would talk about our financial future but we continued to live in the present. When we talked, I shared my worry of how exposed we were because of market conditions and because my income was based on the productivity of a handful of high powered sales people on my staff and the real estate market in general. I knew the risk was great because my team was highly visible on a national scale and were prime recruiting targets for the competition. Because I had the knowledge I was taking steps to guard against it, but I failed to take the right ones.

As a result, I made the wrong investments while my sales team was raided by the competition. Then the market went into a free fall. My income dropped by 90 percent and the businesses I invested in died as well. It was two years before I found steady work again but only after I circulated about 1,200 resumes and gone through countless disappointments and rejections. We cleaned out all of our savings, stocks, and retirement funds to try and save our house, and each time I received a job offer the company would go out of business before I could report to work.

The Darkest Moments

After almost two years of constant disappointment and rejection, I finally lost all confidence in myself and my ability to do anything productive. It was the first time in my professional life that I realized how hard it was going to be for me to find a job. My career in mortgage lending and real estate made me unmarketable in the job market, because many blamed people in those fields for the downturn the economy was taking. A local newspaper ran a front page story about how employers getting resumes from former lenders and realtors were just tossing them in the trash no matter how good they were in their last jobs. In addition to that I had to come to grips with how my age of over 50, excessive weight, and lengthy unemployment from having been out of work for nearly eighteen months also were deterrents for prospective employers. I didn't interview well anymore. I didn't have the confidence I used to have because of how I looked and because of my circumstances.

I lost hope. I could only see the worst, and I thought God was punishing me for my stupidity and arrogance. And if He was, frankly I felt I deserved it. Once I hit that point, I couldn't see an end to the hardship.

I tried to take any job anywhere doing anything I could think of: night accounting at some hotels and motels, I tried warehouses, writing jobs, and sales, just anything that came up with any potential. Trying for jobs in- and out-of-state, I completely dumbed down my resume to exclude that I was a former corporate executive, instead highlighting my years in the steel business but still couldn't generate interest anywhere.

The only people who called me were bill collectors and they were getting nastier. Just before one Thanksgiving, seventeen certified copies of Notices of Default were delivered to our house. One is scary enough, but this company really was bent on taking our home. I can't even begin to explain the flurry of emotions going on inside of me and the deep, deep depression it caused.

I read in the newspaper that the CEO of one of my former companies had been hired to rescue a well-known bank that was also in trouble because of the mortgage crisis. I had had a good relationship with Robert and after discussing the situation with Chuck, one of my former bosses who was close to Robert; it looked like I was going to be able to get an interview but needed to wait about sixty days so Robert could get settled.

Excited, I started to see a faint glimmer of light in the darkness. I marked the calendar based upon Chuck's time frame for me to meet with Robert and I prepped for the interview. Weeks passed until the time finally came to make the appointment, but just a few days before I was going to make the call, I read in the news that the FDIC had been appointed receiver of that bank and Robert was removed to make way for the new bank that took it over.

I was stunned. Until that point, I was holding out hope that I might be able to save my house, that once I secured employment and had steady funds to work with I could negotiate with our mortgage holder to begin a restructured payment plan, at least temporarily. After seeing the news, I had nothing to look forward to. No end to our situation in sight. I had continued sending out resumes meanwhile, but I got no responses and things just looked bleaker and bleaker.

Around the same time I was seeing more and more news stories of fathers who were faced with what I was facing and killing themselves because they couldn't take it any longer. I was supposed to keep taking medications for my heart and blood pressure but I stopped and subconsciously put myself in a self-destruct mode. I was only sleeping a few hours a night and my eating and life habits were getting even worse than before.

Each time I looked at myself, I could only see what a tremendous burden I had become to my family because I couldn't earn a living. I kept thinking about the life insurance we had that would solve their financial problems if I were to die. Since the suicide clause had expired, I didn't have to worry about them getting the payout. With me out of the picture they would have money enough to start over and one less fat mouth to feed. Grappling with these thoughts daily, and each time a bill collector called or an employment application was rejected I got a little bit closer to it. I tried everything including collecting unemployment, which I hadn't done earlier because I never thought I would need it.

While I was looking for any job I could find, I decided to use my professional experience to get a real estate license and an insurance license. I knew the market dynamic had changed and since I had over 20 years in finance and real estate I decided to try and hedge my bets so I could try to make a living by being self-employed.

I managed to get a short term contract with Citi Group in their mortgage division while I was getting my licenses and right after the contract ended and the division shut down, I started a real estate and insurance brokerage. I didn't file for unemployment because I already had about $100,000 in potential commissions in escrow. But the loan money for the buyers dried up and those transactions died which means I didn't get to cash in on those commissions. And despite paying hundreds of thousands of taxes into the system, I wasn't eligible to receive unemployment by the time I applied for it because I waited too long.

My sister-in-law sent me a link to a job opportunity for which I had no enthusiasm, not because I wasn't qualified but because it was a lengthy, cumbersome application process and I couldn't take one more rejection. But I'm not the kind of guy to play victim either, especially since it concerned my family's well-being. So somewhere I found the energy and fortitude to apply for different positions where I thought I might have a shot. But I was applying for positions that I was either over-qualified for like a file clerk, or to positions to which I had no clue of what they entailed, like a Resolutions & Receivership Specialist. I applied to a total of five. Four were rejected which to me was par for the course because of the countless rejections I had already been through. Even though I should have been used to it by now, the rejections still took their tolls. Miraculously I got a call to interview for the fifth one which was a Resolutions & Receivership Specialist in Claims and got a small emotional boost. But I still wasn't very encouraged because I had gone through other interviews that amounted to nothing.

To my surprise I received a conditional offer less than a week after interviewing. The annual salary offered was slightly above what I used to make in a single month, but I was so desperate for a job that it just didn't matter. I was thrilled. When I went in to start the paperwork, the offer was put on hold due to my credit problems. Because the position was in public trust, I had to go under a special security review to determine if my credit problems were something I caused or if there was any fraud involved.

Two months went by before I finally got the courage to start looking into what was happening with the security review. I reached out to the FDIC and I asked Congressman Ken Calvert's office for help in any way they could. I also asked Senator Diane Feinstein's office since she had sent some generic request to my wife asking for her support on something.

About two weeks later it all hit the fan. Congressman Calvert's office let us know that they were able to make an inquiry on our behalf and thought we should be hearing from the special security group fairly soon. That Friday the group let me know that due to my specific circumstances they had to go to a higher authority and it was impossible to say if I would even get approved much less get hired the following week.

That answer shredded the tiniest bit of wishful thinking that I managed to muster throughout the process. It sunk me so low into depression that I sent a written response acknowledging that I would not be working there and thanking them for their time and for the opportunity because I just assumed they weren't going to hire me.

The security packet that I originally sent in two months prior was proof that my credit problems were due entirely to circumstances well beyond my control. I had had many opportunities to lie, cheat, steal, and game the system; all of which might have helped me to preserve some of my credit or even save my house. But I didn't do any of it; I stuck to the high road and accepted the consequences despite having paid hundreds of thousands of dollars in taxes only a few years before.

Managing to get only a few hours of sleep that weekend, Monday morning I was numb and emotionally strung out. It was ironic that a job could have helped me save my credit, but my credit was keeping me from getting a job. I was desperate. It was clear suicide was the only way for me to provide some income for my family. It seemed clear to me God wanted me out of the picture because of what a bad, worthless person I was.

I spent most of the morning with those thoughts hammering at me, and was entertaining the methods of suicide that were available to me. By noon, I had narrowed it down to two. My house was near a mountainous highway, treacherous because of cliffs that, if approached at high speeds, could usually ensure instant death. Option two was to drink some drain cleaner in large quantities. I knew that death would not be immediate but was confident that the local hospital would give me painkillers until the end came.

The mail came while I was still deciding. There were the usual bill collection notices and threats in addition to a letter from Diane Feinstein's office rejecting my request for help. Amazing how many deals she was reported to cut for her husband's companies while she served on the Appropriations Committee, but she couldn't even take the time to make a simple inquiry on behalf of a desperate person with a legitimate need. Then I looked at myself from her perspective; I was broke and certainly not in a position to contribute to her campaign and therefore was obviously of very little value to her. I was also a registered Republican, no doubt making me even less appealing.

Next was the letter from the employment office rejecting my application for assistance because I had been unemployed for too long. A third letter notified us that our house had been foreclosed on and we had to move out. But the letter was from a realtor and not from the bank. How could that be?

I had sent the mortgage holder a proposal in which I would leave the house voluntarily if they would allow us to market it for just a little while at a reduced price so we wouldn't be out in the street. A small commission would have given us some money for a security deposit on a rental. They never responded to my proposal and the real time tax rolls showed that we still owned the house, so as far as I knew the proposal was still under consideration. I was at a loss as to what to believe.

Even though it didn't seem real at the time, I realized that a foreclosure was inevitable now that I had no job prospects. And if that string of bad news wasn't enough, the trash hauler confiscated my trash cans over a $3.00 amount that was left out of our previous payment by mistake. I decided then it was time to end it, and I elected drain cleaner as the simplest method. Years ago I knew of a guy who chose drain cleaner as a means of suicide. It wasn't fast but once he chose that route there was no turning back. Even though it was painful at first, the hospital had given him painkillers until it was over. That's why I elected to go that route, cheap, effective, and no turning back.

A Strange Turn of Events

My family is my life, and by staying around without producing income, I was useless as a provider, as a husband, and as a father.

After more than two years of trying, the message had become painfully clear that things were only going to get worse.

That day my family was gone and I was calm about my decision. Before actually doing it though, I wanted to find a sermon online. Sometimes I would find things that helped through these sermons, and I was desperate for some kind of help. I don't know what I expected to get out of a sermon, I guess I expected to hear something that would validate my choice or push me over the edge. My state of mind was so muddled and confused; all I could think about was what a bad, stupid person I was.

I found a sermon about suicide and I heard the preacher ask the question out loud, "Will you go to Hell if you commit suicide?" His answer wasn't what I expected. He said it couldn't be answered as long as I was alive. As I listened to him speak, I started to think about the hell I had been going through. I began to wonder if I was going to find peace through suicide or was I going to spend eternity living in a worse state than I already was?

Then the sermon took an interesting twist. Instead of pleading for me (or anybody considering suicide) to stop, the pastor said matter-of-factly, "It's your decision if you want to take that chance, but you won't know the answer until you do it."

Huh. I kind of expected to be begged not to do it so that I could be pushed over the edge, but it was almost like he was daring me to do it. It even sounded like he wished someone could come back once they did it just so they could tell him what the final answer was.

This gave me total pause, especially in light of the mess I had made of my life by exercising my free will each time I thought I couldn't lose. More doubt crept in, but so did a tiny spark of faith. I was already a mess, but I had begun to think about what my kids would be saddled with if they saw me give up that way. I didn't want to leave them with that legacy, so I decided to hold on a little longer knowing that I had the means right there if my decision to hold on was the wrong one.

Tuesday I went to our church to do some volunteer work, wondering why I chose to hang on and being totally consumed by how rotten my life was. Sure, I didn't have a job and yes I was going to lose my house. But I still had two eyes to see with, and full use of my body so I could take advantage of any opportunity should one present itself. I wasn't a war torn refugee or in a hospital dying of an incurable disease. None of it mattered to me though because I was busy wallowing in my own misery.

Not long after I got to the church my wife called to say that our son was in a car accident. He was broadsided at a four-way intersection. I left the church in a panic and threw my hands up at how foolish I had been to think that God would help me, and how foolish I was to not have gone through with my plans to commit suicide.

I arrived at the scene and saw the driver's side of my son's car completely caved in, the incapacitated Land Rover that broadsided him, and my son leaning against his car, arms folded and completely unharmed.

What became clear to me was just how much worse my life could have been in a single moment. My son could have been easily maimed or killed, yet he walked away. I knew right away that my life could have been so much more painful. I had been so focused on my depression that I ignored the true gift in my life: my family. Then I thought about all the people who weren't as lucky as me, and who would gladly have traded my misery for theirs. I knew then that things would change, because in that mess God had shown me just how blessed I really was.

Friday morning, I got a call from Ophelia, the assistant in the special security office to whom I'd sent my disheartened email. Ophelia said she saw how bad I was feeling and wished she could have just told me to hang in there. She knew it was going to be alright but couldn't say so because of legalities. Ophelia also told me that I normally wouldn't have gotten the news until the following week, but she wanted to be sure that I knew I had been cleared for the job so my family and I could have a great weekend!

Though we lost our house and were without funds, we were able to negotiate a large enough departure fee for us to have a security deposit for a rental house. The money we got for my son's car helped us come up with the first month's rent on a tiny house within walking distance to the beach. My new job took over from there. I traded my eight pills a day for ten miles of bike riding a day.

Only the Beginning

Once we moved near the beach, we started to settle in but it was much harder than we imagined it was going to be. The house, a 1,600-square-foot, 3-bedroom, 2-bath was tiny compared to the

3,500-square-foot, 5-bedroom, 4-bath custom mansion we had been living in, and it was falling apart. We took our expensive furniture with us, and each piece ended up becoming a painful reminder of how our life had once been.

One of our great concerns was how our sons were going to react to losing their status and having to move out of their very cool bedrooms. We were going from a big house in a wooded area with wide open spaces around us to a tiny house in a crowded neighborhood that backed up to a busy street. Oddly enough though, our sons had actually begun to like living there and much sooner than we expected.

We started to make the best of it. Abby was beginning her real estate career which actually started before we moved but now she was earning some decent money at it, and the boys were having friends over and taking advantage of our being so close to the beach by going there often. Abby was starting to have so much success in her real estate practice that it became obvious that she could have done a lot to help us prevent the financial disaster we had just gone through. Each time she tried to lay blame on me for everything bad that had happened, I simply pointed to her earnings as proof of what she could have done to help us avoid it.

Going into real estate was a promise she had made to me six years earlier, but like most of her promises she never followed through. Six years before and just after our sons got older she had perfect opportunities to build a career or even find part-time work to help us financially. More importantly it could have helped her find the independence she claimed she was looking for. Even though I was making a good living then, my income was based upon sensitive market conditions and my own production as well as the production from the sales teams I managed. There were some months that I would make a lot of money, and other months when I didn't make a dime. Not to mention my vulnerability if my company were to get sold. After nearly losing our house the first time she promised she would find something she could do so we could bank her money to use when things got rough. That was yet another promise she didn't keep.

I didn't lord it over her, but I did become weary of her continuously blaming me for everything. When she finally did go into real estate only a few months before and her earning capacity came to light, she realized that I was right about how much she could have helped to avoid the financial disaster we had just gone through. It bothered her a lot that she couldn't keep blaming me, so instead of pushing ahead to build what could have been a promising career, she just stopped working at it and didn't go any further.

I began working at the FDIC in an office located about forty-five minutes away depending on traffic. The company participated in the train subsidy program which got my interest almost immediately. Through the vouchers they provided I was able to get a monthly rail pass for free. The train station was about a three mile bike ride from my house and the destination station was another mile and a half from the office. Not only was I saving the gas expense, I was getting exercise too. It wasn't long before I had a pretty good system of taking my bike and the train to work each day.

I had already begun to take an interest in losing weight, and because the new job had great health benefits, I started seeing a doctor again to get myself on a better path. I started small at first, in terms of bike riding and exercise but not long after I was up to forty mile rides. I had also mapped out a route so I could do a twenty mile ride home from work at night when time and weather permitted.

Our family life was still tough but it seemed like things were starting to stabilize a little. I found out later just how wrong I was. Once my friend Joel had suggested that I write my story, I decided to chronicle my journey toward better health. Now that I had diabetes along with heart and blood pressure problems, I decided writing about it would help me find a way out of it while helping others out too.

Despite Abby's unwillingness to participate financially after she had promised she would years before, and her unwillingness to accept any responsibility for even an iota of the problems in our marriage, I was still willing to start from scratch and find a way to make up for it. I was still stupid enough at that point to give her the benefit of the doubt.

In the beginning, I would take time in the early morning and write while sitting on the couch and I'd also do research on my laptop. I also had begun to develop some kind of workout routine. So I would usually get a few hours of writing in before anybody woke up, after which I'd spend maybe another hour of doing some exercising then ride my bike to the train or, if a weekend, go on a longer bike ride. At night I walked our dog at the beach to work off dinner. Before I started doing any of this, my appearance had gotten really bad; I was grossly overweight and my ankles were swollen because of the poor circulation. I had dry patches of skin and I was really ugly to look at. Working out helped give me a new glow, but I was still fat as a house.

It wasn't long after I began writing when Abby started having real problems seeing me on my computer when she'd wake up in the morning, accusing me of wasting time. I had forgotten how much time she used to spend looking at women's shoes online back when we were in the black. She wasted so much time back then instead of starting what could have been a promising real estate career as evidenced by her recent successes. It eventually dawned on me that she viewed my time on the computer as time wasted because of all the time she used to waste on her computer.

I never told Abby I was working on a book, and never would. By that point I learned not to speak to her about ideas because of her reactions. She had no vision because she had never tried to be successful at anything. So when I would sit down with her to talk about some ideas whether it was for a new business or even planning a vacation, her answers were always the same. "Just do it if that's what you want to do", or "it sounds great to me", and so on. Or she would stay in the negative. She never offered any perspective even though I was always asking her to be my partner. I had also seen how she treated any ideas that were put in motion. If I had an idea that worked she'd claim at least half, but often full credit for it even though she hadn't put in any effort. But if it failed, it was always my fault. There was no way in hell I was going to tell her that I was working on a book, because of that and because I had begun to change my perspective of our relationship.

I was always willing to shoulder all of the responsibility and yes, take the blame for whatever happened. But I finally saw what I had become because of all the stress I kept taking on for so many years and I hated myself for it. Each time I looked in the mirror all I could see was this fat, hideous blob of a person who I couldn't stand the sight of. It is really hard to describe just how much I hated myself, but it was the kind you might reserve for someone who got away with killing a loved one.

After going to work at the FDIC I began to get some confidence back. I learned shortly after being hired that there were 6,500 applicants for 275 jobs, and I was one of the 275 hired. I found myself working next to former CEOs and CFOs, and other high powered executives whose fates were similar to mine. One of the attorneys I worked with was a former vice president of a small bank that went under during the real estate crisis. He lost over $1,000,000 in retirement and deferred compensation. His new income was about the same as mine, but his commute was an hour and a half each way and there was no train that he could take.

I guess this is where misery loves company. I didn't like hearing that any of my colleagues had gone through such turmoil because I knew many of them felt the pain and frustration as well as the sheer terror I felt during those dark times. Knowing though, helped me to understand a little better that even though I made some mistakes, I had made a lot of good decisions too and had climbed a huge ladder of success. But when the market corrected there was a lot that happened that I couldn't control and there were a lot of people who were smarter than me but who were worse off than I was for the same reasons.

I decided then that I wasn't going to keep accepting blame from my wife who never tried to help or tried to succeed at something while we were married. Worse was how she saddled me with the responsibility of making her happy but wasn't willing to find out for herself what it would take to achieve happiness. She was just as miserable now that we were poor again as she was when we were rich. And she was just as miserable as she was before we were rich, with or without me.

I was tired of it. I had built something that could have lasted us a lifetime if I had had a partner who was willing to commit to working together. After nearly killing myself through stress and bad health in the process, I found myself having to start all over again. I looked back at all the things I had done in my life to make the changes that Abby said she needed from me in order for her to have a better life with me. I made those changes and brought so much more to the table, yet she never made a single change I had asked for in that entire time.

The change I had asked for years before was for her to become independent by developing a career. She was so good in real estate and it could have been a perfect career especially with what I could have provided for her in terms of support and referrals. I wanted to partner with her so we could build something together, but also so she could have an understanding of what my life was like when I left for work each morning. More importantly, I wanted her to really search for what it would take to make her happy and I even went as far as telling her I could accept it if she discovered that leaving me was what she needed to be happy. Once she did embark on her real estate career much later it was already too late for us and eventually quit for the reasons I explained earlier.

I wasn't going to give up my life anymore for a vacuum, but I was still very much in love. As stupid as I now realize it was, I used to get butterflies in my stomach at the thought of being alone with my wife even after twenty years. What changed though was that I wasn't as accepting of the blame anymore, and I wasn't interested in hearing what I needed to do to solve our problems. Abby had shown all of us that she was indeed able to contribute to the solutions to our problems, and now it was her turn to come to the table with her share of the solutions. I had a job that provided the basics including overtime and healthcare, and there were opportunities for advancement. There were also times when I was able to contribute extra by helping her buy marketing media and supplies for her real estate business.

Anything that she brought in could have been used to pay off some of our lingering debt and set some aside in savings. That didn't seem to interest her though; she spent quite a bit on a face peel, eye tucks, and fixing up her car. Looking back at it now, I think she was getting herself ready to find a new man. She completely missed out on the point that if she would have been willing to change herself and contribute to our relationship she would have gotten an entirely new man in me. But she's not the kind of person who can bring herself to make any kind of effort, nor can she see anything beyond herself.

After living like this for almost a year, things were starting to come to a head. Abby wasn't coming out and saying it but the tensions were high and she was becoming more secretive. She had even left the phone book open a few times to pages highlighting local divorce attorneys.

One morning I woke up and had numbness in my arm that wouldn't go away. After about five hours of it, I drove myself to the urgent care where they checked me into the hospital. They ruled out a stroke and a heart attack but determined that I was diabetic and had been so for over a year. Abby didn't come to see me until the next day and her disdain was overt. No surprise that she blamed me for everything that was wrong with my health; and the diabetes was caused in her opinion because I ate mayonnaise on my sandwiches. She had my sons convinced of it for years, and never once mentioned to them how lack of sleep and constant stress over very long periods of time were the likely causes or contributors.

Shortly after I left the hospital, she announced that she wanted to separate.

I found that I was able to get over her being gone much more quickly than I ever expected. What did hurt me the most was being away from my sons, especially my youngest son Austin. My older sons and I had had a lot of time together when they were young, and they had become young men who were getting ready to start their own lives. But my youngest was just reaching that point where we would have a chance to get closer. I was involved with his sports and his music and I wanted to be around to help him grow and keep him safe.

Instead I was faced with what I had recently learned was a deadly disease, and was once again without a home and without the ones who were more important to me than anything in the world; my family.

Like before, my world turned to black. I still had a job, but I was living out of a hotel room and giving up most of my income to my soon-to-be ex-wife even though we weren't going to court at the time. I did it to try and keep my son as stable as I possibly could because the separation was hitting him hard.

All I could do was find out where to begin because I had a life that needed to be fixed. Based on what I had learned from the doctor there wasn't a whole lot of room to mess around.

I started the way I always start a project, I broke it down into small pieces and began working with whatever was at hand for a way to better health, a slimmer physique, and peace of mind. I said in the beginning that I don't necessarily find my story unique. Sure, maybe not everyone who reads this will be hit with stuff like this all at once, but that doesn't mean the impact of those situations will be any lighter. One of the keys to getting past all the dark stuff is being able to sift through it and see the good stuff that still remains.

I often struggled with finding reasons to live because there were times that I thought I was going to lose what I loved the most. But there was also some good stuff that came to light. My going through all of this seemed like Rocky getting back in the ring for the full fifteen rounds only to keep getting pummeled by Apollo Creed. It beat the hell out of him, but he finally won. I have the scars to show for it, but I'm finally feeling as though I'm winning a little bit. And winning for me is not beating down my opponent; it is simply gaining control over my life and finding some peace of mind.

There is quite a bit of reference to my ex-wife and our very ugly divorce, but this isn't a book that attempts to place all of the blame on her. First and foremost, nobody can do anything to you without your permission. My marriage and subsequent divorce were major factors in my overall health and emotional problems because I had devoted my life to trying to make things work. I ended up the way I did, not necessarily because of anything that my ex-wife did, but because of what I took on in order to make things work.

It happened in general because I allowed it to happen for what I thought was for the good of the family instead of everything being about me. But in the process Abby saw my willingness to take on whatever was necessary as my weakness and then decided to exploit them instead of offset them as most life partners might do.

After our divorce I was getting pretty serious with a lovely lady and one day she asked me what I was looking for in a relationship. I answered in the way that I've always envisioned a relationship to be. I've always looked for a real partner, and as part of the partnership sometimes I'll lead, sometimes I'll follow and sometimes I'll partner. It is always based upon how my partner is feeling. I'll never be afraid to make the tough decisions if that's what my partner wants, but out of respect for her would always solicit her input and let her make the decisions if that's what she wanted. I want to be there to celebrate her successes and prop her up at her failures, always willing to show how every failure is simply another step toward success. And that's what I hope a partner would do for me in return. I'm beginning to think that I'm asking too much, because I never came close with either of my wives or later with my girlfriend.

I never wanted my kids to grow up without a father, nor did I ever want them growing up wanting for anything so I set my sights on trying to achieve those goals. All of the other stuff as it related to satisfying Abby's demands were my attempts to keep the peace and to show my willingness to change if that's what I needed to do to make our marriage and home life successful.

Obviously I failed miserably, and twenty-plus years later when I realized I had nothing more to give other than dying, I started doing what I should have done very early in our marriage, which was to ask my partner to contribute. By not doing it earlier, I simply became an enabler. I could have made better efforts to keep myself in shape, both physically and mentally, but I was caught up in a lifestyle that didn't leave enough room for it. And over time I reached a point where I didn't value myself enough as a person to want to do it. That's really where the story begins, when I finally came to realize that I did indeed have something to offer. Once I knew that, I had to decide if I could stick with it because I was going to have to start from scratch again. Given the wreckage that my life had become, I was in for one hell of a ride.

But for me to say it was all Abby's fault, I'd only do that if I decided I wanted to become a victim. She couldn't have done anything without my consent, which she had from day one. That's not to say that I invited her to be the deceiving person on the sidelines that she was, always ready to pounce. I could have taken steps early on to say that I wasn't going to accept it but that meant that I could risk losing my kids. Losing them was something I couldn't bear to even think about, so instead I went through years of hell because of it but I'm satisfied that I did it for the right reasons.

Reliving Buried Emotions

Even though I had changed my perspective on our relationship and had become unwilling to live the way that I had lived in the previous twenty years, I still couldn't see us apart at least at that time. I was looking for some accountability and acknowledgment from Abby so we could both start fresh and rebuild in ways that worked for both of us, but no surprise that accountability isn't part of her makeup. Our youngest son Austin was in the sixth grade then, and he had already been picking up on the tension in a way that was worrying him a great deal.

I didn't want him to worry and did everything I could to compromise and show my willingness to do what it would take to fix things, and oddly enough my reaching out to my wife for help was one of the changes I made. Asking somebody for help was something I just didn't do, and the fact that I didn't was actually a major contributor to my stress load and unhealthy lifestyle.

It was clear that she had no interest once it came to light that she had been making all of her plans in secret. When she announced it was over and was taking the kids we had about two weeks left on our lease at the house. My oldest son Alex decided he wanted to stay with me to help me move everything out. Those two weeks proved to be some of the best times we had together, and really helped him and me to build a solid foundation that lasted for many years. One of the most noticeable things to both of us was the lack of tension now that Abby was gone, and it was liberating.

What I couldn't escape though were the feelings of emptiness every time I saw my sons Andrew and Austin leave and knowing that I lost what had always been the most important thing in my life. I felt some emotions that I hadn't felt since I was a little boy and feeling them brought me back to some very hard periods early in my life. But it also gave me a better understanding of why I was always so afraid of having something I loved taken away from me and why I had always tried so hard to avoid it.

After we separated Abby began a quest to find a new guy and ended up settling on a real gem who I'll call Ralph 1. She went to work right away to try to have him become my substitute while keeping it a secret from me by telling me she wanted to reconcile. Once Alex and Andrew let the cat out of the bag about how she had been seeing this guy for a while, Austin told me about the guy putting him in a head lock. From what my son said, the guy was doing it to prove his strength. It's interesting that he didn't try it with Andrew, a Marine, and Alex, an Army Infantryman. Once I found out this happened, I filed a restraining order on Austin's behalf. Ralph 1 was also involving Austin in text messages and emails over the problems he was having with Abby.

Problems with Abby, how could that be? After all those years of her telling me how perfect she was and that I was the loser, I was really surprised to hear that someone actually found fault with her. Not so funny was what he did to Austin while I was living out of the area; and how Austin was forbidden to talk to me about his mom seeing the guy. It turns out Austin was terrified of him and on the night before I was going to court to have the restraining order put in place, Austin told me how scared he was that Ralph 1 was going to show up with a gun and start shooting at me.

My response? "If the loser shoots, he'd better not miss because if he does it will be a long, long time before he wakes up once I'm finished with him".

I didn't have to confront the individual physically, and I noticed he didn't try and put me in a headlock or even suggest that he could, but I would have welcomed it if he tried.

All I had to do was show up in court and it made him realize he had made a big mistake when it came to his opinion of me and what I might do to him. The judge denied the restraining order because due to Austin's age he would have had to appear in court and I didn't want to bring him into it.

But I didn't need to pursue it anymore because the point got across loud and clear and the guy never went near Austin again. Interestingly enough though was that according to Abby this, in her words early in their relationship, 'great guy', continued to harass and stalk her for at least six months after. I didn't care what he did with her or to her for that matter, as long as he was leaving Austin out of it. She asked me to go after Ralph 1 and beat him up for her which caused my jaw to drop in disbelief. I made it real clear that the only thing I would do is to show up in court with her if she wanted to file charges against him, but unless he was going near Austin I could care less about what he was doing when it came to her.

It probably seems harsh, I know, but there is a much bigger picture here. Ralph 1 sent me a very descriptive email before court, I guess to try and be buddy- buddy to avoid being taken to court. To show why he thought she was a bad person, he made sure to talk about how much fun he had been having with Abby between the sheets and about the games they would play at my expense. The idiot even offered to show me his file which apparently had sexual pictures according to him. The file is why I think she didn't want to take him to court, because of what she thought might be in it and what it would look like if it came out in court. She said that anything he had on her was stuff that he made up and none of it was real, but when I kept offering to help her take him to court for Austin's sake she kept refusing. Hard to say what was real and what wasn't and telling the truth was never one of Abby's strong points.

I had some tough childhood experiences which I go into later, but however rough it got at times also helped me to forge a better path to raising my sons, and was one of the reasons I watched how all of my sons were being treated. And it was why I always struggled with the kind of dad I wanted to become and knew exactly the one that I didn't want to be. I boiled it down to a few simple things:

> *Kids are gifts from God, and all you need to do in life is love them and the rest will take care of itself.*
> *Love them unconditionally; they are imperfect, just like me. But I can have a perfect love for them, and*
> *Never compare them to anyone else, even to each other. Let them know how valuable they are as individuals.*

Those few things are what guided me throughout our lives together. And the way that I used to face a tough world each day was to grab whichever kid was closest to me and give him a little kiss on the head. When I did that I reminded myself every single day that everything in the world was okay and was always going to be okay because they were in it.

I was fortunate to be on the phone with my oldest son Alex for a long time one night, just talking about lots of things like life, girls, and all the way to guiding philosophies. It was incredible for me to hear him say to me out of the blue how much he knew about unconditional love because of the way that I love him and his brothers.

I finally did something right in my life I guess. Now if I could only make a living again and go back to be a dad while getting ready to be a granddad.

I honestly still don't know if they would have been better off with a different dad. I know they could have done worse but I'm pretty sure they could have done better, at least as I'm seeing it through my eyes right now. I should have planned better than simply setting out to not be my father who was never a dad.

So this story is about how I rode through hell over the past six years or so to finally reach a point where I could say I'm a little ahead of the game and looking ahead to a brighter future. This is that story, but amazingly enough, had I not been confronted with learning that I had diabetes I never would have found the motivation to move ahead. Once I knew that I could commit suicide simply by keeping on the same way I had been, I knew I was making a life or death decision much like the day I was about to commit suicide. Yet after learning that by making the right changes in my life and taking control of it, there was a chance that I could reverse it and in doing so accomplish the other goals I wanted for my life.

If I made the right choices, then I could feel and look better again, get my sex life back, and just be healthy. There could have been so many other bad things to happen to me because of the course I kept myself on. Diabetes actually gave me a second chance because I knew that I had caused myself some real damage, but not in a way that I couldn't fix. As I began to focus, I finally found reasons to want to live again, and because I am so goal oriented, the prospect of reversing diabetes became the goal that I needed in my life.

And I also learned that if I succeeded in meeting that goal there was also a chance that I was going to get my heart and blood pressure problems in check but even if I didn't, I would still be better off.

So yes, for me anyway, diabetes was indeed an answer to my prayer. I had kind of been hoping at the time I said that prayer that I would win the lottery or gotten some kind of huge payout that would have just given me all the time and money in the world to work out and fix myself. But it wouldn't have changed the person that I was. I didn't just need a diet and workout plan, I needed my life to change. All the dark times I went through, the terror, and the humiliation over such a long period finally brought home to me that there are no guarantees in our lives and gave me a chance to see what a miserable wretch I had become. No matter how good you think you are, things can change in a heartbeat and foolish pride has no place when making life changing decisions. Be smart and trash the arrogance, learn how to be humble because there's so much more to life than trying to pretend you're someone other than who you really are.

In addition to learning about the disease and ways to combat it, I've also been learning to better deal with some extreme challenges like an ugly divorce, a job that required a lot of travel, job losses, and nomadic living. All of these posed and continue to pose major obstacles to my developing much needed routines, but by sticking to some sort of plan throughout all of this I managed to go from size 48 pants down to 36. My overall health improved too. I still have a long way to go but I've also come a long way too.

So maybe you're not in a job that requires a lot of travel or involved in an ugly divorce, that doesn't mean you're not facing your own significant challenges. By offering my own introspective

I hope that I can give you some encouragement by showing you the light that I found at the end of my tunnel, and more importantly what I did to find that light.

Funny how so much can be derived from knowing that you have a potentially deadly disease, but life has always taught me to find the good in the bad. In this case there is plenty of both.

TWO

The Early Years

How you doin' boy? You here for 30 days.
Get, get, get, get your long hair cut, and cut out your ways

- From 30 Days in the Hole by Humble Pie (Marriott, 1972)

I'm not one to dwell on the past but I can't ignore how much it impacted me, or more importantly, how people and events in my life shaped me eventually for the better. It just took me awhile to figure it out. My life was neither the best nor the worst; a lot of bad happened to me but I can honestly say that much good happened to offset it. Probably the worst thing that happened was how I had to grow up very quickly but in order to do that I had to suppress a lot of emotions. I had to watch my emotional reactions to things that a kid in a normal environment would be able to react to, because I didn't have the luxury of being a kid.

By the time I was twelve I was six feet tall with facial hair and a deep voice, and I was able to pass as a nineteen year old and could buy beer for my friends and me using a fake ID. I also smoked cigarettes in front of my old man at that age which also made me look older than I was. Since I looked that old many people around me expected me to act that old, but in reality I was just a twelve-year old kid who was still trying to grow up.

Even though I did my best to keep myself under control, there were many times when I found myself to be an emotional basket case headed for periodic meltdowns and the disasters that ensued.

This meant that when something scared the hell out of me I couldn't act scared, and whenever I attempted to do a project on my own I often screwed up because people just assumed I knew how to do it. So when I screwed something up I often looked like a total misfit even though I was just a pre-teen who was trying to make a go of it. Fortunately for me though, there were enough good people around me who cared enough to help me make some sense of my life and teach me better ways to do things.

I had a very abusive old man, and way back when my oldest siblings left the house before I went to an orphanage following my mother's death, they were pretty vocal about some of the things he did like molesting some of them and beating others. Instead of changing his ways he had restraining orders put on them so they weren't allowed on his property and we weren't allowed to see them. Losing contact with my sisters and brother that way was my first experience with losing someone I loved and that left a deep emotional scar that I kept running from for most of my life.

In the end, the old man molested four of my sisters, but to their credit and strength they were able to move on with their lives. We all did pretty much, though my brother seemed to struggle the hardest because my mother's death really impacted him and the old man was exceptionally hard on him. He ran away from home at sixteen and struggled until he died. My sisters and my brother not only forgave the old man, they were there at his bedside when he died. I didn't go; I had already made my peace with him but didn't want to go through the expense of travelling from California all the way to New Hampshire just to see him die.

Earlier Years – The Good and the Bad

I'm the youngest of ten, two boys and eight girls. One of my sisters died a crib death before I was born and Rita, the one closest to me in age died when she was nine from a hole in the heart syndrome. My four oldest siblings had already moved out of the house when my mother died of leukemia just before I was three. After our mother died, Charmaine, Mary, and Iris, the three sisters closest to me in age, were placed together in an all-girls boarding school in northern New Hampshire. I got placed in an orphanage closer to home from the time I was three until I was six when I was old enough to go to school.

For me, the orphanage was a pretty hostile place run by some very tough nuns. For the most part those nuns were old and frustrated, and they didn't seem to mind taking their frustrations out on the kids who pissed them off the most. I don't recall making any real friends, but I do remember feeling lonely a lot and sometimes hearing screams from kids getting whipped by the leather strap at night. I was hit a few times as well, but I don't remember screaming like some of the others even though I remembered it hurt like hell. The nuns would use whatever they could get their hands on to inflict the kind of pain that would get your attention if you were a discipline problem, or just being in the wrong place at the wrong time as was often the case with me. I got hit on the hands with big heavy bells and thick rulers; others got slapped in the face or hit in the head by the nuns' hands. The worst offenders got the strap on their bare behinds.

I never really understood why I was at the orphanage or when it would end because I never really understood where my mother went, but I remember the fear and resignation each time my old man pointed the car in the direction that took me back to that place after a home visit on weekends or holidays. I grew to really hate that orphanage while I was there and I was always conflicted in the summer because the place was in the same direction as my favorite ice cream shop. I never knew if we were going for ice cream or if we were just going back to the orphanage.

Once I turned six I was taken out of the orphanage for good because I was able to go to school, and my three sisters came back from boarding school to live at home as well. But the euphoria of leaving the boarding school and orphanage were short lived. Our old man was a drunk and that affected all of us. When he would go on his major drunken binges we would all huddle together and do whatever we could to protect each other and stay out of harm's way until he passed out. We didn't huddle in fear all the time, we'd usually just try to find some fun things to do quietly that could help the time pass more quickly.

I told my friend Jimmy once that my old man was drunk the night before and for some reason Jimmy told him what I said. I thought the son of a bitch was going to kill me. He picked me up by my ears and kept slamming my head into the wall. It's hard to imagine a grown man doing that to a six year old, but that wasn't the first time nor the last time he'd done that, but it was one of the scariest. It wasn't like the old man getting drunk was a big secret or anything, the cops were always taking him back home from the bars and he'd parade himself in the front yard in his underwear while barely being able to stand up.

The next morning after that particular round of head-slamming, I overheard my sister Charmaine tell him point blank that she would have him arrested if he ever touched me like that again, He responded by telling her that he didn't care if he maimed me and would do it any time I pissed him off. Her message got her on his hit list fast but he never hit me that hard after.

The old man was a heavy smoker and drinker and had four heart attacks by the time I was seven. Our home environment caused my older brother and me a lot of emotional and physical problems, not least of which involved bed-wetting. Not only was the old man abusive, he placed high, unrealistic expectations on us from very early ages and was quick to criticize each of our mistakes. Though my brother and I were far apart in age, we had to deal with much of the same thing and the old man never gave us pats on the backs so we never felt as though we did anything right. The fact that he didn't really messed us up emotionally for a long time because we could never celebrate anything we did right. He had us convinced that we weren't capable of doing anything except screw up.

The old man blamed me for causing him stress and cut a deal with Jimmy's parents for me to go live with them full time. Those ended up being some of the best years of my life and led me to meet some people who ultimately got me on a path that saved me from the dark place where I was headed.

So I lived with Jimmy and his seven brothers and one sister. It was a thirty-five room house surrounded by about 200 acres of virgin land that ran along a two mile long creek. At any given time we had as many as five dogs and farm animals like sheep, ducks, pigs and chickens. Most of them wound up on the dinner table, and every time a dog went missing we were always a little apprehensive as we'd sit down to dinner, wondering if the evening roast was our missing pet.

I lived there full time for about five years and over time there were three of us who became pretty inseparable during the time I was there. The trio was Wally, Jimmy's older brother, Eli, a family friend and me. Eli was fourteen, Wally was twelve and I was a pretty old eleven-year-old when we really started trying to find out what life was all about.

During the summers we would camp out in the woods that surrounded the house, and since Eli was the older and most mature of the three of us he tended to give us the voice of reason every time we'd go out on a dare which was pretty often. We raised a lot of hell but we weren't malicious, we were more adventurous. We'd always have two or three dogs with us so we never had to worry about anyone sneaking up on us in the middle of the night. The dogs stayed unleashed and were always in attack mode whenever a stranger would come near.

We built a two-room tree house back in the woods out of sight and earshot from the house and we'd camp there a lot during the summers and weekends. We'd smoke cigarettes and Wally and I would drink alcohol, starting with a gallon of church wine we stole one time. Stealing from a church never sat well with me, but we all agreed the wine was heavenly.

During the camp outs we would navigate the woods late at night under the moonlight and pretend we were marauders from colonial times or just goof around. There were no houses anywhere around us so we were free to roam usually with two or three of our dogs leading the way.

It was a lot of fun but by the time I was halfway through twelve I was living back at home, had hair down past my shoulders, smoked cigarettes with my old man's permission, and had my first real job. The job was as a night waterman at a golf course surrounding our house. It was a country club with a large eighteen-hole golf course and a practice green near the bar. My house was right between the front and back 'nines' and golfers would cut through an easement that my old man granted in exchange for benefits like use of the pool.

The outside of the course was surrounded by woods but there were a few houses lining parts of it. I worked there with Jim Coury who was a couple of years older than me. Coury was a real funny guy and we had a great time together on the job. The work was pretty basic and I was paid $1.60 an hour but the best part was there was no supervisor on site, it was just Coury and me.

The golf course didn't have automatic sprinklers so the boss would set a schedule for us to put sprinklers on the greens for certain amounts of time, change positions two or three times during the night then turn them off, roll up the hoses, and collect all the sprinklers. We couldn't start the job until it got dark, usually about 9:00 pm, and we wrapped it up just before sun-up.

The back nine had some greens and a pump house that were located in areas Coury and I considered scary because they were dark and remote but close enough for bad guys to go and hide or where wild animals could lurk, at least in our imaginations. We didn't really have wild animals though there were packs of dogs from the neighborhoods occasionally. We would run across teenagers and some adults trespassing and drinking so we would have to kick them off the course periodically, but most of the time it was just us playing tricks on each other.

Coury and I would normally split the course to save time rather than ride together in a single golf cart and we would always flip a coin to see who got the back nine. One night I was about a ¼ mile away from my house, about to start my rounds when I heard my sister Iris yell out my name in a blood-curdling scream. Coury heard it too from where he was and got to the house right when I did. My father was a child molester and he was abusive, even though by that time he stopped hitting me since he knew I wouldn't take it anymore. He knew because I told him so the last time he had tried it; and that was the last time he tried it. Still, I was never sure what he would do with my sisters, and Coury knew that my old man was a drunk so when we got there neither of us knew what to expect and we went inside planning on finding the worst.

We found my sisters Mary and Iris and their friend Donna in night gowns, robes and fluffy slippers, their hair in coffee-can rollers, huddled against a wall. My old man was in a wife-beater tank top, which showed just how big his beer belly was, boxer shorts, black socks and dress shoes. He handed me a broom and flashlight while Iris excitedly told Coury and me that there was a bat flying loose upstairs and we had to catch it. They managed to shut the downstairs doors but the bat was free to fly around the four bedrooms upstairs until we found it. Many of the bats in the area were rabid, so it was important that we caught it rather than wait for it to find its way out since we'd all risk getting bitten. The old man was quick to tell me to be careful as he closed the door behind us. We caught the bat and went back to work.

That memory is more of an illustration of the kinds of expectations placed on me because of my size and street smarts. I mean, how many twelve year old kids do you know whose job it was to be out in the woods late at night working until sun up and kicking teenagers and adults off the premises or catching rabid bats? It seems like it might be fun, and overall it was but it also caused me a lot of angst in my younger years because I had the size and look of an adult, but inside I was still a kid. I was expected to act like an adult but I was basing the decisions I was making on the experiences of a twelve year old boy, because that's what I was. I caught on pretty quickly and eventually rose to the occasion, but there were times when I grieved for a childhood that I never got to have. That started me down a path of escaping through drugs and alcohol.

Charmaine, Mary and Iris had moved out before I turned fourteen with Iris being the last to move. A sister moving out might have been welcome news to some brothers, but it was traumatic for me. I always lived with the threat that I was going to lose someone or something that I loved and their moving out felt a little like that. It took me back to those feelings of loneliness that I had while I was living in the orphanage. I also lived with the constant threat that something bad was going to happen like being sent away to a state institution as my old man had tried to do from the time my sisters left because he didn't want me around anymore.

A New Family

Once I was living back home, I was getting more and more street wise because I was spending more time on the street. I had been expelled from Catholic school in sixth grade so I started in public school and in no time was doing drugs, stealing cars and getting in trouble which also got me expelled. By age thirteen I was in reform school for selling drugs and reunited with a few of my friends who disappeared without anyone knowing where they went.

Despite our incarceration my friends and I formed a little gang and became the go-to guys in the cottage that housed us. The way the reform school in New Hampshire was set up when I was in was kind of like an industrial complex with red-brick buildings surrounded by chain link fences topped with barbed razor wire so no one could climb over. In fact, the real name was the State Industrial School; or S.I.S. as we called it. It was set up to be used as an adult prison compound for medium security prisoners, but was in fact a youth prison. It housed youth murderers, arsonists, and armed robbers in cottages within the complex, and some of the cottages had much higher security than others depending on the length of incarceration and the severity of the crimes.

We had a few bad guys in our group, but most of the real bad guys were in the neighboring cottages that housed kids with longer sentences. It didn't take long for me to learn the lay of the land and figure out what I could get away with and what I couldn't. One of our friends, Archie, was a tough kid and a real smart-ass who mouthed off to the director of the compound.

That landed him in Eastwood Cottage, a rotten place where kids would serve 'dead' time, meaning the time they spent there didn't get credited to their sentence time. We knew of kids who served as much as a year in there on thirty or sixty-day sentences. Archie was lucky with only four days of dead time, but he was also handcuffed to his bunk and beaten by the director every day while he was there. Archie still remained a smartass but watched his tongue around certain people. He was fourteen at the time.

We really couldn't speak out because if we got caught trying to let people know what was going on we risked getting singled out and life could get very bad for us. We saw what happened to a guy whose brother had beaten the head guard during an attempted escape months before. The night the guy was processed and landed in our cottage he was mysteriously beaten heavily before being transferred to a tougher cottage, and left with a broken arm. The director claimed he was hurt while trying to escape, but we all knew it was in retaliation for what the kid's brother had done.

But just to underscore the kind of life I was heading for comes in the story of Jeffrey, another friend who was a big fourteen-year-old in our reform school gang of sorts. He was quiet but very tough, kind of a silent but deadly guy and he made sure no one tried to challenge any of us in any way. Unfortunately though, Jeffrey died of a heroin overdose shortly after leaving the cottage.

I was lucky because I only had to serve thirty days. Despite running with the bad pack and raising hell, I learned how to play the game pretty quickly so I didn't make matters worse while I was inside. That is, I didn't get caught. Time passed slowly there and we made do with what we had. We didn't have access to drugs though some of my friends would drink rubbing alcohol and snort dishwashing detergent. Other times we would crowd into a corner of the rec room where the guards couldn't see and we'd hyperventilate until we passed out.

By the time I got out of reform school and back into public school, it was clear that I was heading down a wrong-way path. I didn't sell drugs any more but I went back to doing a potpourri of hallucinogenic drugs and getting high whenever I could, and I was looking to get much higher. After each school day was over, my buddies and I would hang out at Ted's pool hall furthering our street education, and some of my buddies were already experimenting with shooting up coke and heroin.

I had my own needle and although peer pressure brought me very close I'm happy to say I never used it, but I was becoming more and more of a mess. My old man could no longer control me because he knew I wouldn't let him hit me again. And he knew to never try, so I became harder to deal with. Deep down I was still a nice kid, but because of my size I was getting singled out by eighteen- and nineteen-year-olds who were the same size as me and picking fights, so I had no choice but to focus on learning how to survive.

One time just after I had moved back home I was waiting in line in a fast food place, and a guy on leave from the Army came in from behind me and put his hand on my shoulder to get me to turn around. I turned around with my fist in position to throw a punch but he told me to relax because he just wanted to check my height against his. The second I let my arm down he threw a punch that landed squarely on my nose and broke it.

By the time I was fifteen, my old man was working with the local authorities and a judge to have me committed to becoming a ward of the state until I was eighteen. He was in the process of trying to make the S.I.S. my home until I was old enough to be on my own. In retrospect I can't blame him, but he wasn't doing anything to build a life for us either. His drinking hadn't stopped and once all of my sisters left he sold all of the furniture in the house so there was nothing but an empty house each time I came home from school.

I was still close with Jimmy's family so I would stay there for many days at a time but I couldn't live there anymore because I had caused problems when I lived there before. Even though I was close to Jimmy and his brothers, I was going back to hanging out in the street because of some of the emotional problems that I began to go through. A big part of it was I didn't know where my home was, and that created conflicts between me and Jimmy's parents.

My sister Suzy tried to take me in but that didn't work either because of the conflicts I created with her husband Emile. Emile was a really good man and his childhood was every bit as tough as mine if not tougher, yet we were very far apart in terms of life philosophies. We eventually made peace with each other and I'm glad we did. By the time he died I realized how much we had in common and that was a good thing because he was a great family man and provider, but it was unfortunate that he and I didn't get closer sooner. I could have learned a lot more from him.

I found myself once again without a home and waiting for the people to come take me away. I can honestly say if that had happened I probably would have either died very young or still be sitting in prison. God was smiling on me, however. Jimmy's cousin Bob, (by Bob's marriage to Jimmy's cousin Kathy), was speaking in our high school auditorium so I made it a point to watch the presentation. He was a prominent attorney in town and was giving a talk on local law.

After the speech was over I went down to talk with him and we ended up spending quite a bit of time together. I was surprised at how much he knew about my circumstances. He asked me what I was going to do, knowing that my old man was making arrangements to have me turned over to the state. I told Bob there really wasn't anything I could do because there weren't any places for me to go.

Out of the blue Bob suggested I move in with him and Kathy and that floored me. I always had a decent relationship with Bob and took care of his dog while he and Kathy would go on vacations. Bob was a blast to be around, but Kathy was a whole different story. She was a really nice looking queen bitch who scared the crap out of her cousins including Jimmy, and me as well.

I asked him if he had talked with Kathy about it, and he said, "Yes I did, and it will be fantastic because we just bought a place that needs a lot of work so we thought you could help us out with it." I thought about it for a few days, and then after making sure the offer was genuine I accepted. Fortunately it was a sixteen-room house so I had places to avoid Kathy's wrath during those times when I was the subject of her wrath, and the first year was a tough one. Once I got to know Kathy I understood just how much of a truly loving person she was, but she was tough as nails and was quick to cut you down to size if you pissed her off.

I lived there for the next three years, and my life was saved by Bob and Kathy through love, guidance and a variety of freedoms I really didn't know existed. Sure, I had to play by their rules but in return they trusted and encouraged me and in doing so empowered me in ways I never knew.

Bob and Kathy were taking on a lot when they got me and they knew it. I was basically a good kid with street smarts who was accustomed to very little supervision. They gave me some firm ground rules and trusted me to adhere to them. I still got to drink beer and a hard drink once in a while but was never allowed to get drunk. I had to quit drugs altogether but still smoked cigarettes, and I now had a curfew.

While I wasn't perfect I cleaned up a lot and worked really hard to stick to their rules. I was a whisky drinker from age thirteen and never stopped getting drunk but was doing it in more controlled situations, never did it in their house, and did it less frequently. I still hung out with much of my same crowd but to their credit my old crew respected the new me and never tried to push me into anything or give me grief for trying to clean up my act.

My freshman year, before I moved in with Bob and Kathy, I had passed the Honors Algebra class I was in with a really low grade because I was high all the time. The school dropped me into a lower math the next year. After moving in with Bob and Kathy my outlook changed. Early in my sophomore year I finished the new math book independently by November and went into Geometry as I was supposed to, so I didn't miss a beat. I also took two French classes at the same time, so at mid-terms I took my French 1 mid-term and final as well as the French 2 mid-term on the same day. I got straight A's in all of my subjects and made Highest Honors on more than one occasion. I even got invitations as a sophomore to attend West Point, Annapolis, and the Air Force Academy after I graduated but unfortunately I never pursued them. More significant though was finally finding a home where I wanted to be but knowing the home wasn't mine.

During those years the trajectory of my life changed constantly and dramatically. The changes were largely positive but I was often plagued with emotional problems that sent me into deep depressions and I became suicidal more than once. Much of it was over the discovery of a new home life and the internal conflicts and confusion that happened while I tried to learn how to deal with it.

Through most of my junior and senior years I would go to school drunk and leave early to head to the nearest bar and drink some more. At sixteen there wasn't a bar I couldn't go to and most didn't ask for an ID because I had long hair and a beard, and I carried myself like someone in his twenties. Mike Peterson was a counselor whom I had met through one of Bob's friends and who helped me sort out a lot. I think it was over a year that I saw him and during that time I started to understand that I was living with an image that I should be like Clint Eastwood in his movies. Every time I would lose a fight or walk away from one I'd go into these deep depressions thinking I was such a loser. Mike helped me understand the realities around me and helped me put my life in perspective so I could learn to accept what I couldn't change and change what I could.

Conflicting Emotions and New Realities

My time with Bob and Kathy was the very first time that I learned I had value as a human being, outside of being loved by my sisters and brother. Kathy was the first person to tell me I was a handsome young man, prior to that I always thought of myself as really ugly and could never understand why girls would come on to me.

I like to think that they got something positive from me too. About a year after I moved in, Bob and Kathy had a baby boy, Colin; I was their built-in baby sitter and enjoyed every minute of it. Two of my closest friends, Marc and Eli, would come over in Marc's very 'souped' up Olds Cutlass while I was babysitting. Eli was the same Eli when he, Wally and I were tight but though he and Wally stayed in touch I only stayed tight with Eli. Eventually Wally and I reconnected, but that was years later and after I moved away.

We'd break out the beer and cigarettes and play Hearts (we weren't allowed to drink when babysitting, but we set limits to our drinking and I did say I wasn't perfect) and we'd crack up and sometimes argue and raise hell at the card table while Colin slept. At 10:00 pm we'd pause the game and I'd change Colin, give him his 10:00 feeding after warming up the bottle just right, and I'd rock him back to sleep while signing a lullaby. Then Marc, Eli and I'd go back to the game, making sure to quit drinking in plenty of time to hide the empties before Bob and Kathy returned. We never got drunk, and despite our shenanigans the only priority for any of us was that kid.

One of the best times in my life was probably the goofiest. The Cocheco River, which was polluted because of all the local factories dumping into it, was a pretty slow-moving fresh water river that dumped into the Piscataqua River which is a salt water river and has one of the strongest currents in North America. Out of the blue Bob bought a couple of rubber two-man rafts and announced that he, Kathy, and I were going to take a day and float down the Cocheco. Kathy wanted no part in it and kept threatening to call the local newspaper so they could chronicle our folly. She stayed home and planned to gloat, especially if somebody would have had to call the Coast Guard to rescue us.

Armed with a couple of sandwiches and half of a six-pack of beer each, Bob and I set in the river at about 9:00 am and floated. We tied the rafts together and just laid back, talking about anything that came to mind. We marveled at how we would surprise the ducks floating on the river and watched them fly off. After seeing scowling hunters in the woods we realized we were there on opening day of duck season. I'm really surprised that no one took a shot at us.

The day went by ever so leisurely and the beers gave us a nice little buzz. We were really relaxed, that is until the three rivers merged and we found ourselves in the strong current. Damn we were lucky, but we got into a pretty scary ride while trying to figure out how to get to safety. I was a little freaked because some guys I knew from school drowned in that area while navigating those same waters much in the same way that we were, but Bob had it under control and managed to get us safely to shore. It so happened we landed at one of my friend's house whom we were able to persuade to drive us home.

When I was seventeen I spent the summer living on Pelican Island, part of a group of nine islands called the Isles of Shoals, off the coasts of Maine and New Hampshire. Bob and Kathy coordinated a job for me in a big hotel on the island with Eli and a whole group of college and high school kids from the region. For the most part I had a great time, but I still struggled with depression though and would keep going in and out of it until I burned a bridge with the management team and didn't get to go back because I had such a bad attitude.

I lost my virginity there to a college hottie named Susan who had no idea that it was my first time. She could pretty much get any guy there but always found her way back to this skinny guy we called Sheep Dog, who had long hair and puffy bangs over his face. That experience taught me the emotional burdens of loving and dating and I went through some tough times for a while, but emerged much like Hitch, Will Smith's character in the movie by the same name. I decided I didn't like getting hurt and also discovered that I wasn't all that good in picking up women but over time I became very good at creating situations where women would come to me.

Moving Out for the First Time

Shortly after coming back to Bob and Kathy's from the island I graduated high school and decided to move to Virginia Beach where Mary, Iris and Charmaine all lived. It wasn't an emotional exit; I was eighteen and couldn't wait to leave our town because small towns can often stunt your growth and I wanted to become something. I was also beginning to see myself as more of a grown man and I was anxious to get out on my own. I could never have come to that conclusion had it not been for Bob and Kathy, but it was also clear that it was time for their big bird to fly the coup. Colin was getting older and they were a complete family unit and I didn't want to overstay my welcome.

Bob and Kathy did the right thing by making me go see my old man especially on the holidays. Sometimes I'd have a good time with my old man but he was always trying to be controlling and didn't have a sense of humor.

In reality I wanted to stay with Bob and Kathy on the holidays. It was warm and fun at their house and we always had things to laugh about. My sisters lived far away, except for Suzy who I did get to spend some great times with. And for all the emphasis that I've placed on Bob and Kathy saving my life, there is no way that it could have been accomplished without the support of my sisters especially in later years. I didn't like having to spend time with my old man and I missed my sisters. I would visit them while I was on spring breaks and we always had great times, so I decided that Virginia Beach is where I wanted to be for a while.

With Charmaine's help, I got a job at a shipyard and did quite a few different jobs like welding and metal cutting, ship fitting and plumbing, and handling bales of raw asbestos to line smokestacks with. It was a rough and dangerous gig. Two years earlier four people were killed in a massive gas barge explosion caused by their negligence. I drank a lot, did drugs on occasion, was smoking two packs of cigarettes a day plus breathing in smoke and fumes from welding. I was overweight and pasty, but I didn't care. I actually enjoyed the job and some of the people I worked with. I learned a good trade but I also learned how quickly life can change.

Michael was one of my good friends from high school who made his way down from New Hampshire shortly after I arrived. He moved in with me for a while and he and I worked at the same shipyard. One day Michael and I were working with two other guys and had to move two twenty-foot long pipes out of storage. The pipes weighed fifty-seven pounds a foot each and we had to rig them by hand and raise them six feet in the air for them to clear some barriers before getting them to the trailer. The barriers were about ¼ inch too high for us to clear so we had to jockey and manhandle the suspended pipes to push them over. I was on one end and one of the other guys named Tom was on the other end. Tom was a really skilled welder but a real snotty guy about twenty-three years old who was there to fill in since it was a four-man job.

We alternated the jockeying and kept pushing and lifting the suspended pipes until suddenly the rigging slipped and the pipes fell, crushing him at the same time my end pulled me up and caused me to slam hard into the wall.

It took twenty of us to lift a six-foot section so we could drag Tom out, and I could see how much damage he sustained. His hips and legs were all bloody and mashed and he was barely conscious. He lived but he was crippled for life. I knew in an instant that it was only fate that determined him instead of me as the victim. I also started to take notice of what was going on around me and wondered what kind of other hazards I might have to deal with, and what kind of harm could befall me. I worked around explosive gasses and on surfaces that were unstable and could collapse on me, so I was always on edge after that.

That's when I began to notice things that would rile me up for exactly those reasons. I worked for a guy named Wayne, a tough foreman who would just not get off my back. He would assign me challenging projects and then verbally beat the shit out of me every single day. Wayne's counterparts would get on his case because they thought he was being too hard on me even though no one had ever heard me complain. I saw that he was pretty much the same with everyone who worked for him and Wayne had some of the best projects on the site so I brushed it off and just focused on getting better at what I did.

One time however, Wayne singled me out to go to the top of a tugboat's wheel house to grind the welds on a newly-installed panel so it could be painted. The wheel house was three stories high with only a small rail on the outside but not big enough to support anyone. Since I had to grind the welds from the outside I had to be harnessed and tied to the boat to keep from falling to the lower deck three stories below.

Wayne fastened the harness then told me I was good-to-go and started to hand me the grinder, but I tested the harness before I let go of the rail I was holding on to. The son of a bitch didn't lock me in and, had I not tested it, would have fallen in such a way that I would have broken my back or been killed.

It was my turn to beat the shit out of him verbally and Wayne was beet red while he fastened the harness correctly. He was embarrassed at being dressed down but knew he had crossed the line. After I finished the grinding I went back to work below on a project right outside of the tug. Wayne came out and started getting all over my case for something and that pissed me off to no end, especially since he had just made a mistake that could have killed me.

He turned and walked back to the tug entrance and I grabbed a short-handled sledgehammer and shouted out all sorts of expletives as I threw the hammer toward him to get his attention. Fortunately for both of us the hammer hit the steel bulkhead right next to his head as he walked into the tug's lower quarters. The sound was like being inside a large church bell just as the hammer is hitting it, and that was just from hearing it on the outside. Wayne stopped in mid-step when it hit, paused, then kept going inside without looking back or saying anything.

We never discussed it nor did we ever discuss why he was being so hard on me, but I found out later that Wayne only worked with people he felt had talent and despite his temper he kept the ones he liked. I worked with Wayne until I left the company and we always remained on good terms. Every once in a while I think of that incident and realize that if my hammer-toss would have been only three or four inches off I would have ruined at least two lives, his and mine. I started soul-searching.

One night as I tried to fall asleep I heard myself wheezing and couldn't believe that somebody my age was that bad off. Of course, by smoking at least two packs a day and breathing welding smoke and asbestos, what else should I have expected? I had a vision that night where I saw myself as a tremendous success if I quit smoking. I quit the next day and despite going back on occasion, only for a day or two, I still don't smoke.

I became more conscious of who I was and by substituting exercise for smoking lost thirty pounds. I developed routines that kept me in shape and eating right, and I got plenty of sleep.

Part of my focus on health was to quit my job at the shipyard. Through Iris I found a job as a day bartender at a great hotel on the beach. My routines fit nicely. I'd wake up about 8:00 and run to the beach then run about two or three miles once I got there. Since the water there was really warm I'd swim for a little while then lie on the beach to get a short nap before running back home to get ready to start my shift at 11 am. I lived about one and a half miles from work so I walked every day. After work I'd eat, run five miles along the beach, and then dive in for a late swim. [1]

On one of my wilder nights my buddy Michael and I partied very hard in Norfolk and I was stupid enough to climb in my '69 Dodge Charger and fly onto the freeway. I hit 105 mph when a Corvette cut in front of me so I had to change lanes fast to go around it then back in front of it to avoid causing a major accident. When I did, I clipped the Corvette in the front end and sent it spinning into the median.

Fortunately Virginia has wide medians along their highways so the Corvette just kept spinning in circles until it came to a stop. The great news was the driver was unharmed and no one got hurt. An off-duty cop watched the whole thing happen and got the police there quickly. I really felt bad and was pretty drunk still, so when the officer came over to find out what happened I was upfront with him. I said I had been drinking and speeding and the whole thing was my fault.

---

[1] I did that until I saw Jaws which changed my whole outlook because we had sharks at our beaches. It took me years to feel ok about going into a bathtub much less the ocean at night.

He got me and the driver of the Corvette into his car to get our information. She was a gorgeous blond who sat in the back seat just bawling her eyes out. The cop asked her if thirty was her correct age and apparently I must have thought that was so incredibly old because when she said yes, I went "Wow, you're 30? You look so fantastic!" She managed to say thank you in between sobs.

That night was the first time I landed in jail as an adult (not the last though). My sister bailed me out the next day and I chose to give up driving for a year. Although I can't remember the driver's name, she and I actually hit it off though I was too young and unseasoned to figure out how to take it to another level. Shortly after the accident, I called the driver to apologize to her and asked if there was anything I could do. She told me it would help her tremendously to get money to pay her deductible so she could get her car fixed. We agreed to meet at a coffee shop a few nights later where I gave her the money for her deductible and we stayed awhile. We had coffee and talked a lot, and it didn't take long for her to understand that I was genuinely sorry for what had happened. It was also becoming obvious that there was a definite attraction between us except I wasn't quite sure how to handle it, and I don't think she was either.

I had a court date and was represented by a good attorney on the criminal charges, though he was really mad that I had opened up to the cop the way I did. The driver of the Corvette had to appear as a witness and we sat together and were pressed close against each other, almost like we were on a date. She applauded when my attorney got the case dismissed on a technicality, and we left together. She and I went out to lunch to celebrate but we never went beyond that I'm sorry to say. She was recently divorced and I think she too may have had trouble knowing what to do next, especially with someone twelve years her junior.

One of the things I chose to do on my own was to stop driving for a while, and it ended up being over a year before I drove again. Instead I hitchhiked almost everywhere I went, and that led to an interesting event. Once when I was hitchhiking to a neighboring town the arresting officer stopped and gave me a ride in his cruiser.

He knew who I was and asked how I was doing. I remembered him to be very meticulous and said I was really surprised that he would make the mistake that he made in the documents, I don't remember it exactly but it was something like getting a date wrong.

I only paused for a moment then I thanked him and he said "You're welcome." He wouldn't say it but he tacitly acknowledged this kind of error was unlike him for a reason. He had cut me a major break but couldn't say so. He knew the harm a conviction would have caused me but he also knew that he wouldn't be arresting me again under those circumstances. In retrospect though, I don't think I ever would have caught the break had I not been straight forward on the night of the accident and then changing the way I had been.

Thinking about moving on

Although I had a fairly idyllic life there at the beach I was far from satisfied. I was fit and healthy, lived within walking distance to one of the best beaches on the eastern seaboard, and my life was pretty laid back. I was also pretty naïve when it came to women, and frankly I sometimes still am I'm happy to say. I think there is a lot of fun to be had through discovery.

Iris lived further down the strand but equally close to the beach so I'd often ride my bike down there and hang out. She had a roommate named Patty who was quite hot and she was one of the main reasons I would go there. We'd hang out and smoke pot, joke around and go to the beach. One day I showed up and Patty was lying on the enclosed porch topless and invited me to sit with her, never bothering to put her top on. I knew she was dating a guy so I never caught the hint until Iris told me years later that Patty wanted to go out with me but didn't think I wanted to go out with her. That was her invitation to me. HUH? I hate looking back and seeing all those missed opportunities.

Another time I went to Michael's house, also near the beach, where he lived one floor below a couple of other hotties. He wasn't there so I figured I'd wait for him so we could hang out and go drinking later. While I was waiting I found a golf club leaning up against the house so I grabbed it and was taking practice swings using the nuts that fell from a tree in his backyard. As I was doing this I looked over and one of the hotties was standing there in a raincoat just staring at me but with a smile on her face. In lightning speed she opened the raincoat and flashed me her naked body. Bear in mind I had never met her though always wanted to, but I guess I was too shocked and didn't react soon enough so she turned and left before I even knew what to do next. What stinks is now that I know what to do in those situations nobody ever bothers to flash me!

If you have never lived in or visited Virginia Beach, it's a beautiful place in southern Virginia with incredibly warm water. In the summer it's a major tourist center for people coming from as far north as Canada. All summer long you battle traffic, crowds, long lines and a lot of aggravation. In the winter everything comes to a halt and many places shut down. Not a good place for someone prone to depression because the place becomes downright depressing in the winter months.

The weather is often really cold, it rains a lot, and every once in a while it will snow, causing work and schools to close.

I had a lot of trouble dealing with my emotional problems then; I was taking hard looks at my life and wondering what I was going to do with my future. I was also looking back and seeing all the lost productive opportunities and wasted time that was my life up until that moment. It was paralyzing me to the point where everyone seemed to be giving me unsolicited advice and telling me to get it together. All they were really doing was showing how much they cared. I couldn't see that way at the time and was becoming emotionally unstable, to the point where I was afraid to leave my apartment because I felt that everybody was laughing at me and judging me.

A strange thing happened during that time and I can't really explain what prompted me to do it. I woke up on a gray day in the fall, not hot and not cold, and at six in the morning I walked outside and just kept walking. I walked in a full circle covering three cities and arriving back at my house at eight thirty that night only making stops to eat and rest a bit. I saw some great things and some great places but I also went through some very tough neighborhoods where friends who knew the areas told me how lucky I was that I didn't get attacked. I had run in to some rough characters but I was neither a challenger nor a subservient person. I simply carried myself on the assumption that I had every right to be there and remained cautiously but not overly friendly. I was amazed at how much peace I found that day and how much clearer my head became.

The Road Trip

Not long after that experience, I just decided to move on. I quit everything, gave up my apartment and piled the few belongings that I had into a crappy VW and headed north to New Hampshire.

I stopped in New York to visit Michael who was there visiting his sister then made it in to New Hampshire.

Once I got there I realized that I had no home. I saw Bob and Kathy, friends, and my old man and aunt, and while all were genuinely happy to see me, none got too warm I presume out of fear that I might have asked them for a place to stay. I was there only for a couple of days and met up with an old friend from the island named Holly who I thought at one point that I might want to marry. We spent a night together and that changed my mind. I got a chance to see what marriage to her might be like through certain interactions, and in my opinion she would be a great friend so that's where we left it.

The next day we went out to a real dive bar in the late afternoon in January and talked about what I was going to do. I didn't have a plan so I decided I needed to go out and learn about life by getting away from all the advice and responsibilities just so I could see what would happen. I remember that day, January 20 at about 4:00 pm. It was just starting to snow but I had made up my mind with a little help from Holly. She told me point blank if I was going to do something, that moment was as good of a time as any.

So I gave her a parting hug and kiss and set out. I decided I would hitchhike and left with nothing but what I was wearing and only a quarter in my pocket. I managed to survive passing through Boston at night during the snowstorm and found a trucker who was going to New York.

Even though I didn't have a long-term plan, I was heading back to Virginia to pick up a final paycheck so I would have travel money. The trucker let me out in the middle of a tunnel in downtown New York at 1:00 in the morning; and I can assure you this type of thing is not for the faint of heart. Not sure what to do next I decided to keep hitchhiking. I wasn't naïve enough to think that I was going to be safe but I had no choice.

It wasn't long before a guy stopped to give me a lift. Before I got in I looked him and the car over to make sure no one else was in there and to see if I would have a fighting chance if he tried to overpower me. I asked him to drive me to a rest stop on the next highway that I would be taking because I knew it was pretty close.

He told me he would but asked if I would mind if he made a quick detour before dropping me off. It wasn't like I had many choices so I agreed. Mentally marking landmarks, I noticed that we were traveling in circles and realized the purpose of the detour was a ruse. Tired and hungry, I didn't protest when he invited me to grab a bite then offered the couch at his house if I wanted to crash. I accepted and after talking a little more once we got there I took up his couch offer.

No surprise that I woke up not long after to a hand running along my leg. Fortunately I'm a very light sleeper and woke up immediately. Asking him what the hell he was doing, he told me he thought we were going to have a date. I asked him where he got that idea then made it pretty damn clear that he wasn't going to be dating me, not now, not ever. I went on to say that if it was a condition of my crashing there then I would pack up and head out and he would be very wise to let me do it. To his credit he was apologetic and let me sleep uninterrupted. In the morning he dropped me off where I wanted to be.

It was at that moment that I formulated a guiding philosophy to carry me through the trip. First was to not get into a car with someone that I couldn't defend myself against if needed. Second was not do anything my kids (if I were to have any) would be ashamed of, like dressing up as Little Bo Peep or something. The third was to find a legitimate way to pay my way every chance I got. I decided to make my way to California to see my brother whom I hadn't seen in at least ten years, but I was going to stop and smell as many roses as I could along the way.

The Southern States

After New York, the trip back to Virginia was pretty uneventful and included another overnight stay. A rich hippie type of kid picked me up and let me stay at his house which was really comfortable. He and I barely spoke during the entire ten hours or so that we were driving together, and after eating breakfast together he drove me to the freeway where we parted company. I stopped and picked up my check; without saying anything to my family I just hit the road. My biggest concern was if I stopped to say goodbye they might have talked me out of it. There was a whole lot of unknown waiting to happen and the uncertainty made me vulnerable so I would have been susceptible to changing my mind if I was subjected to a heartfelt speech.

This was in the mid-seventies and the movie Deliverance was fresh in my mind, especially the part where the Tennessee mountain men made Ned Beatty squeal like a pig. I wasn't about to have any of that, so as luck would have it a ticket on Continental Trailways Bus line to anywhere in the country was $50. Rather than become part of the fabric through that part of the south I watched it from a bus window.

Somehow a rider who sat next to me managed to fill me with enough doubt to cause me to want to turn back. Instead of going forward I got off at the bus station in Columbia, South Carolina, with plans to turn back. Neither the bus going back nor the bus going forward was due until the next day so I sat in the bus station the entire day and night deciding what to do while being bored stiff. The experience did me some good because I made up my mind to finally go with my gut and start having some faith in myself. The next day I hopped on the bus going south and landed in New Orleans. I spent time looking for a little work there and took in some of the sights. After spending a couple of nights I hit the road going east heading to Florida, deciding it was something I wanted to try.

When you're close to a city, especially on a weekday, a lot of people are commuters and won't pick you up so I started walking along the 10 freeway. A car pulled over pretty far ahead and just stayed there so I thought they might be having car trouble. I had an idea that I might be able to help them fix the car in exchange for a ride. It turns out it was a bored housewife. There was too much traffic for her to back up so she just decided to wait awhile to see if I'd show up. Needless to say I got a ride, and then she drove me to the outskirts where it would be easier for me to get a lift heading in to Florida.

The next ride that I got was from a lady weighing about 500 pounds heading into a place called Apopka, Florida. She kindly offered me a place to crash for the night which I accepted since it was late, and because thankfully she wasn't looking for anything in return. She seemed nice enough so the next morning I accepted her offer to have breakfast with her family and possibly get help finding work with her brother. That's where it got weird. I met her mother and brother and ate breakfast with them, the whole time her mother was staring at me and saying how much she wished her husband was there. Her brother was missing quite a few teeth, and it soon became evident that much more was happening than met the eye.

It turned out that the girl who gave me the ride was married and in a really rocky relationship. She had a habit of bringing boy-toys home with her and her family thought I was one of them. The brother was a professional mooch and his efforts at work were to do everything he could to con advances out of his boss while habitually calling in sick. I was polite enough but figured it was time to go so I made my way outside. He and about ten of his equals followed me, forming a circle around me. The conversation stayed reasonably friendly but I was making it real clear to them that this scene wasn't intimidating me, even though I suspected they hoped it would.

Then the toothless brother popped the question; though I won't repeat what he asked here, let's just say it amounted to something much worse than dressing up like Little Bo Peep. He got a quick answer and they quickly made room for me to pass as I went on my way.

The fat lady tracked me down and was apologetic while still trying to get me to stay, though I'm not sure what made her think I'd want to unless I was in a coma or dying, and even then I would have had other thoughts. She got me to the freeway and I decided to keep going south. In my mind, the fat lady had sung.

Florida is kind of a mixed bag, it's a beautiful state but at the time it was a blend of families like the one I was with in Apopka, to the filthy rich, and plain and simple folks. It is also a hot and humid place but fortunately I was traveling in the late winter and early spring months so the weather was pretty good for the most part.

I had some interesting experiences there, from encountering a whole group of rednecks in a bar who clearly wanted to make me their entertainment, to being shot at from the roadside, to landing in jail once again and being let out in the swamps in the middle of the night without even the moonlight to help me see if I was going to step on a snake or an alligator. I made it out of the swamp that night untouched, but almost became breakfast for a pack of dogs that spotted me on the road. I didn't even realize it until a car came to a screeching halt with the door open and the driver screaming at me to get in. I turned and saw what I was about to get hit with and at least three of them were German Shepherds. Earlier in the month I had heard some news reports about some hikers and hitchhikers being killed by dog packs but that was in New York and I didn't know it was a possibility in Florida.

One of the more memorable experiences there was when I

worked with some migrant workers for a few days picking fruit. I was getting a ride heading further south in Florida and asked the driver if there would be any work where he was letting me off, and he was pretty sure there wouldn't be. As we were driving I noticed some orange groves and asked him to let me off. It was about three in the afternoon and he looked at me like I was crazy but I got out anyway. That was the assertive me going with my gut.

I climbed over the fence and saw there were quite a few people picking the oranges but I couldn't find anyone who could speak English and I couldn't speak Spanish. It would have been great if there would have been French-speaking fruit pickers, but alas I couldn't catch a break.

My objective for that day was to pick enough fruit so I could earn some money to buy dinner for the night and a little food for breakfast the next morning. Through my hand gestures, a tiny bit of the Spanish that I knew along with the little bit of English they knew I managed to pick enough fruit so I could earn the money I needed. The people were very kind and invited me to stay with them in their camp which was concrete-floored shacks provided to them by the corporations that owned the groves.

One of the teenagers living there spoke English so we talked and he was able to convey my objectives over the next few days. I went to work with them for two or three days, making $5 for each tub of oranges I picked. These weren't ordinary tubs, each was large enough to fill with water and use as a pool for about 15 little kids.

The teenager observed me on the first morning and immediately straightened me out by showing me how to shake the tree to get all of the oranges on the ground then quickly scooping them in the tub. I averaged about four tubs each day compared to their six to eight but I was satisfied.

It turns out they were a family from Texas that traveled to different states during each of the destination state's picking season. Everyone worked, and at lunch grandma would light a fire in the grove and make homemade burritos for everybody. I watched them and saw how well they did for themselves. They made a good living, they lived in a nice house when they weren't traveling but chose to stay in the corporate shacks because they were free.

They lived clean lives, the kids were educated and they drove around in a brand new truck. And they were paid in cash. I didn't know if they were legal or not and frankly I didn't care. They were a good family that worked and played together and helped others in need.

On the morning I left, they drove me to the freeway and the dad got out. We weren't able to talk but we had developed a mutual respect for each other; me through my observance of how he and his family were together, and him through my communication with his son. We shook hands and thanked each other then went on our way.

Later that day a rich white redneck picked me up in his Cadillac and made a comment about migrant workers being lazy and dirty. I quickly set him straight, but like a true piece of white trash he started looking at me the same way he saw them instead of considering an alternate view.

I decided it was time to head north then west and reached a part of the freeway where no one was going to give me a ride. Despite being clean and kempt, I saw every hand and finger gesture known to man and occasionally had to duck bottles being thrown at me. After walking a while I saw a broken down VW in a rest area. Unfortunately the driver wasn't a bored housewife; instead he was a crusty old redneck who really was having car trouble. It was a broken throttle cable which I managed to fix in exchange for a ride out of there. Unlike some of the other people I'd been with this guy could not wait to get rid of me and dumped me out without so much as a thank you.

On my way west I headed to New Orleans again, only this time it was Mardi Gras. That was the one night I abandoned my no heavy drinking rule and cut loose. Hard drinks were five cents in cheap glasses that you could take with you to the next bar. I couldn't find a hotel room to save my life but after a hard night of partying I managed to find a hostel and for $2.00 I could sleep on any piece of floor that I could find. I ended up sleeping in a sitting position with my back to a wall at the top of some stairs.

The next morning I set out without any idea of where I should go. As I was walking along the French Quarter I noticed how empty the streets were and started to turn in to an alley when a sailor stopped me. He told me he had seen somebody go down the alley the day before and get attacked by someone with a 2x4 for no apparent reason. I didn't see anybody in the alley so I wasn't all that worried about it, but we got to talking anyway. He was a pretty friendly guy who really seemed to know his way around the area. Once he knew I was looking for work before setting out on the road he talked me into going with him to a place called Morgan City which is southwest and quite a bit further from New Orleans.

By this time I carried a backpack and sleeping bag, a change of clothes, toiletries, as well as a very large and very sharp hunting knife. Guys would ask me about my sex life on the road and although I'm far from reserved I had no interest in talking with anybody about it. Then they'd ask how I defended myself when I got in to a tight spot. That's when I'd pull out the blade and show them. I never had to use it but I'm pretty sure the fact that I had it was exactly why I didn't need it.

It took us about a day and the trip down was the only time that I got into a car with people I might not have been able to defend myself against. The knife wasn't going to help me with the guys who picked up the sailor and me. They had rifles in the trunk, were drunk as skunks, and hit speeds of over 100 mph at times. It really surprised me that we made it alive.

Once I got to Morgan City I knew I wasn't going to be there long. The sailor was right about finding work there but had failed to mention that Morgan City was a modern-day equal opportunity slave camp. Oil companies hired laborers to work the fields moving and connecting pipes. You earned minimum wage while living out of their bunk houses. They provided you with white bread baloney sandwiches but the charge backs from the room and board were right above market rates and that ate up most of your minimum wage, the rest went to taxes.

I left the same day I arrived. My sailor buddy was pissed off but I wasn't interested in what they were offering. Making my way northwest, I hitchhiked through some very nice but humid places. Once in Texas I again had no particular plans and a boat captain who picked me up apparently hitched cross-country only years before. He convinced me that I should be looking for work on some boats and after a very long day of driving he dropped me off in Freeport, Texas, a boat town on the east coast of Texas and south of Galveston.

It was already dark by then but I went knocking on boats to see if I could find a place to stay. I couldn't find anyone that would answer but found an empty boat where I bunked for the night. The next morning I walked around the yard and found work on a shrimp boat that was about to sail.

There was the captain, the first mate, and me on this boat. Shrimp boats have tall 25- to 30-foot-long arms, or outriggers. Once the captain identifies a shrimp area, he lowers the outriggers which have big wooden things called doors on the ends. Attached to the doors are metal leaders that look kind of like anchors. So the leader is dropped in the water, followed by the door, which then takes the net down so the shrimp can be caught.

As we were setting out, the captain was testing the equipment and lowered the outriggers while we were going to the open ocean; that is, the shark-infested Gulf of Mexico. One of the leaders was jammed so he looked at me and told me to get out and fix it. After checking both my to-do and bucket lists and noting that climbing out on a pole thirty feet out over the ocean while the boat was moving was not on either of them, I did it anyway and freed the leader.

The fact that there was a hurricane only a few days before made the first night and the rest of the trip unbearable because of the waves. I got incredibly seasick but there was no sympathy and I definitely had to pull my weight. A big part of my job was checking the sample net, a small net used to gauge the percentage of shrimp in the haul. For some reason, it was important that I check the sample net between two and three a.m. If the net was thirty percent or more of shrimp, I'd have to hit the signal so we could stop the boat and haul in the catch.

Once the nets were up we'd dump them on the deck and see all sorts of things in addition to the shrimp. I can't remember all of them but we had sea turtles, snapper, and rock fish to name a few. We'd throw all of those back in the water and pop the heads off the shrimp before throwing the bodies in the coolers below.

After the shrimp were processed and stored, it was my job to clean and hose down the deck. I used something similar to a big squeegee to gather the heads and dead fish so I could sweep them off the boat into the water through the holes along the sides. I was in effect 'chumming' the water; typically there would be sharks along the side of the boat catching whatever I was throwing over. One day in particular I was extra sick, throwing up over the side of the boat and could see about six or seven sharks in the water swimming in the chum.

It was pretty unsettling seeing them in feeding mode as I leaned over the boat right above them. At one point I leaned over again to get sick and just as I did a strong wave hit the side of the boat behind me and knocked me off balance. I was really lucky to have caught the rail otherwise I would have gone over the side and become the main course for those sharks.

What we were paid was a percentage of the haul along with room and board on the boat at no charge. I ended up spending eight days total out at sea about 24 hours away from land, and never did get over being sick. Worse, our shrimp hauls were really bad so I ended up making a total of $32.00 for all eight days of work.

I decided to keep moving and made my way further south to a town called Rockport. I was still in the 'get-a job-on-a-boat' mode and landed one as a deckhand on a tugboat that serviced the oil rigs nearby. That job was a dream compared to the shrimping experience and far more lucrative too. Other than having to retrieve a loose barge during a hurricane to keep it from hitting the derricks, it was a pretty tame experience. I made about $350 for two weeks work and lived on the boat while eating like a king. I only stayed the two weeks before deciding to keep moving on.

After getting my check and leaving Rockport, I went further south and stopped for lunch in Port Aransas Island. The weather was beautiful and so were the girls, and unbeknownst to me I happened to land there at the beginning of spring break. Port Aransas is at the north tip of Padre Island and back then spring break there rivaled Fort Lauderdale. I stayed there long enough to have plenty of fun and with money in my pocket was able to enjoy it.

When spring break was over I kept heading south to Corpus Christi and Brownsville which are at the very bottom of Texas. I remember being depressed by the surrounding areas. I stayed in a pretty seedy part of Corpus Christi and as I encountered tough guys during my travels I decided that I had to appear tougher than they were in order to survive. Fortunately for me, no one called my bluff otherwise I would have been in a world of hurt. It wasn't that I couldn't handle myself, but some of these guys looked like they were pretty experienced at being tough.

After a few days there, I headed north on the west side of Texas to catch the 10 Freeway heading to California. I landed in a few small towns where I'd hit some bars and pool halls, and I'd knock on doors to see if I could find work for a few dollars. Walking toward one house I noticed a pen around a pond, and then realized there were alligators in the pond. From the house a good sized Labrador Retriever came at me at full speed with teeth bared, ready to rumble. Patting my legs and calling him to come over, I surprised the hell out of him. The Lab stopped mid-way and came to me, allowing me to pet him.

I gave him a good rubdown and we became fast friends which I don't think excited the owner. There were a couple of long-haired guys in their forties and after talking for a little bit they made it very clear they didn't have any work for me so I went back on the road. A few minutes later a car pulled over to give me a lift, and I recognized the driver as one of the guys in the background at the alligator pond place.

He kept asking me a lot of questions about what I was doing there and why. I asked him why he had all of the questions. Once he was comfortable that I was just a traveler he gave me some insights. Apparently the group I left was drug dealers who had just gone through a major bust. When I showed up out of the blue looking for work, they thought I was an undercover Narc trying to get established with them to take them down again along with their network.

He then went on to tell me that one of the things they talked about before sending me on my way, was putting me to work before beating me up and throwing me in the pond for the alligators to finish. I thought the guy was kidding at first but his face had paled as he described it which told me just how lucky I was that they let me go. The reason he came and picked me up, he told me, was to make sure to drive me far enough away so they wouldn't come looking for me in case they changed their minds.

A couple of days later I found myself in another small town and was stuck in a light industrial section watching cars go by but never stopping. There was a guy leaning against a Jeep talking to two girls the entire time I'd been there, and they would all glance over at me pretty regularly. I hollered over at them and walked up to ask why I wasn't getting a lift. The guy looked over at the girls then explained to me that just a week before a drifter came to town and for no reason hacked the woman postmaster to death with a hatchet.

Like it or not, he told me, I didn't stand a chance of getting a lift because the townspeople all liked the woman who was murdered and I represented the guy who killed her. He went on to say that if I was still in town by sunset I would probably be confronted by groups looking to cause me some pretty serious harm. I didn't need any more convincing and got him to agree to drive me out of town. I also got him to agree to give me the cheeseburger on the console.

I continued to head north back to the 10 Freeway and was starting to see some landscape that I had only seen in movies, and I liked what I saw. The trip north was pretty relaxing for the most part, and although I had become cautious in light of some of the things I had just gone through I had become pretty relaxed and at peace with how far I had come to that point. I started the journey in mid-January as a mixed up kid full of self-doubt, and by the beginning of April I was more at ease and not so afraid of the unknown because I was learning to think on my feet.

Once I hit the 10 Freeway, I caught a lift with a guy who was a little older than me but we had a fair amount in common. It was clear neither of us was going to take crap from the other; we developed a mutual respect that worked for both of us. He was heading to California and welcomed the idea of having company and being able to alternate driving so he could get some rest without having to stop.

We got through New Mexico and in Arizona where at some point I realized that I was looking at landscape that I had only seen on Wild Kingdom and in movies about the west. I grew up in lush greenery which I always found beautiful, but the desert held a different beauty for me. I think it was because while I was growing up, places like the desert and Disneyland were places I never thought I would see so seeing the desert at that moment was almost like a dream come true.

We came across a pretty lonely section of the freeway overlooking some very large hills in the desert terrain. I shocked the hell out of the driver when I asked him to pull over and let me out. He thought I was crazy when I told him I wanted to go hiking out there, and he was actually a little pissed off that I was leaving him. His parting shot was to remind me of the dangers I would likely encounter like rattlesnakes and scorpions. Maybe even a Gila Monster or two. I didn't care though, that was the first time I had ever seen a cactus and I wanted to see more.

I was in shorts and hiking boots so I found a long stick to use as a precaution to ferret out snakes if there were going to be any. Miles from the nearest services, very few cars on the road, and without a first-aid kit I would have been a goner if something poisonous bit me.

Cautiously, I took a long hike away from the freeway and completely enjoyed what I was doing. I had read somewhere that you could find water by cutting into a barrel cactus and going toward the root so I gave it a try. I did find some moisture and squeezed it to drink a few drops, and then I ate the cactus meat. Growing up in

New Hampshire, I knew some of the basics in terms of not eating vegetation from the woods because of the various poisonous plants you were likely to encounter. For some reason I didn't exercise much caution in the desert probably because I was enthralled and maybe a little overwhelmed at what I was seeing.

Eventually I made my way back to the freeway. I was a little disappointed that I didn't see any snakes or scorpions, but I did see a road runner and some hawks, neither of which I would have seen where I came from. When I got to the freeway I stood under a white billboard, blank except for what some poor soul had written in big bold letters: **HELP ME PLEASE! I'VE BEEN STANDING HERE FOR 44 HOURS AND I NEED A RIDE!** I got a ride in less than forty-four minutes. I was surprised when the driver told me how energetic I looked for having stood there for that long! As good fortune would have it, he was going straight to California and within a day I would be seeing my brother for the first time in many years.

THREE

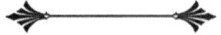

California: Part 1

The trip from Arizona to California was fun but uneventful. I was riding with a guy who was paid to drive a car cross-country for a family that was moving to California from the east coast; the driver was on a mission to get there as fast as he could. He had a flair for adventure so we hit it off real well. It wasn't long before we were belting out California Girls as we crossed the state line and played road games with a lot of those California girls on the freeway. A few girls did some pretty wild things to get our attention like flashing us, and two cuties even went so far as to pull us over and give us their phone numbers.

I knew I had come to the right place even if I hadn't been coming to see my brother. Yet I was really anxious to see Joe, a big strapping man with a heart of gold, somebody I had admired since as far back as I could remember. After not seeing each other for so many years, his first reaction was to reach for a club to come at me with, thinking I was an intruder. Once Joe realized it was me, we locked into a huge bear hug, and from that moment on we had a blast. It was also the first time I had met his four boys and we all hit it off right away, and not long after my sister-in-law and I became close.

Joe and I were inseparable; he got me a job where he worked through a temp agency. From there we were on a mission to get drunk and raise hell every chance we got, something we ended up doing very well. While I was a guest I made it a point to chip in by fixing things, paying my own way, and making sure to not become a burden. That is a philosophy I still embrace today. Monitoring the tone and ambiance, after a couple of months of camping, barbecuing, and lots of drinking while staying at his house, I decided to leave for a while to stay with my sister Mary in Hollywood before moving on.

When I arrived it was another warm welcome although she and her boyfriend, Marty, visited with us at Joe's a lot. Hollywood was a great experience, and sharing it with Mary was a blast since she was also a hard partyer. She lived in a singles complex and it was only a matter of days before I knew just about everybody there and was introducing Mary to people she lived near for years but never met.

My funds were getting low so I was on the prowl for some work. Mary let me use her car, a 1962 Ford Fairlane pimp-mobile with a faulty gas gauge. I used it to go to downtown Los Angeles where I thought I could find work but ran out of gas instead. I managed to push the car into a parking garage where I talked the owner into letting me keep it there overnight so I could get enough money to get it out and get gas.

I had no idea how I was going to achieve that goal, but there was no way in hell I was going to borrow from Joe or Mary because I had no way of knowing how I was going to pay it back. The good news was Mary didn't use the car at all so she had no idea it was missing. The next morning after she left for work I decided to go out and start knocking on doors to see if I could get some handyman work for cash.

I didn't get a single bite after knocking on more than one hundred doors that morning, in both commercial and residential sections of the area. The last place I approached was a boarded up building that had building debris on the outside and didn't appear to offer much promise. The debris was wallboard and wood, like someone was gutting the building. There was a faded American Legion sign on the top of the outside wall like an old advertisement and there were three entrance doors around the building, so I knocked loudly on all of them. Walking away after knocking on the last door, I heard a low grumpy voice behind me calling out and asking me what I wanted.

I turned and saw this big, tall, ugly looking guy named Csaba (pronounced Chaba), who I apparently woke up, unusual considering it was late morning on a weekday. I offered to take away all of the trash around the building for five dollars on the condition that I could get it up front so I could get my car and put gas in it. Eyeing me suspiciously, Csaba provided the five dollars and told me he would give me another five if I came back for real and did the job.

I would have done it anyway for the five dollars I'd asked for but it was a nice added incentive.

Armed with his advanced funds I was able to pay a partial parking fee with a promise to come back the next day to pay it in full. Leaving my overnight gear as collateral, they let me take the car so I was able to finish the job. I still hadn't gotten out of my travel mode so I was always taking my back pack and road gear just in case I got a notion to leave town, even though I really wasn't expecting to go anywhere. Gas was about fifty cents a gallon then so I had enough to haul the trash away and collect the rest of the money. I also made good on my promise to pay the parking garage fee.

Csaba owned the American Legion building. He was a tough guy who had escaped from Hungary during the revolution in the late '50's, after watching when his eighteen-year-old brother was shot to death in the street by the Russian KGB. Impressed with how I managed to get an advance out of him, Csaba asked if I would like to work with him on the building. He was in the middle of building a recording studio and financed it by working forty hours each weekend as an X-ray tech at UCLA Medical Center. He hated the job but managed to do all forty hours in a single weekend every weekend which worked out for his medical colleagues too. He got his weekdays free to build the recording studio, and they got their weekends off while he worked.

The pay I was getting from Csaba wasn't much but it included room and board there at the recording studio. Over the next few years I not only helped build the studio along with Csaba and Alex, the studio engineer, I ended up becoming the General Manager and bouncer. One doesn't think a recording studio would need a bouncer but rock-and-rollers can get rowdy and others needed incentive to pay their bills. There was also a leg-breaker on the payroll, but that was a secret side that I barely delved into, in part because I didn't need to know what all was going on and in part for survival. Sometimes it's just better not to know everything that goes on around you.

The leg-breaker was a friendly ju-jitsu expert with a massive chest who stood about 6'6". He had been in prisons all over the world mainly for political crimes, many of which were trumped up according to him. Despite being friendly, he had no trouble casting that warm-and-fuzzy part of him aside when it came time to fulfilling a work order, particularly when he needed the money.

The studio was located on the east side of Hollywood and had one of the best sound rooms in the city. Csaba was a master at finding unique equipment and buying it dirt cheap so it wasn't long before word got around about our studio. Though we lacked some of the recording equipment that the big record companies wanted, bands liked us because they could play around with different sounds in our studio before going to cut tracks in the big Hollywood studios. We played hosts to bands including Cheap Trick, The Runaways (Joan Jett), Devo, Toni Basil, Jules and the Polar Bears, and others affiliated with well-known acts. By hosting the bands, large groups, and rich kids who wanted to lay tracks, we were booked around the clock.

Despite the fact that there were drugs all around me and they were always being offered, I never did most of the available drugs while I was there in the studio. The road trip cured me of wanting to do them and I liked staying straight for the most part, even though I was still a hard drinker on occasion. I only smoked pot once in a while if the girls I was with wanted me to, and I'd do some coke with some friends and my sister once in a while too. By the time I turned thirty I quit pot and coke and haven't done it since. And up until I turned twenty-eight I was still getting myself in jail periodically and for various reasons but I had reached a point where I was really trying to clean things up.

A lot of work for little money, the studio was a great experience overall. I made good friends, developed experience that helped me in later ventures, not to mention rubbing elbows with famous musicians and actors, as well as dating some very attractive women. There were also fun adventures, or at least some interesting events.

One time I was riding down Sunset Boulevard and pulled up next to a car bearing New Hampshire license plates at a traffic light. Our windows were open, so I got the driver's attention. The exchange went like this:

> Me (excitedly while looking over at him): "Hey, I'm from New Hampshire too."
> Driver (Middle Eastern, not smiling and looking over at me): "Good."
> Me: "Uh, where are you from?"
> Driver: "California."
> Me: "But your car has New Hampshire plates."
> Driver (just as the light turned green): "I know, stolen car."

Another time I was using Csaba's car, a 1963 Mercedes with a four-speed on the steering column. The car was in great shape overall but with one big problem: every time you would shift in or out of first or reverse the horn would honk, and it was a loud horn. Without realizing it, I pulled up at a stoplight behind a biker gang and shifted into first. That horn blast got me quite a few dirty looks. After the light changed and I shifted gear, the second blast had them surrounding me and telling me to pull the hell over. I learned how to talk real fast that day.

One of the more memorable events stemmed from an on-going feud between us at the studio and those at the little theater across the street, run by a big-breasted air-headed lady who liked me and I liked her. Members of her cast kept parking in our lot and taking spaces reserved for our customers. We tried asking her to ask them to stop and that didn't work. We'd leave notes on their cars that got progressively worse telling them they'd have consequences if they didn't stop. That didn't work either and we were getting more and more irritated.

One night we only had a small recording session going on yet our lot was full. We recognized one of the cars as being from the theater. I was manning the studio myself while Alex and Csaba were out on dates. Thinking that Csaba was already gone, I found him letting the air out of the offending car's tires. He said the obvious, that he was pissed the car was there. Csaba then told me he had a loaded .38 in his desk drawer and said for me to feel free to use it if the car's owner went ballistic, though neither of us knew who the owner was or what he or she looked like. He then looked at his handiwork with great satisfaction and left to go on his date.

Not surprisingly I heard some angry yelling outside the front door later on so I went outside and saw this big bruiser of a guy voicing his displeasure at his deflated tires. He had to be at least 6'5" and probably weighed 240 or 250 pounds. Our stoop was three steps high and as I stood on top of the stoop and he on the ground, I noted that we were looking at each other at eye level. That was indeed one of those proverbial "Oh shit" moments we all hope never to have.

It became clear to me that the only way for me to survive the upcoming exchange was to go through a battle of wits which I desperately had to win. He didn't have to worry about his wits because there was no way I was going to be able to pummel him or make it to the gun before he beat the life out of me.

I stood there looking into his beet-red face watching the froth seep out of his mouth but stayed surprisingly calm. The question on the table was what gave us the right to let the air out of his tires? The answer I gave him was how many times were he and his buddies told not to park there? Just then he started to raise a fist high enough in the air like he was going to pound it hard on my head, so I said the first thing that came to mind:, "Buddy, you come close to using that and I'm going to cut you in half where you stand." I had no idea how I would do it or with what, but I knew it was something Clint Eastwood would have said and it seemed appropriate at the time.

Motionless for a minute or two, neither of us said a word until he turned and started to walk away. As he did, I hollered over to him "Hey asshole, get your car out of here or I'm having it towed." Nothing like slapping the bull on the ass, but I was on a roll and wasn't about to stop. He had some kind of pouch strapped to his shoulder, almost like a purse with a shoulder strap. He turned to me, clutched the pouch, and stomping his foot on the ground, shouted "Ooooh!" before hurriedly walking away. Shortly after, his car was gone and that was the last time we had trouble from him and his fellow actors. Sadly though, I never did get to see where the big-breasted air-head and I were going to take our mutual attraction because she stopped talking to me right after.

Around this time the Hillside Strangler[2] was terrifying the community. Csaba and Alex had a good friend named Melissa who was a lesbian psychologist and far more emotionally messed up than any of the patients she was treating. It didn't matter that Melissa was gay; I simply bring it up to show that our intentions for Melissa were sincere and without ulterior motives like trying to get her in the sack. Melissa was terrified over the Hillside Strangler because she worked in the area where he seemed to be striking. Her house was in Mt. Washington near Pasadena but she wasn't going back until the strangler was caught. So we fixed up a private room for her in the back of the studio so she could live with us for a while and we mapped out her route to our place from her office in Hollywood while she lived with us.

This was in the seventies so there were no mobile phones, everything was by pay phone. At her request, she would call us

---

[2] Hillside Stranglers Kenneth Bianchi and Angelo Buono were apprehended January 12, 1979 and October 22, 1979, respectively.

every night before leaving work and we'd note the time so that if she didn't get home to us in the usual amount of time we would get a search going and would know the exact route she was on.

You might think it was overkill, and frankly, we felt that ourselves until the police discovered one of the victim's bodies in Melissa's backyard in Mt. Washington. That experience brought it home, and even though the victim appeared to be placed there at random, we knew her fears were justified. We stuck with her and held her close until the stranglers were caught.

Still, we weren't without some mischief. At times we were rotten bastards in a good natured way. One night a few weeks after the body was found in her backyard, Melissa and I were taking a walk near the studio and she was unloading about the things that were bothering her, not least of which were the Hillside Strangler episodes that terrified her. I let her vent for a while and was showing genuine empathy and I even put my arm around her shoulder to give her comfort and security in a brotherly way. Then I stopped her and looked her in the eye, hesitated a moment, and in a concerned, breathy voice told her I was the Hillside Strangler.

I learned new curse words that night. I'm not sure what possessed me to do it but I couldn't resist because it seemed so right at the time. Melissa shoved me out of the way and screamed what an asshole I was; then flew past Alex and Csaba to lock herself in the bathroom, screaming the whole time.

Csaba came out and asked me what was going on so I told him, and then in his thick Hungarian accent he proceeded to tell me just how low of a jerk I was and called me every name in the book. He wanted to know how I could have done such a thing to someone who was obviously so fragile.

He got to me so I crawled back to the bathroom apologizing profusely through the bathroom door while begging forgiveness. It took a minute once I paused and she shot back this comment, at the top of her lungs I might add:

"It wouldn't have been so bad if that asshole Csaba hadn't done it to me just an hour before you did! What the hell is wrong with you dickheads?" Csaba mysteriously had to leave after hearing her complaint.

Meanwhile, the Hillside Strangler events had another weird twist for us while everyone was desperately trying to find him (them).

We had a very attractive girl named Virginia booking time in the studio and she quickly had my and Alex's attention. And she'd play us pretty well, taking turns kissing us and giving us attention at different times.

Alex and I decided we wanted to take her out on a double date and we flipped a coin to determine who was going to ask Virginia. We actually had thought about both of us taking her out at the same time to see what would happen, but decided we didn't know her well enough. I lost the coin toss and took Jeanne, another one of our clients. We all went to dinner and then to the Laserium Show up at the Griffith Park Observatory. That was the longest amount of time we spent with Virginia and despite the fact that she was with Alex, she was still taking turns kissing each of us. However, the time we spent with her caused Alex and me to independently come to the conclusion that something was amiss. She just seemed a little strange so neither of us dated her after or even talked about her again.

Some months later, I was eating lunch and watching TV when Alex came in the room and asked me if I had seen the news. When I told him I hadn't he suggested I turn on any news station to catch up. There was our girl Virginia, in handcuffs with the police somewhere in the Pacific Northwest. She turned out to be Kenneth Bianchi's girlfriend and had been caught trying to strangle a woman so the police would think the Strangler was still out there. You just never know with people I guess.

Life at the studio was constantly evolving and we had a revolving door of friends, girlfriends, and band people on a regular basis. Eventually I became involved with a former girlfriend of one of the band members who used our studio a lot. She and I moved into an apartment right off the Sunset Strip and we had a grand time.

Carol was, as my nephews put it, 'smoking hot' but, on a maintenance scale with the highest being ten was a thirty-five. Despite having dated quite a few girls it was the first time I ever had a steady girlfriend and I noticed that in a short time I had put on over twenty pounds. I was active so I wasn't sure what was happening.

Our relationship was incredibly passionate, with her picking fights at least once but up to three times a day and then we'd rush to the make-up sex. She was wild and we did some wild things. She brought a lot of things out in me, most of them good in terms of passion but she also used to push my anger to the limits. I almost felt like she was trying to take me to a place where she knew I would never go, which was to hit her, just to see if she could do it. I never did but it disturbed me even more once I found out that her previous boyfriend had beaten her so badly she was in the hospital for three months.

We had a strong passionate relationship for about nine months and lived together in the apartment her father paid for. My life was pretty cool given my circumstances; gorgeous girlfriend with a rich father, a job at a recording studio and going to the beach just about every other day. Despite the passionate make-up sex that always ensued, the emotional strain had become more of a problem. After a while the sex wasn't offsetting it anymore.

And I was getting tired of the recording studio that I helped build. Csaba started working with a guy named Israel who made it his mission to point out every wrong thing I did in order to make himself look good, and Csaba was buying into it. One day I walked in to Csaba's office with Israel in tow and told him point blank that the two of them deserved each other, so they were going to have each other. I left and never went back, though a year or two later Israel sought me out to apologize and to tell me he was wrong about me. I accepted his apology and we ended up becoming friends.

At that point I was looking to try and find what one might consider a normal life, which to me was a career path with a steady paycheck. I was still living with Carol at the time, but I set out on a quest to find a career. I started looking, and the only thing that was available was a sales job in San Gabriel Valley with a company that distributed structured metal products, like shelving, racks, and lockers.

My mode of transportation was an old van that I got while I was at the recording studio. The van had been completely refurbished but was in an auto garage when the entire garage caught fire. When I picked it up all the paint was burned off, and the windows were blown out, not to mention a whole lot of other problems. I got windows for it and drove it long enough while at the studio to identify some of the other mechanical and electrical failures, like having the brakes fail, and the brake and headlights blowing out by me just stepping on the brake pedal. I drove it long enough to where I thought I had everything fixed, though I didn't get it painted.

On the morning of my interview with the storage equipment company I put on my business suit and drove the van to the company that was about twenty-five miles away from our apartment. For some reason it decided to rain hard that morning so I turned the windshield wipers on, something I hadn't done since I bought the damn van. At that moment I wished I had used them sooner because the entire wiper arm on the driver's side flew off while I was on the freeway.

Had there been a passenger with me they would have been able to see just fine because that wiper was intact and working, but I couldn't see at all. Since I didn't know the area and only built in a fifteen minute buffer for my appointment time, I had to improvise by sitting on the engine compartment between the driver and passenger seats in order to see the road ahead. Ridiculous was that it rained the entire way until I pulled up to the interview site and got into the building yet once inside, it stopped raining and was sunny for the rest of the month. I got the job and after about two months I got a company car and was able to get rid of the van.

I continued living with Carol for about six more months before she decided to move to Colorado. We packed some of her stuff in her van and I used her father's station wagon to haul the rest of it. We used walkie-talkies to communicate and had an enjoyable trip. This happened during the gas crisis so gas was often scarce depending on where you were and it had gotten expensive, though nothing like we have today. Fortunately though, her father paid for everything.

I stayed with her for a few days to help her get settled and then had to get back to LA for work and to get her father's car back. I'm not sure what town it was but there was a sign at the gas station just before crossing into the desert that said 'Last Gas Stop for the Next 105 miles!' I was low on gas and the car was a gas guzzler so I stopped and filled it up.

Gas pumps today usually have concrete poles to protect the pumps from damage. Back then there weren't any of those poles. As I was finishing my fill-up I watched a van with a full load of people pull up to the island right next to me. A guy jumped out and was shouting something in a foreign language as the van was backing up to the pump. His shouting got louder and faster and I looked over to see the van back into the pump and knock it right off the island.

As it did, the tailpipe passed over the pipe leading to the underground gas tank and caught it on fire. I watched this expressionless and thought, in anticipation of the explosion that was surely about to take place, "they're going to bury me in five different states."

I marveled as I watched these numbskulls run around frantically in circles yet doing absolutely nothing. Fortunately the fast-acting attendant had seen the whole thing from inside and ran out to hit the Emergency Shut-Off switch in time to keep that whole part of town from blowing up. About a year or so later I began seeing the concrete poles being put in at various gas stations.

I didn't want to follow Carol to Colorado. We carried on a long-distance relationship for a while, and since she was working in Vail I went out there once or twice, got to stay for free and skied all day while she worked, then partied at night when she was off. By the time the relationship ended, I had moved to the Los Feliz section of Los Angeles in the apartment complex where my sister Mary lived.

Los Feliz is a great place near Griffith Park where many health conscious or nature-loving people go for peace of mind. I started running there and it didn't take me long to take off the extra weight I'd gained while I was living with Carol. Once I did, I spent the next six years developing a pretty enviable social life and was incredibly relaxed as a result.

I mentioned earlier that I was never good at "picking up" women if you will. I was the kind of guy who wanted to spend time getting to know someone and I tended to move slowly, sometimes so slowly that I'd miss what clearly could and would have been fun opportunities. What I did observe and ultimately focused on was that if I stayed in shape and just kept being myself, women, in fact, would come to me.

Once when I was heading out to play tennis with a buddy I walked out to my car and a very cute girl waved to me from across the street. She had a really pretty smile along with a great body, so I smiled, waved back, and then got in my car to go to play tennis. The next morning as I was getting in the car to go to work, I found a note on my windshield from the girl with her phone number on it. Needless to say we connected.

Another time I was in San Diego on business and while sitting down to dinner at the TGIFs I couldn't help but notice a very attractive girl at the bar. I saw that she was with two guys so I decided that I wouldn't be getting to know her that night or any night for that matter. After ordering dinner and wine, I started reading the paper I had brought with me. Not long after, the waitress brought up a glass of wine from the girl I had been looking at. She was a stewardess there with some friends, and we hit it off well, indeed.

That was pretty much my life those six or so years, working out, excelling in my job, and dating. The funny thing was that if I wanted a date, the best thing for me to do at any time was to not try and get one. I was turned down more times when asking women out, yet it was very common for me to be with four or five different women in a week because they found me approachable.

I had never been healthier and more relaxed than I was during those years. At twenty-four I became sales manager for the steel storage equipment company and covered the area from Central California to San Diego, Palm Desert, and Las Vegas. I bought a condo in Orange County, California, overlooking a pool in a largely singles community that was surrounded by great places to run and exercise. In the summer I did a lot of swimming, running and working out, and in the winter I did a whole lot of running and skiing on top of going to the gym. I bicycled all year long.

Despite dating so many women during those years, I was different than some of my friends in that I got to know the women I was dating and made it a point to make the relationships something more than just sex. There was no question that sex was a big part, but we took a lot of time to laugh and have fun. One of my favorite dates was a midnight movie after a night on the town. I would always get my dates to bring large purses which we would stuff with bottles of wine to drink while watching the movie. Then we'd go out to breakfast at two in the morning and find ways to crack each other up.

I tried to incorporate healthy living with dating, even though it wasn't required of the women I was dating. But still, the fact that I did made for some pretty fun dates like skiing, sailing, horseback riding, bicycling, hiking, and beach picnics. It wasn't always healthy though, sometimes it was just plain fun like bar hopping and staying in bed all day long. Even though I was dating different women, I was very careful to never bring anyone else into the conversation, even when asked. Out of respect for my dates, I focused only on them, not as a game or as a conquest but because I learned enough about them, and they about me, to know that we could enjoy our time out together.

From the time I was about 19 to 27, I was enjoying myself immensely. Bit by bit though, I found myself looking for more. I realized that while I had no trouble getting dates, I had no one to be a couple with when I'd go out with my friends who were couples. I was also looking for more at work. I felt like I was in a career that anyone could do, and despite being good at my job I was in a tiny company with limited opportunities. I learned to listen to those little voices telling me to look for more. Professional motivational speakers say the only way to move ahead is by being willing to leave your comfort zone.

Forming a pathway to success is one reason for leaving a comfort zone, but another is from a tenet we learn in business which is that non-growth is the first step to stagnation, the step right before a decline. If you don't try to improve and move ahead, you risk outliving your value as an employee. Much like the way I never wanted to overstay my welcome when visiting friends and family, in business I decided I might need to seek opportunities to grow or I would never get ahead. A case in point was shortly after I came to that conclusion one of the manufacturers we represented had a job opening. I had decided that I wasn't going to see any growth where I was so I approached them and they offered me a job. I took it and worked there for about six months until my former company came back and offered me a sales manager's position at a significantly higher pay scale.

That lasted for a few years but again felt like I needed more so I started sending out feelers and even studied for a real estate license because I wasn't sure where my quest would take me. Around the same time I was starting to feel like I needed something more from my relationships with women, or lack thereof.

Jeff was a salesman working under me at the steel company who became one of my best friends. We always had a blast together and admired and respected each other. Despite our friendship, I set expectations quickly and clearly so Jeff could see the lines that couldn't be crossed. He knew that our friendship was built on our business relationship and one of the keys to staying friends was to do our jobs the way we were supposed to. Jeff also knew that our friendship wouldn't stop me from firing him if he chose to try and take advantage. But with Jeff, that was never a problem nor was it ever a real concern.

Jeff and I did a lot together both professionally and as friends. Surprisingly, he made it a point to introduce me to his sister who was stuck in a nowhere relationship. It was surprising because he not only knew my reputation with ladies but he frequently saw it in action. He did know the kind of person I was though and I think that's why he was comfortable introducing me.

At one point, I agreed to go out on a double date with Jeff and his girlfriend Marsha who later became his wife. That's when I met Rachel, Jeff's sister, and she and I hit it off right away. Although I continued to see other women for a while, Rachel and I started seeing each other more and more until we became a couple and later moved in together. The fact that Rachel and I were living together was a big problem for her parents since they were traditional. She was also a born again Christian trying to figure how to assimilate into her faith while living with me so she was conflicted on a number of fronts.

As for me, I was trying to move ahead while trying to figure out how I could stay faithful to Rachel in light of the freedoms I had given up, like freedom to exercise when I wanted and date who I wanted. I also had observed that I was starting to put on weight again.

Meanwhile, I was still at the steel company but one of my feelers landed me an interview for a management position with one of my company's competitors. As we were getting down to the point of an offer my company caught wind of it and interviewed me for the general manager's position heading three companies they had bought in the San Francisco Bay area. Eventually my company made me a great offer but required that I relocate to Northern California, which proved to be a little more difficult than anticipated. The bay area is beautiful with lots to do, but my support network was down south and the weather in Northern California left a lot to be desired compared with Southern California.

At twenty-eight, I accepted the promotion and had no idea what lay ahead of me as I set out to run three divisions with a group that had problems with its previous owners. I had experience in selling but not in pro forma management nor did I know how to manage such a large group. Worse, the group had a bad reputation for not completing their jobs and I had to take on some large contracts that were underbid by the corporate office.

I went ahead and got an apartment in San Leandro which is a little south of Oakland on the East side. The apartment was nice and brand new, but the area I was in was industrial and depressing.

I had a nice big office but the job was a ball buster because I had to go in and re-write the rules that were opposite to what the staff was accustomed. The company was comprised of three divisions, one was a major subcontractor that sold and installed lockers and storage equipment and marketed directly through major contractors on a variety of construction projects. The second division distributed the shelving, racks, and lockers through a dealer network comprised of about 250 dealers. The third division sold the equipment directly to the end users.

We also had a top security contract to provide equipment and staff to one of the laboratories in the area. The security contract meant that we had three employees on our payroll whose only job was to service equipment in a highly classified section of Lawrence Livermore Laboratories. Their security clearances went back to when and where they were born and took over three years to complete.

The staff at the main office was used to being run by managers in each division who were more interested in being friendly than they were in performance. I was just the opposite and made it clear on the first day that I wasn't there looking for friends. I was a new manager and had a lot to learn, and in retrospect I could have and should have blended a little of what the other managers did into my style, a technique I did in later years.

It was a busy place and I was focused on getting all the work completed that was not yet done and tying up tens of thousands of dollars in hold-back funds. I was also cleaning up the warehouses to try and find thousands of dollars in lost inventory. During my second week the owner of the company was up there and we were having in-depth meetings with my other managers when we heard a loud crash and felt the entire building shake. One of the crew had tipped a loaded forklift over. Fortunately for us no one was hurt.

We had a few characters there, not the least of which was my secretary Freda who was a very shy individual in her late forties who had many quirks; one being was her message delivery. She would stand in my doorway while I was conducting a meeting until I'd acknowledge her; once I did ask her what she needed, instead of simply telling me, she'd walk across the room and hand me a note that would say something like "John is on Line 2."

I caught a delivery company paying bribes to some of the warehouse staff and got them out of the picture which landed me threats to start watching my back and some vandalism to my car.

Others just didn't like my direct style so one-by-one some people left. One surprising supporter though was my Ops Manager who not only warmed up but we became good friends, and he also became a great sounding board. Don understood my style and came to appreciate it because it got the results that he would try to get but couldn't. He had a great eye for detail so Don was able to ferret out significant items that I would often miss.

He and I made a great team. The other thing that he came to respect was that as part of my leadership style I assumed all of the responsibility for the actions of my crew when they messed up, and we had some doozies. That didn't mean that I took things calmly, just the opposite. I was a son-of-a-bitch when it came to certain things and I probably would have knocked the hell out of me if I had to work for myself.

But it wasn't my style to throw them under the bus, nor was it my style to find blame. Regardless of the mistake, like when Don caused a major job to shut down over a mistake, we would analyze it in simple terms after first fixing the immediate problem: 1) how did it happen, 2) is it something that can happen again, and 3) what do we need to do now to ensure that it won't happen again?

Our relationship went deeper. One weekend when Rachel was visiting not long before she moved up, I took a chance and asked Don if he and his wife, Sheila, would like to meet someplace for dinner and drinks. We ended up at a Japanese restaurant and after a few minutes of small talk Don let out some of his goofy side which in turn unleashed mine, and for the rest of the night we couldn't breathe because we were laughing so hard. The funnier thing was that Rachel and Sheila didn't quite get what was setting us off but they were laughing hysterically because of how hard we were laughing.

That was a fun-filled friendship that lasted quite a while, but one problem we had was when we sat facing each other at work, regardless of who was there or what we were working on, Don and I would break out into hysterics. It got to the point where we couldn't face each other because neither one of us could control it.

Although Rachel and I were living together in Southern California, she decided she was going to move up with me and that really caused her parents some angst though we didn't talk about it much. They had already accepted our living together, but were now having to face their daughter leaving the area. Jeff and Marsha had no issues with it, and for the most part it didn't bother me except that I had a lot of respect for both of Rachel's parents and I didn't like seeing Rachel under stress.

As I settled in with the company and the area, Rachel was still winding down her things in Southern California which had lasted for about six months. I was either driving or flying down nearly every weekend and that was getting old. I knew she was still struggling, not only with us living together but because she was leaving everyone she was closest to so she could go live with her boyfriend in a crappy area far away.

I'm not sure what prompted me to do it, but on a Friday morning before heading south to see Rachel, I called an airplane company and arranged to have a marriage proposal written on a banner and flown over our barbecue that weekend. I signed the contract, called Mary to tell her and ask that she get in touch with my brother and his kids and their girlfriends to come to our barbecue, but no one was to know why. As far as they were concerned it was just a get-together. Then I called Rachel to ask her to ask her mother if we could have a barbecue with both our families at her parent's place.

Fortunately everybody was amenable and said they wanted to come. The day of the barbecue everybody was there except for Rachel's dad who was out golfing. I pulled her mom aside and asked if there was any way she could get in touch with him to get him to come home. I had to tell her why but made her promise not to say a word to him or anyone about why he was giving up a perfect day of golf. Her poor mom was useless from that point after. The anticipation and the gag-order were far too much for her to handle and there was no soothing Rachel's dad once he arrived.

The setting was perfect. We were all outside by the pool talking and joking at the time the plane was scheduled to fly over. My plan was to look up and point to the plane while asking if anyone could read what the banner said. As luck would have it, the plane was late and the clouds rolled in making it cold so everyone went in the house.

I had to make up an excuse about why I was staying outside, which was strange to them because it was my party, and because I was always the one keeping everybody going. They watched me laying on a lawn chair and kept wondering what was wrong until finally the plane flew by to which I could say, "Hey, look at that!"

The event made the local newspaper but in a year's time we were already working on a divorce. What set the wheels in motion for the break-up was Rachel's unwillingness to compromise.

She was from the Country Club set and didn't really have to worry about money or support, and I'm a working man who's easily consumed by the tasks-at-hand. I'm pretty demanding of myself, more so than I am of others. The first problem, though not Rachel's fault at all, was that the time off for the honeymoon ended up costing my company a major client. There wasn't anyone in the company experienced enough to deal with the problems that happened on the contract while I was gone, and by the time I got back a small problem had turned into a big one. I fixed it and got us back on track, but it cost us and the client a lot of money and they weren't very forgiving. Because we were such a small group of divisions we could hardly afford the loss. But that's not why we would be heading for divorce.

On the personal side once Rachel and I settled in, in the spirit of compromise I agreed to do my share of the housework while at the same time refurbishing the house we were planning to buy from her parents. The house needed a ton of work, including a new roof, new flooring, and new paint, which I did when I wasn't working or out on jobsites. My field work sometimes included weekends. Rachel went to school four hours a day to be a hairdresser, and decided it was too hard on her to go to school and work at the same time. I was okay with it as long as she wasn't complaining about money or my job, so I didn't see any reason to argue.

It didn't take long once I was married to put on close to thirty pounds of extra weight, and so did she. We enjoyed ice cream sundaes a little too much and we also enjoyed eating out at bad-stuff restaurants but never seemed to enjoy walking there and back. One of the reasons I used to play the field so much and avoided steady girlfriends was because I would put on weight each time I was in a relationship. I was terrified of marriage mainly because I was afraid of getting fat since most of the married guys I knew were fat, yet here I was becoming what I had feared most; a fat married guy.

After about a year, my company got a shot at attaining the client lost during my honeymoon. Right after the job started though, the state safety rules changed concerning one of our installations. We had to scramble to comply and meet the deadline for completion or risk major penalties. We were also starting a new job with the federal government at the same time; those two events caused my crew and me to work twenty-one consecutive, sixteen-hour days until we were able to get them finished.

I got home at midnight on a Sunday after finally finishing both jobs, hoping to get a few hours of sleep before having to go into the office the next morning for another full week.

Rachel was asleep so I was very quietly going to take a shower, and that's when I saw the last straw. There was a can of Comet sitting on top of the toilet tank with a dry sponge and a note to me. It said, "Here's a reminder that you haven't been doing your share of the housework and I don't appreciate it."

It went downhill from there and we never did recover, though we eventually parted on decent terms. I'm not sure that we ever would have made it mainly because our differences were too great and there weren't any common areas to help us offset them.

It took a while but over time the company was also taking a turn downward and we began to consider its future and even looking at winding it down. Even though we had good successes in turning things around in terms of profitability and efficiency, the market was changing for the worst. Construction bids were producing less and less profit until they were making no profit at all. Our retail network was down and fewer jobs and product orders were coming in, and our direct sales were gone for the most part except for small orders here and there.

There were a number of problems like the market was smaller because the growth of the companies buying our products was stagnant, so more and more manufacturers were selling directly to the end users and cutting us out of the picture. Ours was the type of business where anyone could be a distributor out of their home and operate on a lot less.

I looked at getting into alternative products and services, areas where we were equipped and capable but it was too late for us to develop anything to transition to in any reasonable time. I was also looking at my own future and seriously questioning whether or not I still wanted to be in this industry and where I wanted to focus my future.

I took a look at people who had been in the industry for their entire career paths and didn't like what I saw. The distribution networks were changing, and ours were products that companies only bought because they had to and not because the products were going to do anything to increase their productivity or profits. This was during the late seventies and early eighties when many companies were closing their doors so our customers were able to buy our products used at dirt cheap prices.

For me the picture looked pretty bleak. Somewhere in my early years, I had decided that I wanted to have five million dollars or more to my name at some point in my life. I didn't know how or when I would get it, but I did know I wouldn't be getting it by staying in the steel industry.

I was also emotionally strung out due to work and my home life, so I wasn't at my best. I was performing but it was becoming more and more by rote rather than as an enthusiastic quest. I went to see my boss and gave him six month notice.

He was gracious at first but soon became skeptical by thinking that I might be leaving to join a competitor. It wasn't hard to get him to understand because we had mutual trust and respect for each other, and because I had no such plan. In fact, I had no plan at all. I had been with the company for close to ten years, starting as a salesman and finishing as general manager. The problem was I had no outside training so even though I had a good title and a decent salary with perks and benefits I still didn't have the skillset companies outside my industry were looking for.

I had planned to move back to southern California once my employment ended and go to college to get a degree. I kept the condo that I bought in Orange County before Rachel and I were married and rented it while I lived up north, and my brother was my last tenant. I had been taking a loss of $500 a month by renting it out but I didn't want to sell it yet either because I felt like the market would turn at some time and I might be able to make a profit. So even though I didn't have a job, it was still cheaper for me to move back in.

My boss decided to simply close the company and lease out the building. I made sure that we got out of there correctly and without anything left undone. He helped me by providing me with side jobs so I could generate some cash while I was getting re-established.

Once I moved back to Southern California, Rachel and I were already in a type of separation called Disillusionment. It is for couples who don't have kids or assets and want to terminate the marriage simply and without attorneys. To Rachel's credit, she did all the research and gathered the paperwork which we signed then filed. Since I bought condo before Rachel and I were married, we agreed that it would stay mine. I think the big motivator there was that there was no equity in it and had the potential to become a big liability.

One of the conditions in the Disillusionment was a six-month reconciliation period so the divorce isn't legally final until that period passes but you are legally separated during that time.

Once I was single again, it didn't take me long to drop the

weight and for a little while Rachel and I started dating again. She also dropped weight and started looking really hot, and our sex life was better than it ever was. Rachel also made it a point to apologize about four months into the split. It seems she had moved in with a roommate who was exactly like her so she was able to see what she had been like to live with. As soon as we started talking about possibly reconciling though she fell back into her old ways so that ended all hopes of reconciling, at least for me anyway.

I enrolled in a local community college to get my GE requirements out of the way, and I landed an undercover security job at a Bullock's department store in the mall across the way from my condo complex. I was able to re-establish my running regimen, but I also rode my bike to school and work so I could incorporate exercise into my daily life.

It was a struggle for a little bit but it wasn't long before I was back in my dating mentality and enjoying myself. I was a little older and more mature, but I was still getting hit on by the kind of women I wanted hitting on me so I was doing ok.

I was enjoying school and the job was ok, nothing that I wanted as a career. It was only paying $7.50 an hour so I was broke on a regular basis and knew at some point I was going to have to make some changes.

I ended up selling my condo at a $5000 loss which was salt in the wounds since I spent about three or four years taking a $500 a month loss each month in hopes the value would rise. I found a pretty cool townhouse to rent in a town much further from school and my job so that interrupted my biking and workout routines. My nephew, Dan, and I became roommates since he relocated to Southern California after we closed the company, and that offset some of the expense plus he always kept me in hysterics. We had fun for a while.

Dan and I were always close and we were always doing goofy things that usually rendered us nearly comatose in hysterics, mainly because he was incredibly good natured but always ended up messing up in the most hilarious ways.

An example of that was when he lived with me and worked for me in Northern California. He was an installer but also made deliveries for us, and despite being somewhat shy he always made the effort to be friendly and strike up a conversation if the opportunity presented itself. One day Dan was picking up an order for us and had to wait about ten to fifteen minutes for it to be ready, so he struck up a conversation with the guy behind the counter. They had a few things in common and the conversation stayed pretty fluid until the order was complete.

As Dan was leaving he thought he should say bye to his new found friend but unfortunately blended the two most common goodbyes, which at the time were "Have a good one" or "Take it easy". Dan called out in a loud voice to make sure his friend could hear him say goodbye and said: "Hey buddy, take a good one!"

Of course with Dan, that only scratched the surface and I lost count of how many times when driving I'd have to pull over because my eyes were tearing up so much from laughter that I couldn't see.

Then life got to be boring. I was going to school full time and working full time so there wasn't much time for socializing. Unlike my previous bachelor days the townhouse I lived in had no female prospects so I was confined to whomever I could date at work or anyone I'd meet in the various social events I might be attending.

My job at Bullock's was in undercover security which meant that we had to catch shoplifters in the act. There could have been worse jobs so I didn't mind it much. Because of my school schedule I worked the shifts that were the most boring because there weren't any shoppers most of the time. There were a lot of pretty woman who worked there so even though we weren't really allowed to socialize with staff, it was really too hard to resist.

The company had an incentive plan where employees could report on each other, and if we caught an employee committing a crime on their tip then the company would pay the tipster $300. The security people weren't supposed to mingle because it could create a conflict of interest if they were friends with an employee who was reported on. Our boss frowned on fraternization but there wasn't much he could do because he was madly in love with one of the cosmetics managers and he couldn't hide it. He was a great boss so we didn't give him any reason not to trust us.

One day I was given an assignment to start watching one of the sales girls in cosmetics because someone had reported that they thought they saw her stealing. I started watching her and was having difficulty because she not only was very pretty but had a great ass and great legs to boot. Ironically, she worked in cosmetics but never used makeup to make herself pretty.

I tried to hide my interest, but I caught her noticing me too. I reported honestly that I did not see her doing anything in violation of company rules. When we looked at the complaint more thoroughly and talked with the person who filed it, we found out that I had been watching the wrong girl.

Here's how that happened. Other than security, all of the staff was supposed to wear name badges. When the employee reported the suspected theft, she didn't use the person's name but simply pointed her out to one of our fellow security officers. He went over for a friendly chat and to read her name badge, but no one realized that she had borrowed the badge from Abby, the girl I ended up watching.

Once I knew that, I didn't have reservations about getting to know Abby better. It seemed to be mutual because Abby's boss, the one my boss was so in love with, set Abby and me up on a date. Actually what she set up was an impromptu party at the bar across from work. We barely had a chance to talk which I thought was due to all the noise and activity in the bar. It turned out that Abby wasn't great at conversation and chose to mostly answer yes or no without any elaboration but at the time I thought she didn't want to compete with the noise. I invited her to a movie a few nights later and started seeing her regularly soon after.

Since Dan and I were living together and were close, we would often take Abby out for brunch, lunch, or dinners and we could get ourselves going simply by playing with the words on the menu items or bringing up past hilarities. Despite Abby's seemingly quiet demeanor we were able to put her in a laughing coma on more than one occasion and got her to come out of her shell.

I'm not sure why I fell in love with her so quickly but I did, so much so that I ignored red flags that ended up working against me in later years. We became a hot item in a very short time; in that short time I caught her in at least three lies that she never came clean on. I wrote it off as shyness as I've seen some people choose to lie to save face rather than just deal with the truth.

I learned later that this detail was very much a part of her family's make up. Despite that however, I couldn't help myself and was falling madly in love with her. We had only been together for about a month when we started talking about babies and raising a family. I was pretty adamant that I wasn't ready for a family because

I was still working on my general education credits and didn't have the kind of job to be able to raise a family on.

She tempted and pleased me in all sorts of ways as I did for her, and I was naïve enough to think she was doing it out of love because that was how I was doing things, out of a passionate love for her. I learned many years later that love had nothing to do with it; she was simply looking for a way to get out of her parent's house.

After a few close calls, she let me know one day that she was pregnant. Her excuse was that she lost track of the calendar. She asked me what I thought we should do and for me it was a quick answer, we should get married. She then asked me what I would do if she simply got an abortion as she had done with another guy some years before, and I replied that I couldn't see her again if she did. We agreed to get married, except there was a teeny problem. The disillusionment from my previous marriage wasn't going to be over for a while and I couldn't get married until it was.

We took a little time to try and work things out in terms of what our future life was going to look like. My school load was heavy, my job clearly would not support a family, and my vehicles were starting to fall apart and were becoming liabilities. The beautifully tricked out 1970 El Camino I'd purchased while up north was getting to be more trouble than it was worth.

In the first couple of months after realizing what was about to take place, it was beginning to weigh heavily on me. I looked back at my own childhood and wondered what kind of father I was going to be. I looked at my financial mess and wondered what kind of provider I would be. I looked at my past exploits with women and wondered if I could be a faithful husband. I was faithful in my first marriage, but now I was looking at a really long commitment. It's not that I wasn't in the long haul in my first marriage, but now that there was a child soon to be in the picture, I knew I would no longer have the luxury of thinking about my own needs.

As I was thinking about this at a stoplight, I noticed a guy about my age in a ratty old car in front of me just yakking up a storm and laughing like crazy with his little daughter. This guy looked easily as broke as I was, yet there he was having the time of his life and really seemed to be loving life.

And then it hit me like a ton of bricks! I was wasting time worrying about all those other things, when the only solution I needed was to love my kid with all my heart. He or she didn't ask to be here, and they weren't going to care where they were as long as they felt loved. I knew from that moment that as long as I loved my kid, all the rest of the stuff I had been worrying about would fall into place.

Once my family knew my plans they were extremely supportive. Bit by bit, Abby had let her sisters know and introduced me to them, and she let her mother know. To them I was the married man who got Abby pregnant. Abby was still living at home with her parents so she could never stay with me overnight, and that was something that I really wanted. I began looking forward to getting married just so I could be with Abby, morning and night.

When I met Abby's mother, Mrs. Frazier, she came across as supportive. Mrs. Frazier's parting question to me that morning was when did I plan to tell her husband about our plans? We agreed it would be the next night. Abby was beside herself in a panic and kept asking me all sorts of questions she knew I couldn't possibly have the answer to, but that was the kind of person she was. She asked me what I would do if her father rejected us, and my answer was pretty simple. "If that's his choice then he won't get to see his grandkid. I'm not the kind of guy who is going to have my kid aborted just because it may be an inconvenience for someone who might not approve."

That fateful night came, and all of Abby's sisters were there as were her mother and father. Abby introduced me to him and we shook hands, but it was pretty clear he wasn't a warm and fuzzy guy. A retired LA Deputy with a whole bunch of loaded guns in the house, Mr. Frazier had a perpetual scowl on his face. Worse, he loved being the center of attention but that night it wasn't him and that was already getting us off on the wrong foot. The sisters had put us all in a sitting room and sat me next to him; then her mother and sisters sat as though they were in an auditorium watching a play. I think they secretly were wondering what their father was going to do to me once he got the news.

Here's how it went: "Mr. Frazier, I have something important to tell you. I love your daughter and plan to marry her. She is carrying our child, but I can't marry her until my divorce is final."

FOUR

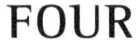

California: Part 2

Abby and I made plans to be married. Despite her family's display of putting their best feet forward it was obvious they didn't like me nor did they care for the situation. Abby and I moved in together which at the time was like a dream to me because I was really in love with her. We ended up moving in together because once the baby started showing her mother was embarrassed and tossed Abby's clothes on the floor, then threw her out of the house saying she wished we would have just decided to get an abortion. Abby and I moved into a tiny one-bedroom apartment overlooking a very busy freeway and we joked that the loud traffic noise was a simulated ocean sound.

My divorce from Rachel was finalized on the day before our second anniversary. Three days later, I was married to Abby and a month later our son was born, satisfying Abby's need that Alex was not born out of wedlock. Shortly after Alex's birth we moved into a slightly larger two-bedroom apartment with a fireplace and a little backyard in a neighboring town. We traded loud traffic for noisy neighbors and cockroaches.

We lived across the street from a well-known Catholic church which held dances on Friday nights that were supposed to end around 9:30 pm but would last much longer. The dances were really noisy and would keep waking our son up. We'd have trouble getting Alex back to sleep which was really troublesome because of my work and school schedules.

Abby called the priest to talk with him about it, appealing to him because of the noise waking Alex but he quickly dismissed her saying there was nothing he could do. We both observed the priest's lifestyle which was dramatically different from ours. He had a housekeeper and his bills were paid by others, he always drove a

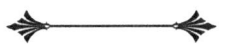

new car, and he had minimal demands on his time because that's what he chose for himself.

He didn't know what life was like when trying to raise a family and earn a living, so of course he was unable to relate to what our lives were like. This left us both with poor tastes in our mouths knowing that a priest's job was to minister yet was too selfish to consider others in need. In his total comfort he ignored those of us who didn't have much comfort; and didn't seem to care that he was actually making things worse.

I was still in school full time but had found a job selling cabinetry on a straight commission basis because there was no way I could support us with the job at Bullock's.

For a while I did well, even though the job was often seven days a week. I didn't get benefits and if I didn't sell an installation I didn't get paid. I was fine with Abby's choice to be a stay-at-home mom, but was often stressed at how little she would contribute in financial terms. Abby was eligible for disability because there were complications with Alex's birth, but I had to beg her to apply for it and it took weeks before she finally did. It wasn't much but it helped buy groceries or pay for gas and utilities in between commission checks.

Over time, the company I was selling for began cutting territories and adding more sales people. Unfortunately they were cutting from people like me who were closing sales and giving leads to others who weren't. Worse, the people they had answering the phones weren't taking down information correctly so it was common to be unable to contact potential customers for an appointment. It was becoming harder and harder to earn enough money to survive.

I began an extensive job search and landed a night manager's position at a blueprint company while carrying eighteen units at school. I continued my cabinetry sales job in between and on the weekends. My schedule went like this:

4:00 a.m. to 6:00 a.m. – Study
7:00 a.m. to 11:00 a.m. – Classes
12:00 p.m. to 2:00 p.m. – Lunch and Sales appointments
2:30 p.m. to 11:00 p.m. – Night Job

On Saturdays I would have a full day of cabinet appointments and generally no more than a couple of appointments on Sundays.

The night job got more difficult in a very short amount of time. I found out that I couldn't go home if there was work to finish. We started getting some larger jobs plus the day crew was also leaving their big jobs for us at night, so I was starting to get home between two and three in the morning.

Something else I did was get up with my son at night, change his diaper, hug and kiss him; then bring him to Abby to nurse. It was one of the few ways I could try and lighten Abby's load and also how I could spend some time with him since I had little time to spare. I was in love, bound and determined to not only build a life for us but I was consciously trying to fix everything Abby was saying was wrong with me. And don't kid yourself, as much as I want to make myself out to be a saint, there was plenty wrong with me and I accepted that and approached the fixes without complaining too much though I did complain some. I had a lousy temper especially when I was under stress and because of it I wasn't easy to live with. My heart was in the right place, but there were a lot of times when my head was up my ass. What can I say? I'm human.

When I was a kid I used to watch commercials or look at the table settings on cereal boxes and wish that my life was similar to the lifestyles that were depicted in those scenes, like a nice home and nice surroundings. My cereal bowls were reused Cool Whip containers and our plates looked like they were a thousand years old. I had lived with a drunken, mercurial father who couldn't be bothered spending time with his kids. When my kid grew up, I never wanted him to experience that feeling of want nor did I want him to have an absentee or disinterested dad so I took it upon myself to see that it didn't happen.

It's funny but when all of my kids got older they would tell me sometimes that I didn't have to tell them I loved them all the time because they knew it already, but good luck trying to get me to stop telling or showing them. Like that will ever happen.

My night schedule seemed to get worse; with a forty-five minute drive to get back home each night from my night job since it was so far away. Sometimes I'd get home at one or two in the morning so exhausted that I'd fall asleep in my car after parking it. Abby would come out to wake me up and as I'd open the car door she'd hand me a bag of trash that she'd want me to take out. I'd sleep on the couch because of how uncomfortable it was so that I wouldn't oversleep and miss my first class.

In the meanwhile, Abby's parents continued to put me down because I wasn't giving their daughter the comforts that they felt she should have. Abby saddled me with debt, unknown to Mr. and Mrs. Frazier, which I had to pay off because she stopped working and had no money saved. One day Mr. Frazier and I were arguing about my financial state and he was implying that I was a big loser. In truth, had I been not paying Abby's debt off I would have been very close to paying off my own and our situation might have been a little better. But in his eyes Abby could do no wrong and I could do no right.

Despite all of that, I made it my mission to build a life for us amid whispers from her family that we should just accept being, in essence, poor white trash. Ironically, one of Abby's sisters and her husband lived with Abby's parents for about nine years rent-free but carried themselves off as yuppies and were very condescending toward me. I was always looked at as the loser because I was struggling to raise a family while going to school and working two jobs yet was broke all the time. The husband didn't work while living there and going to school, but Abby's sister did work though they didn't have kids or anything else to support. Of course they always had spending money and nice clothes.

I didn't waste too much time worrying about their opinions of me; I was too busy making a living for us no matter what it took. I also employed something that has helped me well over the years and that was to kill them with kindness. That didn't mean that I felt lesser than them, to the contrary actually because I saw them for who they were. But I also saw that when they were at their best they could be a good, loving family but just had very strange ways of showing it and they weren't at their best very often. We were always broke but somehow we'd manage.

Abby's way of contributing was to call me every time there was a problem, even if it was a problem that she could fix. We had agreed that she could always come to me with a problem and I stuck to that agreement but there were times when I wished she would have made some effort to lighten the load. The night manager job was proving to be too much so I looked for a different line of work. Right around then, nine months after Alex was born we found out that Abby was pregnant with our second child. Kids, as many of you may know, don't really care if their presence is convenient for you; they simply let you know they're coming one way or the other.

Well, my second kid lucked out because if it was left up to Abby and her family he wouldn't have made it out. Some of her family focused on Abby by questioning if having a second baby was really the right decision given our circumstances and suggested that she consider having the fetus aborted. Of course none of them had the balls to have that conversation with me because they knew how I'd react, especially because to me it was my child and not simply a fetus. My response to Abby was I didn't care if I had to work fifteen jobs but I would figure out how we were going to survive, and no matter what we were going to have that baby.

Right before Andrew was born I found a job in Corporate Sales with a uniform company which was a nice step up from the night manager printing job. It came with a company car, a salary with an option for commissions, benefits, and the hours were much better. I had accumulated enough units in my general electives to work on an undergraduate degree, so I took a break from school to work regular hours at the new job.

I continued to work selling cabinets as my second job on evenings and weekends but it was a breeze compared to what I had been going through, and the timing was right because having two little ones who were seventeen months apart was no picnic. And for all the grief I give Abby on these pages, I cannot ignore the one thing she was exceptional at and it was being a mother and paying attention to their health and needs, at least back then that is.

I complimented it by being a father and husband who loved them all unconditionally and would always try to put myself in last position to ensure I was putting them first and doing whatever I could to solve whatever problems were facing us. Abby and I would take walks with the stroller in our neighborhood which was near a little golf course that had some beautiful homes around it. I began to form visions of where and what I wanted our life to be.

For me, setting goals always included visualizing where those goals would take me. As I continued in my second job I started paying attention to my clients, their homes and what they did for a living. I found that a majority of the nicer homes I was selling cabinets for were owned by people in the mortgage industry so I started setting my sights on what it would take to be a loan officer.

The uniform company job wasn't working out as I'd hoped, in part because of the territory but also in part due to the salesman, me. Despite the nicer working conditions and the perks, I was conducting negotiations for contracts amounting to nickels and dimes a week. It was very hard to envision earning more than $25,000 a year much less the six figures I was beginning to set my sights on.

I started researching the mortgage business and after a few false starts I landed with World Savings, a savings bank that put me through training on how to sell their somewhat unique products. Their school was a four-day offsite event where I learned the skills I would need to go out and sell. It was a very intense training event and each day was twelve hours long. Most of us knew nothing about the lending business so we not only had to become experts in those four days but also had to formulate marketing strategies to make ourselves successful.

Our graduation required each of us to present our products and expertise in front of senior management while being video-taped. That was a tremendously rewarding experience that I used throughout most of my selling career. By getting to see myself on tape, I was able to understand what other people were seeing so it helped me improve my presentation skills. From that point on, whenever I would develop a new presentation, I always tested it in front of a mirror.

When I graduated from the four-day training I reported to work without a territory but was spending time on the phone and being mentored by the other loan officers. The pay was a small draw against future commissions (which had to be paid back from commissions) plus the commission, and bonus plus benefits, and with that I hit the ground running.

Right about that time, Abby and I moved into a nice little three-bedroom house to rent in Riverside which we had been hoping we would get. The office I was working out of was in a town about sixteen miles away from our new residence. It didn't look like I would get the Riverside territory anytime soon because it belonged to a seasoned agent who seemed to be doing a good job. However, about a week later the Riverside loan officer was caught bringing in fraudulent documents and was arrested, so I got his territory. That was an eye opener for me as I began to shape my business philosophy, which was to do things by the book despite any temptation to do otherwise.

We were starting to become a family with a nice little house in a decent neighborhood and I was starting on a second career path instead of just working jobs that I found once I left the steel business. I finally ended my job selling cabinets and just devoted my time to building my lending business and spending time with my family.

My relations with Abby's family were slowly starting to improve as they saw my commitment to making a life for us. They didn't particularly like where we lived because of the distance but more because of the smog. Riverside was incredibly smoggy, so much so that there were frequent warnings in the summer for residents to avoid going outside.

When we were able to go outside I'd pack the two little guys, Alex and Andrew, in a trailer on the back of my bicycle and I'd load them up with books, drinks and snacks and I'd take them out to the bike trails. Other times Abby and I took them to the beach or the mountains for doses of clean air.

I began to focus on significant visions like actual paychecks and the kind of house we would buy. I focused on a vision of getting a single net paycheck of $10,524.00[3] and got one within a year which we used to pay cash for a used Taurus wagon that was in great shape. Taurus wagons were the hip thing with moms then, and that was part of the attention I paid to my family, but there was something in it for me too. Abby's previous car was a little Honda Civic wagon that ran great, had good air conditioning but I could barely fit in it especially when we went grocery shopping.

The Taurus was a huge step up and was great at the time we had it. I continued to drive my old Toyota Celica which hadn't had air conditioning in over four years. Riverside, in addition to being smoggy, is normally in the low 100s in the summer. I would have liked to use the Civic because it had air, but I had too much trouble fitting into it so we sold it and kept my car.

Part of my job as a loan officer was to make sales calls on a regular basis while wearing a suit. Most of my competitors drove air-conditioned BMW's or Mercedes', so I had to get very creative when showing up for midday realtor gatherings in the sweltering heat, trying to look cool. To compensate I made sure I knew what I was doing so when people talked to me they knew they were talking to an expert instead of someone who had only been in the business for less than six months.

---

[3] I was only off by a few hundred dollars from the amount I had in my vision, but it was close enough for me to realize the visions worked.

Almost immediately after being assigned to the Riverside territory I set out to be the only person to call by calling on real estate offices incessantly. There were eighteen top offices in my territory and on any given weekend you could go in to any one of them and see my business cards everywhere. A top office meant that those offices accounted for much of the sales activity in the area on a percentage basis. There were other offices, but the bulk of the local business came through those top offices.

Not only were new referral sources getting to know me, so was my competition. My value proposition was pretty simple, call me first and I'll let you know quickly if I can help you. If I can't then I'll help you find someone who can.

In the loan business, especially back then, we made our money by either getting realtors to refer us to their buyers or refinancing homes with existing loans. The banks I worked for wanted us to focus on new buyers because it meant bringing in new customers for them.

Realtors on the other hand just wanted a lender who could be relied on to close a transaction when and how they said it would close since their paychecks were contingent on that promise. It was pretty common for inexperienced loan officers to package a loan incorrectly only to have it declined the day before it was supposed to close. Other times buyers would be lying to you but often wouldn't get caught until closing.

Realtors didn't really care about the bells and whistles some companies tried to feature; they simply wanted to be able to call somebody at night or on the weekend who could meet with their client, take the loan application, and close the loan. That was the guy I was working hard to become. And believe me, I paid my dues.

The Loan Business

While in training we were warned to avoid using jargon since it might confuse the borrower, but some loan officers would use it at times in order to appear seasoned. I'll be the first to admit that I was one of them. In the loan business we used a few different ratios to determine if a borrower could qualify for the loan. Two have to do with the property itself and two were based on the income and debt. In the income ratios, we used the Front End Ratio or "Front End" which is the ratio of gross income to gross house payment. The second is the Back End Ratio or "Back End" which is the gross income to gross house payment plus outstanding debt payments.

My first loan application was at the home of a very pretty lady in her mid-thirties. I was by myself and a little nervous being that it was my first time taking an application but I was careful not to let it show. The lady was very friendly and seemed to have a nice disposition. After a few minutes of talking about what she was looking for we jumped into the application. I got everything completed and started to check the ratios and other calculations when she asked me what I thought.

Without thinking, I used a little jargon to compensate for my newness. "Well, we'll know how everything else looks after the appraisal, but your Front End and Back End look great." Just then I realized what I said so I kept quiet and didn't look up from my notes, hoping she didn't notice.

"Huh, I didn't think you were paying attention. But what do you think about my loan?" she asked with a good-natured laugh just as her big bruiser of a husband walked in. That taught me a lesson I'll never forget.

I was on a career path and, despite the frustrations of the job, I began to see the benefits for my family especially if I stayed focused on being successful. I made it a point to learn as much as I could about all of my products, the industry itself, and the products with which I was competing. World Savings had some niche products and could do wonders that no other banks could at the time but my competitors could reach so many other prospects because they weren't relegated to niches.

I pursued my territory very aggressively using whatever legal, legitimate means were at my disposal. I targeted a highly-visible office which had some good, productive agents. It was extremely hard to get into because the company owned its own mortgage company and, as I found out later, the manager was married to a sales manager with another mortgage company down the street.

Most professional real estate offices back then didn't dictate who their agents could use but they encouraged them to use company owned mortgage companies and restricted other mortgage lenders from coming in to their offices. In Lisa's case, the real estate manager, her situation was even more precarious because she had to encourage her agents to use the company-owned lender and didn't even allow her husband's mortgage company to have access to her office. The odds really were against me but I was still very determined.

My bank, World Savings, was running an ad in the local paper talking about how we were launching a new campaign that buyers could use to make home-buying easier. I circled the part in it that said Realtor and wrote a note saying that I needed to meet with her so her agents would know what to say when customers asked about the ad. I attached my card and left it with the receptionist.

A couple of days later I received a call from the real estate manager and managed to convince her to allow me to speak to her agents at their meeting the following week – unheard of because of their relationships with the other lenders. I made enough of an impression on her that she told her husband to recruit me for a job with his company, Profed Mortgage, which was part of Provident Savings, a well-known bank in town.

Leaving World was a tough decision but I ended up making the right choice. The new bank paid me a bonus to join them and they had a product line that allowed me to reach so many more clients. In less than a year's time I was earning more than my previous company's top earners. I was also introduced to more ways to do business and was given great opportunities, mainly in recognition of how hard I was working.

One of my quirks was how I could tune in to people's body language and voice tones. I could uncover objections to make the sale by observing if the customer was unhappy, allowing me to work on diffusing whatever the problem was and keep them from canceling. This quirk did not go unnoticed by upper management.

Somehow they figured out that when the president or the executive vice president of the company paged me it would send me into turmoil until I was able to talk to them and give them what they needed. I simply was one of those guys who jumped when customers or the executives called.

I found out much later that the president and executive vice president, two of the smartest people I ever knew in the business, were also a couple of wise guys. Sometimes when they were looking for a break in their routine one of them would say, "Hey, let's page Gardner so we can mess with his head." They'd have little bets to see how fast I'd call and how much of a panic I was in. It drove me nuts.

On the flip-side, it was because of my responses and hard work that they would refer some of the top banking clients to me and when they went into a joint venture with a home builder they named me as the onsite lender. Those two benefits provided me, a commissioned loan officer, with the closest thing possible to a salary and I enjoyed it.

The joint venture was in a town called Rancho which has gained quite a bit of notoriety over the years. It's a great wine-country community and one of the few clean-air places in western Riverside County, situated about halfway between Riverside and San Diego. I began spending a lot of time there and was beginning to know the place pretty well, but Abby didn't know it at all.

I had to do a late document signing in Rancho on a night before a holiday and decided that it would be fun to take Abby and the boys with me to have dinner when the signing was over. Alex was about three and Andrew was about one and a half, and that made the signing a bit of a challenge but it still ended up being an enjoyable night; Abby fell in love with the locale. We started fantasizing about living there, though I wasn't sure how it could work since it was so far away from the territory I needed to be in to make a living.

Fate decided for us. Alex had been experiencing severe allergy problems and had his tonsils and adenoids out shortly after his second birthday. Prior to that, he got pneumonia in the summer and then again in the following summer after he turned three. Alex's doctor let us know it was because of allergies that were probably made worse due to the smog, and pretty much wanted to keep him medicated all the time.

Neither Abby nor I could handle it; there was no way we wanted our little boy to be medicated all the time. We visited Rancho a few more times and found that Alex didn't have the reactions nor did he need the medications when we were there. We decided the best thing for us to do was move. I talked with the president of the company and told him the circumstances and, because of our need to move, I would probably have to quit my job.

The president told me it wouldn't be necessary to quit since they were looking at opening new mortgage branches and this would be a mutually beneficial situation. What a relief that was, and an exciting opportunity as well. I was promoted to Branch Manager and the company opened the new branch in Rancho. Abby and I found a great three-bedroom, two-story house to rent near kids who could become great friends for the boys. It was an eighteen hundred square-foot, three-bedroom, two-bath place, and it had an association pool. It also had a wide, open field where we would later fire off rockets and run and play with our two new 'watch' dogs, Timex and Seiko, also known as the Barker Sisters.

Rancho proved to be a great move where we made a lot of friends and flourished. It was also a place where both Alex and Andrew saw puffy white clouds for the first time for the lack of smog. They thought they were in Care Bear-land.

Like before when I opened the territory in Riverside I plastered my face all over town so people would know who I was. After about nine months of being in a territory where I hadn't been before, it wasn't uncommon for me to be referred to the same client by two or three competing realtors with different companies. I used every opportunity to speak in public and in realtor meetings so I would get noticed.

I borrowed from something I had seen someone else do in a different meeting just a few days before and it really opened some doors for me. I found two front page newspaper headlines only days apart from each other; one headline said "Mortgage Rates Could Rise" and the headline two days later announced "Mortgage Rates Could Drop". Our realtor meeting, always well-attended, happened to be on the board-sponsored "Crazy Hat Day" and I was wearing one of my favorite fun baseball caps with an eighteen-inch visor. Despite being the newest guy there knowing no one, I took the opportunity to make a special announcement, a mortgage rate update.

I showed both newspaper headlines and said, "I went ahead and checked the market with our top experts based on these news reports. The experts told me they officially concur with these headlines, and yes, mortgage rates could likely be going either up or down now or in the near future."

It cracked us all up and a realtor grabbed me in the parking lot after the meeting to give me a lead. The realtor confided that she liked my presentation and wanted to see what I knew about the business. Once we had a few minutes to talk she was convinced and we ended up doing a lot of business together.

Another time I saw a little blurb in the paper about a soldier who was getting a special award, so I cut it out and put it in a congratulatory card telling the mom how proud she must be of her son. I had recognized her name as being an agent in an office that I could just not break into because it was so exclusive. I dropped the card off at her office then went back to check on her a few days later to make sure she got it and I was so surprised at the response.

She came out and vigorously shook my hand. Apparently, she had no idea her son was getting that award. That in itself was hugely satisfying to me. We formed a business relationship where I made over $15,000 from her in the next few months plus I got into the office and made even more money on transactions with other agents.

I also started writing press releases and had a few feature length articles published in the local newspaper, though I wrote under a number of bylines because of the nature of the particular articles I'd be writing about.

All of that happened once Abby and the kids and I settled in to our new town and our new home, but the first few months were tough. Our rent was higher and it was taking a while to build the business up to where I could get back to making a steady living. On the day we moved in, I had to come up with the first and last month's rent and security deposit but my paycheck for the month was twenty-four dollars due to a couple of cancelations but mainly because my loans got pushed back into the next month.

That didn't stop Abby from walking me through her list of everything I needed to buy for the house, not to mention that I had to put in a new back lawn as part of our agreement to get our move-in costs lowered. It was great that we had such a big back yard, but it took a tremendous amount of work to put it in. I was rototilling and seeding every day after work so I was doing fourteen-hour days because I didn't have enough money to hire it out.

It's hard to imagine that I was able to stay motivated after spending so much money to move into the new place while spending all the time and money for the lawn but only earning twenty four dollars for the month. That's how the business was sometimes, and despite my temptation to give in to the pitfalls of what some might think was too tough of a business, in reality I usually made more by closing one loan than I could have by working all month in an average hourly job.

Most of my colleagues survived the financial ups and downs of it because their wives contributed in various ways while still being great mothers and great partners. Some wives worked full time, others worked as real estate agents and picked when they wanted to work but still closed sales. Others learned the loan business and helped their husbands with the phone and packaging the loans. Unfortunately, Abby had no interest in helping me at all despite how easily she could have.

The life of a loan officer back then meant that you had to go out on sales calls to build relationships with referral sources, mainly real estate agents. Most of the offices had barriers that restricted access to their agents so we loan officers had to devise creative ways to get exposure in order to get them to give us a try. Other offices had in-house lenders which meant that we had no access to their agents even though some of them wanted to give business to an outside lender.

As a commissioned loan officer it was especially tough when opening up a new territory because you might call on a territory for a month and not get a single lead. Calling on a territory meant stopping in real estate offices to talk with agents and showing up where agents show up. In the early stages of developing the territory often the only leads you got were the ones that the known lenders couldn't do because the buyers were so poorly qualified or the properties they were buying were so bad. I would get these leads knowing that I couldn't do anything either, but would use that time to leverage my exposure to demonstrate my level of service and depth of knowledge while bargaining with the agents to give me their next lead.

It might be forty-five days before I would get a single lead out of a new territory, and once I got it, I had to make sure the buyers and the property qualified, and once they qualified I had to wait until they got an accepted offer. Then I'd have to take the application and get all of their supporting documentation so I could package it to submit it for underwriting.

Once the loan was in process, I had to hope the buyers didn't lie to me about their debts or income, my processor didn't make my agent or the buyers mad enough to find another lender, the underwriter would approve the loan, the clients didn't lose their jobs or go out and buy a new car while we were in the process of closing their loan; that the clients didn't find some fake rate that was lower than mine and threaten to cancel; and that the appraisal came in at the value they bought it for, something that was often tough in a declining market.

For every transaction, I had to keep at least seven people apprised of its progress on a regular basis, sometimes getting hit with questions to which I didn't know the answers. If the transaction survived all of that in the forty-five to sixty day period (at that time), I would have to wait another fifteen to thirty days before I got paid.

In a new territory, it might be four months before I got a paycheck from a lead with commissions anywhere from five hundred to twenty-five hundred dollars per loan. Obviously I had to close multiple loans in order to make a living, and since not all of them closed I had to get as many loans in my pipeline as possible. Often I'd carry between twenty to thirty loans in my pipeline, closing from six to ten a month. With an average of seven people to talk to on each loan, I had to stay in touch with about one hundred and fifty to two hundred people a month while getting whatever else I needed to get the deals to close because I had no assistant.

In that whole mess of stuff, I still had to find the time to go out and make sales calls because in our business, the reality was that as loan officers, we were only as good as our last deal. If we messed one up, we usually didn't get another for a while, or at all, and if the agents didn't see us in their offices they gave deals to the people they did see. It was a constant battle.

This was a seven-day-a-week gig whether I liked it or not, and sometimes while I would be doing chores, I would get called to meet with clients. I would have to drop what I was doing and spend time with the clients. It was extremely frustrating each time I had wiped out a Sunday afternoon only to have the buyers go with another lender or not buy at all.

Life In Rancho

Over time Abby and I got settled. I was in a career that I was enjoying despite its many frustrations, and despite being on straight commission, in general I was earning a good living. Abby still didn't contribute financially nor did she seem to feel it necessary to make any attempts to lighten my load in any way, but I think I may have been making it look too easy.

We had our kids in a private Christian school and we attended a great community church and loved the fact that the pastor was married and had kids and grandkids. The pastor and his wife lived in our world and we respected their guidance when they gave it to us. This was the pastor of a community church versus the priest at a catholic church, and the contrast could not have been more noticeable. The pastor understood the trials of raising kids and having to work for a living whereas the priest knew nothing of the sort because it wasn't required of him.

From the time I met her and throughout the first three or four years of our marriage, Abby was very shy but by the time we moved to Rancho she began to come out of her shell and began to socialize with other moms. Like with many environments, there was some competition going on between them; for instance did you own or rent, what kind of car did you drive and more important what your husband did for a living? Some of it was brutal because of the egos but we tried to minimize it so I continued to work on the business, and Abby continued to take care of our kids.

Despite my often twelve hour days and weekend work, every other Saturday I would do all the laundry, clean the entire house and that included washing the floors by hand on my knees because that's how she claimed she wanted it done and I couldn't stand to see her do it. When that was finished I'd go outside and do yard work. Since we lived on a ¼ acre lot that too was a challenge; especially because I had to pick up the dog poop for two big dogs. If I got paged to see a client, then I'd have to drop what I was doing so I could see the client then come back and finish where I left off.

I did all of this out of respect for Abby's time with the kids. I knew it was a tough job so I would do it so she would have a break, and usually while I was doing that in the hot sun she'd be inside on the couch reading a book or talking on the phone. My fault for taking it all on, because what I really expected was that we would share the workload and get things done twice as fast, like other couples do. But back then I didn't mind doing it because frankly I thought over time she would reciprocate in some way by looking at what I was taking on to make our lives better.

On Sundays I'd spend the day with Abby and the boys; we'd go out on outings and have some fun. I started night school around then so I would do my homework in the early mornings while they were all asleep and spend time with them during the day. There were times when I had projects that would take up the day, but I managed to keep those to a minimum.

In the early years of my two oldest boys' lives Abby and I managed and built our lives around them. We went through some really tough times in the mortgage business and it always seemed like my earnings would drop around Christmas which would create so much anxiety for me because I wanted to give them what they wanted yet often I was just short of what I needed to make everything happen. Abby and I finally worked out a plan to start buying in the late summer and having all of our Christmas shopping done by Thanksgiving. That went miles toward easing some of the anxiety.

My relationship with Abby was okay and it seemed like we were developing some common goals when it related to the kids. When it related to the household things, like finances, Abby never wanted any part of it. She simply wanted to spend when she felt like it and when I'd protest over the timing of the major expenses she'd pout and entice me with sex. I'd ask her to try and understand what impact it was having on us, particularly me, when I'd have to bear the stress of whatever we had to sacrifice in order to get her what she wanted. She wasn't interested and she'd pout and entice me until I gave in.

I'm a guy; and a monogamous one at that when it came to being married so it wasn't like I was going to turn down the sex. From my perspective under those circumstances, it became obvious that my only solution was to figure out how to make more money, regardless of what it might do to me. By the time we had our third son, Austin, I had pretty much abandoned any thoughts of my own health and welfare. I was on a mission to earn as much money as I could to give my wife what she said she needed and the kids what they thought they needed.

I worked long hours and endured the stress and just kept driving home the need to earn more money. Even though I was earning a decent living after a while, it was straight commission and the business was cyclical which meant that some months would be great and others would be dismal. Even though we were living in a nice house we would still have our utilities turned off once in a while. The only break I would get during those years was when I would sleep; as long as I knew my kids were in a good place I slept well.

My focus remained on making money. I was very aggressive in my territory and was notorious for knowing more about my competitors' products than they did and because of it I would often get the call first. Sometimes agents would call me when they were forced to use a lender their client insisted on but wasn't getting the job done. They knew they could count on me to analyze the problem and very often I would school the lender on what they needed to do to fix the problem. Sometimes the problem would be with their bank so I would get the deal as a result, and of course those realtors would keep me at the top of their list.

The community was small so I remained highly visible and earned a good living as a result. Over time the market changed and it was harder to make a living because of low property values and depressed sales. There were months where I'd close eight or nine loans yet my total paycheck was five hundred dollars.

I stuck with it and continued to circulate because I was committed to the career. I'd joined certain groups that might include other lenders but the groups were usually comprised of top realtors. Being in those groups was a great opportunity to showcase myself. Even though I was an aggressive competitor, I also offered myself as a resource to some lenders that I felt were top notch and I'd even give them leads that I wasn't able to do for some reason relating to our policies.

Each time I'd go into a territory I'd do informal interviews with referral sources to see who they were using and why. Then I'd research who these lenders were and what products they were offering, and based on what I'd find out, I determined who I was going to target as my main competitors. There were a few lenders known for supplying phony documentation so not only did I cross them off the list, I didn't pursue business from the realtors who were using them because expectations of phony documentation was something I had no interest in delivering on. Others were top notch and by competing directly with them we learned a lot from each other and often developed mutual respect, and believe it or not, it was good business.

One of my top competitors was a sweet kid named Myrna who was also strikingly beautiful. She was designated Mrs. Rancho for a few years running, and she owned much of the business in town until I showed up. At first people looked at me as some scummy broker until they saw me close deals and at times work magic, and after a while I had taken a lot of her business that she wasn't able to get back.

Myrna was one of the loan officers that I gave a little business to at times and we liked each other professionally. I'm not sure how long it took but somebody in her company began recruiting me. In terms of product line I had more to offer with my company than they did, but Myrna's was Home Savings of America, a Fortune 500 savings bank that paid their loan officers a salary plus offered other attractive perks like marketing budgets and high visibility.

My company was also going through some changes I didn't like.

After a series of interviews I accepted a position with Home Savings. What was surprising at first was that they assigned me a territory thirty miles away despite how well-entrenched I was in my territory. Myrna eventually admitted that she was the one who asked her boss to recruit me to get me out of her territory so she could get some of her business back. Despite its initial appearance, this had a major positive impact on my career path.

At first the transition was a little tough. Despite the fact that I was now with a Fortune 500 bank, I was amazed at how far behind they were in terms of products and underwriting methods. This revelation ended up being the catalyst that sent my career into a positive orbit.

From their perspective, that is the managers at the new bank, I was an unknown quantity and in their view I was a mortgage broker who had to earn their trust. I was actually a mortgage banker and was careful to remind people of that because at the time in that area, mortgage brokers did not have the best reputations. A mortgage banker is one who funds loans with company money, versus a broker who shops loans with various banks and mortgage bankers. Both provide valuable services, but many brokers in the area were thought to be unscrupulous at the time. So management viewed me as somebody they had to keep an eye on. As for me, I was the same guy I always was, cocky, aggressive, but above-board.

I went to a two-week training and while I was really excited to be part of the organization, it was painful to have to listen to inexperienced trainers teach about the products I was skilled at. Especially since they were teaching them all wrong. I offered what I could in terms of assistance but I was also aware of the setting so I kept quiet for the most part during the entire two weeks. I didn't want to blow an opportunity.

Once out of training I hit the ground running making this now the third new territory that I was opening. The salary helped plus the company had some great marketing strategies that I was able to use to generate business quickly, and it had a great benefit plan.

Whenever new loan officers would join a company they were on pretty strict probation for the first ninety days but especially for their first five to ten loans. Operations managers and processing staff would rate you based on how complete your applications were and how well you documented your package.

Since I processed and pre-underwrote all my loans from the start of my career, I was miles ahead of the average loan officer which raised red flags for added scrutiny to make sure I wasn't turning in fraudulent packages. Once again, I acted the same way I always acted, and because I was working with a real estate agent who wanted me to take a loan application but didn't want me spending much time with her buyer, that raised a red flag of my own.

After reviewing the file I assessed what else we would need and I advised Tina, the real estate agent, that I would need two years of the buyer's tax returns. Normally I would have been having this conversation directly with the buyer but the real estate agent insisted she would take care of it. Something she said in that conversation made me a little uncomfortable so when I gave the loan managers the updates on the file I cautioned them to scrutinize the tax returns once they came in because there was something that didn't feel right.

A few days later the assistant loan manager called me into his office to share a conversation he had just had with the real estate agent. The tax returns had come in and based upon my recommendation to scrutinize them he was able to locate the fraud. It took a while but there were two years of returns and the borrower was claiming to own nine properties but his mortgage interest deduction was exactly the same for both years which is something next to impossible.

When the assistant loan manager called the agent to ask some questions, she asked about the file and he advised her that they found the returns to be fraudulent.[4] Her first response was to tell him that I was the one who dummied up the returns and she would get the correct ones. The assistant loan manager responded by saying in general he would have believed her but couldn't because I was the one who called it to their attention.

That event became a hallmark of my career, not only with that company but throughout my entire mortgage and real estate career. Had I not caught it and advised them of it my entire professional life would have been ruined over a false accusation because there would have been no way that I could have proven I didn't do it. Since I had no history with the company they would have had to take the agent's word for it. An accusation like that would have meant my immediate termination, but worse, I would have been branded for committing

---

[4] That was something they were allowed to say back then but can't any longer.

fraud and would have been barred from working in any areas dealing with public trust, such as banking, securities, insurance and real estate. I can't imagine somebody brazen enough to kill someone's livelihood with a false accusation but she never gave it a second thought.

A couple of years later we had a nimrod who quit and filed a wrongful termination suit against the company, naming my boss and me as the contributing parties. Before the company chose to fight it, they had their attorneys conduct a six-month investigation of our management style, and not only did we look very good because of the way we managed; that incident with the bogus agent came up as evidence of integrity.

Adapting To Family Life

While this was happening, my kids were getting bigger. Out of the blue one of my friend's from our kids' school called me and asked me if I wanted to join him and a few other dads in forming a Cub Scout Troop. It didn't take long for Todd to talk me into it, and there wasn't a whole lot to convince me of. The thought of doing fun things with my kids was great, but my concerns were that I didn't know much about scouting[5] and because in my referral business I wasn't in total control of my hours. I had to be available when my customers needed me to be.

Todd had me in as the treasurer which was pretty easy and I agreed to be a co-Den Leader with Scott, another friend from our kids' school. Scott had scouting experience so it was really easy to follow his lead. In a short time we had a full pack with all the dens filled. As a pack we did something that I think was a bit unusual in that we took the kids camping more than normal for Cub Scouts because of their young ages, but we also opened up to entire families.

As a pack we did Pinewood Derbies, Rain-gutter Regattas, Adopt-a-Family, and things like kayaking and water skiing merit badges. We also organized orienteering outings during the campouts, so teams would have to use their compasses to find clues until they got to the end of the trail.

We liked to live a little. My friends and I would take Starbucks

---

[5] My experience with scouting amounted to learning the bastardized mantra that my friends and I would recite with great frequency when I was a kid: "on my honor I will do my best, to help the girl scouts get undressed".

coffee and a karaoke machine to the campouts, and at 6:00 a.m. sharp I would yell into the microphone 'Good Morning Camp RCC Troopers' in the style of Robin Williams doing 'Good Morning Vietnam'. Then we would blast out the song 'Shout' to get everyone in the camp moving.

That proved to be a fun experience for my two older boys, Alex and Andrew. Austin is nine years younger than Alex and seven-and-a-half years younger than Andrew so by the time Austin came into the picture, we were already winding down from Scouts.

Earning a better living, I was able to hire a housekeeper and landscapers which lightened my load at home. Abby did a great job making sure the boys had what they needed. Before they were in school, she got them crafts tables and table-top easels so they always spent time during the day being creative. Avid readers, she and I both read to them every day. Abby was great about organizing play dates for the boys with the neighbor kids and it was always fun for me to watch the kids interacting.

For my part, if it had to do with any of the kids, I found a way to make it happen and I rarely questioned the need for anything relating to them except on very rare occasions. I also tried to pay attention to what Abby wanted too. When we were first married she complained that her father was so stingy. She let on the first time we went Christmas tree shopping that she always loved Noble firs but her father wouldn't buy them at Christmas because they were usually twice the price of regular firs. Until the time we had to stop buying real trees due to the boys' allergies, I bought only Noble Firs because I knew she loved them.

But enough of me talking about what a saint I was, and if you believe that then I have a bridge to sell you. I talked earlier about my temper and although I have worked very hard to get it under control I look back and see things I'm not proud of. I can make all kinds of excuses and try to blame Abby, or my father, or my long hours, but the truth is at times I was a total dick. And for that I'm truly sorry.

One of the things I tried not to be was my father and I think overall I succeeded in that. It took a while to finally understand that I needed to control my temper. Once I became a banking manager, certain people would push me the wrong way and I'd yell so loud that I could be heard at the other end of the building, which was a long way down. Other times, I'd have to have another manager sit with me when I'd talk with certain people just to be able to help calm me down if I got going.

Abby would take advantage of that at times, but other times I would fly off the handle and put on these ridiculous displays which my kids learned from me. I didn't realize how ridiculous they were until I saw my kids doing it and I was ashamed when I realized that it was me who taught them. Most things in our lives can be reversed, but I don't think imprints left by our parents can be reversed very easily.

What I did know is that during my twenties I had no temper to speak of once I left the shipyard because I was relaxed and enjoying life. As my kids were growing up and I was building my career I was enjoying life but had no opportunities to relax. We used to joke that when it came to Abby, we had Mother's Day week and Father's Day minute. We'd go all out for Abby making sure she didn't lift a finger, but on Father's Day I'd do the cooking or take them out somewhere and I'd be the one walking the baby if he got fussy.

I can't blame Abby entirely for that because over time I accepted that position and ended up enabling her to keep going. I lived for my family which meant that I never wanted to put myself first; and that became my undoing over time. But I had a long way to go before I would be undone.

For me, the only place I had left to go was up, at least financially that is. I had a great family (at least I thought I did), a nice house and a decent job but there was no way in hell I was going to let myself get comfortable with that. No matter how good things seemed to be the fact of the matter was that I still had to work for a living and that meant I needed to find a way to make more money.

Back when we lived in our little two bedroom apartment, I started to focus on how many dollars a year I was making then playing with the idea of doubling what I was making. That idea stuck with me, I didn't know how I was going to do it but I knew that I had to find ways to do it. So when I started doing that, I was lucky to make about $20,000 a year and by the time I reached my comfort zone about three or four years later, I was making about $65,000 a year.

The solution was simple; my next goal was to be making $130,000 a year. Only this time the pressure was on. It wasn't just the doubling of the money, but I needed to find a way to do it in half the time. Nothing like slapping the bull in the ass yet again, but once I got fixated on that goal I had no choice but to go after it and that's what I did.

FIVE

The Corporate Ladder

The four levels of (increasing) competence:

1. Unconscious Incompetence: You don't know that you can't do it well.
2. Conscious Incompetence: You know you can't do it well.
3. Conscious Competence: You do it well, and you think about the work as you do it.
4. Unconscious Competence: You're so successful it's "automatic" – you do it well, without thinking about it.

"Kirkpatrick Model" by Donald L. Kirkpatrick

Over time my expertise grew to a point where the loan business and how to generate income from it became second nature to me. By the time I was opening up my third territory, it wasn't taking me as long to generate business but I was performing more by rote rather than enthusiasm. I was an Unconscious Competent, but this was a concern to me because a key part of my success was the creativity that was borne by my former need to stand out and be noticed allowing business to come to me.

I found myself falling back on my laurels; though I'd seen what that did to long time veterans who forgot more about the business than I would ever learn. They were still loan officers in the field even after twenty-plus years and lacked enthusiasm for the work they were doing. I decided that I'd be taking a different path so I wouldn't be stuck doing a job I no longer had a passion for. The savings bank that recruited me was Home Savings of America which was a Fortune 500 company with 10,000 employees and many offices nationwide.

It didn't take me long to realize the opportunity I had before me. Earlier I said I had embarked on a career which means that I was looking at a life plan rather than simply working at a job. I looked around me and saw that people working inside this company really didn't have a vision beyond showing up for work every day, which to me was a perfect opportunity to pursue my career path. What I saw was a large company that had grown without me and would continue with or without me, but I had skill sets that could help while propelling me upward to places I wanted to go.

It didn't matter to me that others didn't share my vision because I knew I was onto something. I set out first by learning what I needed to know about corporate life. The second thing I needed was to find out how I was going to stand out. Subconsciously I was approaching the corporate hierarchy in the same way I approached a new territory; when you think of it from that angle it really was a new territory.

A Quick Guide to the Loan Business

A lot of people don't really understand the relationships between bank deposits and bank loans. It took me a while before I had a decent grasp, but it was something I had to learn because I was in the business of making loans with those deposits. When a bank takes money in as a deposit the money it takes in becomes a liability to the bank. The bank needs to give the money back to the depositors when they ask for it, and it costs money to service those accounts for the depositors.

When the bank lends money out the loan becomes an asset to the bank. The bank earns interest on the loan, and the money is usually secured by collateral such as a house, a car, or even business inventory depending on the type of bank. The bank and its management have options relating to how they want to lend the money out provided they demonstrate proper stewardship of the money to the regulators.

When a bank lends money it has to fund the money out of what it has on deposit but it also has to utilize various mechanisms to access cash in order to keep from running out of money. Money on deposit always has to be available in case a customer wants to withdraw. If you saw the movie 'It's a Wonderful Life' you might remember Jimmy Stewart explaining how a lady's deposit was in a neighbor's house and the neighbor's money was in someone else's house and so on. Thankfully certain mechanisms, like the Federal Reserve, secondary markets, mortgage-backed securities, and GSEs were put in place to lessen the risks of banks running out of money but it can still happen in theory.

Most of us have heard of Fannie Mae and Freddie Mac. These are known as Government Sponsored Enterprises, or GSEs. Fannie comes from the Federal National Mortgage Association (FNMA) and Freddie comes from the Federal Home Loan Mortgage Corporation (FHLMC). These two enterprises essentially operate money warehouses or money distribution centers using protection and credit lines from the Federal Government. The protection means the GSEs will continue to operate because of government intervention in the event of a crisis, and the credit lines are available cash from the government to keep them operating.

One of the mechanisms for a bank to access funds is through the secondary market which consists of a number of organizations including Fannie and Freddie. As long as the loan is underwritten according to Fannie or Freddie's guidelines, a bank can sell the loan to Fannie or Freddie after having made fee income from it and get cash to lend again. The fee income is part of the profit they make, and the cash is what they sell the loan for which is the amount of the note, plus or minus interest. Fannie and Freddie in turn package these loans and sell them to Wall Street or other banks as mortgage-backed securities (MBS) in which individuals also invest.

Some banks consider Fannie and Freddie guidelines to be too restrictive and will choose to lend according to their own guidelines and keep the loans. I started my lending career with World Savings, a portfolio lender that was later bought out by Wachovia which was later bought out by Wells Fargo. Portfolio lenders have their own rules for lending, provided of course that they follow all of the federal lending laws. Working for a portfolio lender is one of the reasons I was able to service niches when I first started my lending career.

Back when I started, if a real estate investor wanted to keep buying investment properties, Fannie and Freddie would only lend him or her money as long as he or she had less than four mortgages unless the mortgage was their principle residence. World Savings on the other hand would allow the investor loans on up to ten properties as long as he or she could demonstrate that the loans were going to get paid back.

There are other banks like Wells Fargo that originate loans to sell to the secondary market but also have portfolio underwriting, especially for their more affluent clients. Originating a loan simply means taking a loan application and putting it in process to help a client get the funds he or she needs to buy or refinance a property. Portfolio underwriting or Secondary Market underwriting (GSEs) are where a loan officer looks to get the client what he or she needs based on the client's financial circumstances as well as what the client can document. The underwriting guidelines are what determine what the client needs to document in order to qualify for the loan.

I started at World Savings, at one time a Wall Street darling; then I was recruited by Provident Savings out of Riverside, California which originated loans for sale to the secondary market. Not only was Provident Savings a great bank, but in 1993 Fannie Mae had it on its Top Ten Lenders of the West because of their loan quality and innovation. Being associated with Provident Savings, I not only learned a lot but saw them open up doors within Fannie and Freddie that other secondary lenders didn't know were available.

Becoming a Corporate Manager

I joined Home Savings after leaving Provident Savings when Home was beginning their transition from being a portfolio lender to a secondary lender and instituting a new computerized originating program, both of which were causing their top loan consultants to think about leaving. The loan consultants (sometimes called loan officers or loan agents) thought of leaving because not only were the new loan programs to offer customers hard to learn, the new system was even harder.

My frustration was mainly because I knew what loans could be approved for the secondary market and would package them that way, but the underwriters and managers didn't know enough about it and kept driving me nuts by declining my loans or asking me for things they didn't need. Underwriters are the ones who approve or deny loans based on the programs applied for and based on how well the customer qualifies, or on how well the loan agent documents the loan to prove the customer's ability to pay it back. Managers oversaw the loan agents and underwriters and could sometimes override an underwriter if the case was compelling enough.

When I was with both World and Provident, I would package the loan correctly and turn it in, and my closing rate was about ninety-eight percent; the two percent loss was normally due to low appraisals or buyers changing their minds.

I still had a high closing percentage when I first joined Home Savings, but it was taking me two to three times longer than normal because I had to educate the underwriters and managers. Those delays greatly impacted my service model and almost created opportunities for competing loan companies to take my business.

At Home Savings, the bank was divided in terms of business models. There were the savings branches that took care of the depositors and there was the lending division which took care of homeowners and home buyers. Each of these divisions wanted to claim rights as being the most important to the organization, kind of the heart versus the brain argument. In reality each was equally important. Each division was broken down into regions and then broken down to branches or centers within those regions.

On the lending side, each was run by a Regional Vice President of Mortgage Production who was responsible for sales and bringing loans in, and Loan Operations had counterparts who were responsible for processing, underwriting, and then funding the loans.

I started as a loan consultant with Home Savings and I worked out of a bank branch in Corona, California that had a satellite loan office attached with about five other loan consultants in it. We loan consultants would cover our territories from there, and our loans were processed and underwritten in Rancho, about twenty miles from my loan office. My territory was another fifteen miles northeast of the loan office. For a while it worked out pretty well and I was able to help my colleagues out by taking their packages with me and dropping them off since I lived very close to the loan operations office in Rancho.

Our regional manager was a great guy and one of the best sales people I've ever known, a man in his sixties with incredible charm. He was also the father-in-law of the CEO of our company. That didn't mean that Chuck didn't earn his keep, he was a great manager with field experience and was the kind who always had your back provided that you merited it.

At first I didn't know what to make of Chuck because he was at times difficult to read. Over time we developed a mutual respect for each other and became good friends. I was always amazed at Chuck's energy and marveled that he started in the loan business around the same time I did and yet he became one of the top loan officers in the country for Home Savings. His son-in-law being the CEO no doubt opened some doors to clients that otherwise might not have been opened, but simply because the door gets opened doesn't mean success is guaranteed. A person still has to earn it by being willing to do what it takes and performing with excellence. I knew from talking to and observing him that Chuck was a high caliber performer and earned his success with his clients.

That is something I caught on to early on whereas some of my colleagues chose to make fun of Chuck behind his back, implying that he only made a lot of loans because of his son-in-law. They also complained about the company rather than embrace the opportunity they had right in front of them. I was fortunate in that I knew both sides of the fence, meaning I had experience with other lenders and knew what benefits the company had that offset what it didn't offer. I didn't judge my colleagues for their complaints but there were a few times when I asked them why they just didn't leave if they hated it so much. They never really answered my questions, especially when I'd point out many of the great things Home did offer, I also gave them a birds-eye view of the other lenders and showed them that the grass wasn't all that green on the other side.

I built my territory and though I was friendly with most of my colleagues, I kept my distance, especially if they were complainers. I wasn't about to kill my career by absorbing or participating in all the negativity. Instead I went to work on a spreadsheet program to make it easier for me to do calculations and print out sheets that I could give to my customers so they could take the information home and decide for themselves which decision would best suit them. I was still working on my Bachelor's degree and that program ended up being my Bachelor's thesis for which I got an A.

The program did more than just get me an A in the course. One day Chuck was making the rounds and stopped in our office to check in on everybody and yuck it up. He came into my office and asked me what I was working on. I showed Chuck my spreadsheet program and demonstrated that other loan consultants could use it for the new government loan programs that Home Savings had just acquired. The calculations were very complicated and many of them didn't know how to do the calculations by hand and weren't interested in learning because it took time away from their main businesses.

To my surprise Chuck was impressed. To my bigger surprise,

a few weeks later Chuck told me there was a new position being formed to support Regional Vice Presidents and suggested that I apply. I did.

On the day of the interview I was in front of Chuck and a guy named Tom, the Loan Manager. Tom and I had a good relationship and respected each other so I felt pretty good about the interview. I had had an opportunity to review the position; in anticipation of the interview I drafted a business plan as to what opportunities I saw in the region, what goals might be achieved, and how I would go about supporting the Regional Manager to achieve those goals.

Chuck was an excellent administrator and grilled me to see how well I knew my mission as well as his own. The interview didn't last very long and Chuck closed it by asking me how much I needed to make. I thought to say $4,500 a month but when I glanced at Tom, who'd blocked his face from Chuck's and mouthed $5,000, I suggested $5,000 per month and left.

Everybody else seemed to know it before I did, but by the next week I was the new Assistant Regional Manager (ARM) covering a very large territory, after only having been with the company for six months. Not only was I Myrna's new boss, I was new boss all of the loan consultants in our region, including my former colleagues who'd spent their time complaining and bad mouthing our Regional Manager. The loan consultants were very concerned about how I was going to treat their antics, and while they didn't want to ask I brought it up at the appropriate opportunity.

This is when I started to adopt a new style of management which I alluded to when I talked about my days in the steel business. I could have been a real drip and lorded it over them or tattled to my boss but neither would have served any purpose or add value to the company. Instead I set their minds at ease by declaring their comments would be relegated to the past. I then set expectations to ensure they saw me as a manager who could be their friend but who fully expected them to perform. They respected that and we got along well.

Similar to how Bob and Kathy saved me from a life in prison and set me on the right road of life, Chuck was my corporate mentor who was only too happy to take me under his wing. Not an easy achievement given that he was considerably shorter than me. Chuck had a goofy, fun side to him and it would crack us all up when he'd come out into the loan operations office wearing my suit jacket having grabbed it from the back of my chair. It looked like it could have fit six of him in it.

It didn't take Chuck and me very long to bond, and that bond was tight. I'd be lying if I didn't say that his being father-in-law to our CEO didn't have some bearing, but that was more so in the beginning. We became close friends over time as we worked together. I was also cognizant of what I called "Conversations at the Holiday Dinner Table" meaning that I made it a point to make my boss shine whenever possible in case I might become a small topic at the dinner table when Chuck and his son-in-law would be at family gatherings. That just followed my marketing technique throughout my lending career which was to get positive exposure whenever and wherever I could.

In truth, Chuck and I needed each other. If you've ever seen the movie 'City Hall' with Al Pacino and John Cusack, our relationship was like theirs where Cusack was the messenger who did the deeds, ran the errands, and delivered the powerful messages. Chuck was like Pacino, the Godfather who had the muscle and was the enforcer who made people stand at attention. That was Chuck and me.

The transition from being a portfolio lender to becoming a secondary lender was becoming increasingly tenuous because the work was getting harder and there weren't many loans getting closed in time. Loan consultants were working twice as hard but earning so much less. It was a product line that I understood and Chuck didn't, at least not as well at first. Chuck gave me a lot of latitude and in return I protected him by making sure to help the loan consultants be successful while minimizing loan errors that might lead to customer complaints.

Defining Moments

I designed training programs, and continued to develop my FHA / VA loan program tool which I copyrighted as EzGov© once I completed my bachelor's thesis. I also taught the loan consultants how to package their loans the right way because of the new dynamic happening throughout the lending divisions. In the past because the company was a portfolio lender, loan consultants (they were called loan officers back then) met with clients, helped them choose the right program then took the loan application and turned it in to a processor who then did the rest. Not much documentation was required.

In the secondary market environment far more documentation was required and the loan consultants needed to get that documentation when they took the applications. They also had to review what they were getting to ensure nothing was fraudulent and they had to do calculations to make sure that the borrowers qualified.

Over time the loan consultants changed their ways but it wasn't without conflict. We had a top producer named Rich who I would be proud to call a friend but back then it wasn't like that. He was a former cop and very tough, his loan packages were the crappiest anybody had ever seen but his market share was unheard of compared to anyone in the company.

The way Rich used to break in new managers was to give them a few days to settle in then he'd seize on some conflict, important or not and literally put the manager up against the wall to let the manager know who the real boss was. Rich didn't do that with every manager and not with Chuck because Chuck would have eaten him alive. Though small, Chuck was a tough old guy and of course had the resources within the corporate hierarchy to back him up.

Rich was also best friends with Eli, a UFC fighter wannabe and barroom brawler who was also a loan consultant. From their perspectives the jury was still out on me but I knew it was only a matter of time before they put me to trial by fire.

One day I put out a new requirement for all new loan packages to include certain forms that weren't required when the company did portfolio lending but were needed in the secondary loan programs. The form was something that was easy to get from an applicant and the loans couldn't be approved without it. Rich walked in to the regional office and lit his match by getting right up to my face and screaming that he didn't want to do it and wasn't going to do it. I didn't budge but looked him square in the eye and screamed right back, "I don't give a fuck if you want to do it or not. I told you to do it and it's not negotiable. Otherwise don't let the door hit you in the ass on your way out."

This shocked everyone who saw what happened because nobody ever talked to Rich that way. Rich looked over at Chuck to see if he was going to step in and realized Chuck wasn't. Rich decided to do it in order to meet guidelines but for a while it created a lot of tension. He turned the corner though once he saw me fighting for his loans with underwriting managers who were trying to require more than what was needed on his loans. I also intervened when other loan consultants would try to take Rich's loans or steal his customers. Those were fights I didn't lose. Once he saw that Rich realized that I was an ally and not his adversary; we ended up with a good relationship over the years.

Eli was also one of my buddies from the branch loan office days and he had a temper that rivaled mine. He and I had a similar showdown after one of his disturbing episodes but he left knowing which lines not to cross or he'd be out of a job. We never had a problem after that and we too became good friends.

I, along with Selma who was our very resourceful administrative assistant, was tasked with designing training and information programs, and strategy planning meetings for the loan consultants. Chuck empowered us to select the locations and design the meeting agenda. We always designed them to keep the group entertained to help offset being forced to sit in a meeting. Nothing is worse for a high-powered producer to be sitting in a meeting getting paged and missing opportunities to do business.

One of our meetings dealt mainly with teaching the loan consultants tricks to knowing their new loan products so they could make quick decisions on how to package their loans and get them funded quickly. I asked a mid-level loan question and when the first person answered it correctly, I gave him a ten from the $300 approved by Chuck, shocking the group. It was fun to watch how quickly the group learned to navigate their loan manuals. We made sure that each consultant got one of those ten dollar bills; by the end of the session, the loan consultants knew all the basics and their frustration levels dropped tremendously.

I didn't know it but Chuck was grooming me for executive status, something for which I'll always be grateful. Chuck was a former bank president and had run some banks for the Resolution Trust Corp (RTC) during the 1980s when many banks were closing. He drew my attention to things like corporate etiquette, grooming and management hierarchy. I in turn researched his projects and wrote memos and responses, and Selma and I developed methodologies for training, budget review and report development.

Chuck also recognized that I had an intuitive ability and would use it to his advantage which ultimately was our advantage. Once our bond became tighter, Chuck would have me listen to certain voice messages for analysis based on words used, how they were used and intonation. While some might view that as paranoid, it was a legitimate concern because there were quite a few people who were willing to lie about things or try and trip him up so they could embarrass him.

As part of my grooming, Chuck had me do presentations in front of senior and executive managers. He would also have me develop proposals to submit to the executive office, proposals which not only showed me as an author but yielded ventures to which I would be assigned. It didn't mean my job was fully protected though.

My job as an ARM came with a salary and bonuses on production, and my income had steadily climbed because of the successes we were achieving with the loan consultants. Even after making my mark I was dealt a major blow. The company went through major changes in the appraisal department that left a lot of people without positions. As a consolation, the company offered the ARM positions, including mine, to any of the displaced appraisal managers wanting them.

Because we were on at-will contracts, those of us ARMs stood to lose our positions. Chuck called me in once he found out what was taking place and reluctantly told me that he had tried to protect my position but couldn't. That was one of the worst weekends I spent while I was there; knowing that I could be out of a great job and powerless to do anything. On Monday I was able to breathe a sigh of relief when I found out there was only one person who was eligible for my position but she didn't want it.

The corporate world was a different environment, especially in a Fortune 500 bank. The fact that we were so visible to the public meant that regulators were often shopping us to see if we were doing anything wrong. If they caught a bank our size doing something wrong and penalized us for it, the ripple effect would cause many smaller institutions to take notice and clean their acts up without the regulators having to do anything.

When we were in the corporate headquarters we couldn't walk around without our suit jackets, and we always had to be mindful of who might be in the restroom stalls while we were using them. Some of them could have been bank executives or bank regulators, so I had to learn to stay quiet on corporate trips. Chuck and I would often be at offsite corporate meetings and I also learned in a hurry to be careful of what I did and said in public. Our contracts had clauses letting us know that what we do after hours could impact our positions and possibly lead to termination for things like bouncing checks, drunken driving, and obnoxious conduct. I also knew to be careful in hotel elevators at the offsite meetings because we might be in one with an executive or regulator we didn't know.

There were all sorts of horror stories of people who didn't pay attention to the rules and found themselves without jobs the very next day. Chuck taught me a lot about it, and though we socialized with our colleagues we set our limits and got out before things would get rowdy, a rule I continued to follow in general throughout my career.

Even though the job came with a steady paycheck we still had struggles at home but managed to live through them with very few scars. My father-in-law and I had settled our differences by then and were beginning to form a bond of our own. Mr. Frazier drove an old Buick Century that had a little less than two hundred-thousand miles on it. He offered to sell it to me. This was a quandary I didn't care to find myself in; I agreed to buy it for $2,000 mainly because I knew he'd be offended if I didn't.

To Abby's credit, she spotted that her dad was playing on my soft-heartedness and let him have it; then she had him price it fairly to $1,300. The car was copper-colored and the body was in pretty good shape except for the taillight that was held together with duct tape. It looked like a company car which regional managers got, and it was a step up from the old broken down T-bird I had been driving, yet it wasn't without its challenges.

The Buick had no air conditioning but I covered San Diego County where the weather was tolerable for the most part. The headliner covering the ceiling was falling apart and because I had to drive with the windows down it would nearly beat me to death any time I was going faster than 30 miles an hour. The radio used to work fine, but the antenna motor had a problem that kept the motor running which would kill the battery. A mechanic disconnected the motor which left the antenna up and the first time I took it through a car wash the antenna bent at a 90 degree angle.

That was also the first time I learned that the car windows leaked, but only at the front drivers side when a large splash came through the window and got me soaked. That was on a day suits were required and I was on my way to a regional meeting, dressed in my thoroughly soaked suit. I had fun explaining that one at the meeting.

Abby and I began calling the Buick the BT for Brown Turd, but since we didn't use that language in front of the kids, we told them it was the Brown Terror because it was so fast and powerful. For all the grief the car gave me its plusses far outweighed the negatives. The car never needed maintenance and ran great even with that many miles. Since people with my position got car allowances, and because of the miles I was putting on I was making another $1,000 to $1,300 a month in mileage reimbursements, so the car more than paid for itself in the first month and a half. And I sure didn't have to worry about wear and tear ruining the car because, hell, it already had 200k miles on it!

There were some dark sides to the job being that people will lie, cheat, steal and file false accusations if they think they can get away with it, much like the real estate agent I talked about earlier in Chapter 4. We had a prima donna in our region who was harassing a fellow loan consultant and slandering her with false accusations. When the prima donna didn't like the results of the independent investigation, she quit then filed a wrongful termination suit against the company. Only in California, right? The company looked at a quick settlement of $150,000 which the lady turned down but the company investigated our region for six months and decided to fight it because of how we managed the region. Emotionally it was tough, especially once we went to court. The prima donna won her case but didn't quite get what she was looking for.

What was interesting was the jury's response when our attorneys polled them about why they came up with their decision. The original suit was for $10,000,000 but the plaintiff got $500,000. The jury said they didn't like the individual but all of them had a problem with their bosses at one time or another so they thought she should get something. The irony for the plaintiff though was that in order to prove she was harmed, she didn't work for two years. Out of that award she had to pay the attorneys $300,000 and the income tax on it was $200,000 which meant the idiot got exactly what she deserved, nothing!

My First Big Promotion

Chuck was a great teacher and mentor, and I was an able and willing student. His mentorship paid off in less than two years. Chuck was promoted to the Area Office which was a senior management position in charge of all of the regions in that area. He didn't want the Area Manager's job and took the Assistant Area position instead because he didn't want the pressures of being that high up now that he was nearly seventy years old, but he also wasn't ready to leave the company so the Assistant position was a perfect job. I was promoted to Vice President and Regional Manager of the Inland Empire Region, which was the lowest region in the country in terms of performance, quality control, and profitability. I had my work cut out for me to say the least.

The region was run by a guy named Steve who was a former top producing loan consultant, and somebody who was a jovial guy but definitely not a manager. He had no controls in place and told his consultants that he didn't want to hear about complaints. In doing so, he ignored that his region was getting twenty to thirty serious complaints a month. Steve and his operations counterparts were in adversarial relationships so it was nearly impossible to get loans approved, and the region's morale was in the tank.

When I got the promotion, Steve became a loan consultant under me and he saw no reason for his demotion. In his eyes he had been a great manager, so he was quite bitter about it in fact. Out of the forty or so consultants and staff he had organized more than half to bet against me staying on as their new manager much less succeeding. The bet was that I would be gone in less than two months and he was going to do whatever he could to make that happen. His hopes had been to send me packing so he could get his old job back.

Meanwhile, I was in charge of our old region, the region that I managed with Chuck. Chuck had already settled in his position as Assistant Area Manager, and I was now the new Vice President and Regional manager for both my old region and my new region. There were no assistants in either region, so I had one hundred people under me with no assistant, and I had a former manager making plans to undermine my role. And if that wasn't enough, because of my new salary and bonus structure, Abby had us buying our first house.

My first month as Regional VP was a tough one to say the least. After only one week, I organized my new region's first meeting at our company headquarters. That meeting served two purposes: to set expectations with my new group, and to build bridges with the operations center and my operational counterparts.

Making Changes

Steve was notorious for letting people show up late for meetings, something I had observed while I was an ARM at executive gatherings.

That was part of what ended up working against him when the decision to demote him was made. I had no tolerance for tardiness and made sure everyone knew it. The morning of the first meeting, four of the loan consultants were late; these were four of the five I worked with at my old loan branch in Corona when I first started as a loan consultant. I had everyone sit in the meeting doing nothing until the four arrived more than thirty minutes late. Once they realized the tension they caused, they were extremely embarrassed but that was the last time anyone ever showed up late for a meeting.

A great lady named Jackie was my loan operations counterpart and she and I immediately hit it off well. She not only found me to be a willing ally, she knew I knew the loan business and we started closing loans. The loan consultants began to respond, and despite my initial abrasive style, they quickly learned that they could come to me for help on a loan. I'd walk them through the packaging, and once they delivered it they saw the approvals coming in.

The loan consultants also saw an entirely different approach to handling complaints. Whereas their previous manager wanted nothing to do with a complaint and left the consultants to deal with it on their own, I was just the opposite. Complaints, when handled correctly, are opportunities to build customers for life. But when handled badly those same complaints become major lawsuits. The region was heading for lawsuits and the complaints were getting to the federal regulator; which is something that should never happen because if the complaint is bad enough the regulator can impose heavy fines or even shut the bank down.

I had all new complaints routed to me immediately. I would speak directly to the customer to hear their concerns and ask them what kind of resolution they were looking for. After talking it through, I would set expectations with that customer, meaning I would share some of the due diligence I would need to pursue and would give them a timeline so they knew when I would be calling back. Usually I would build in twenty-four hours before they would hear from me so I would schedule a next call time for within forty-eight hours or sooner, and I would also review with them whether or not what they were looking for was achievable, and if not what some of the alternatives would be.

I would talk with the loan consultant about the issue and require by early the next morning that they give me a memo describing the issue and what they felt caused the problem. I would use that opportunity to coach the consultant as to how to avoid the problem in the future, and ninety-nine percent of the time I never had a repeat problem.

I would also involve my operations counterpart to discuss the resolution and gain a commitment so that when I talked with the customer I could give them guarantees. Once the loan closed I would send the customer a thank you card and a $50 gift card to their favorite restaurant. Not only were the complaints disappearing with more loans being closed, in less than three months we became the number one region in the country for customer service.

Within the first six weeks of my promotion, I was able to help usher in the manager of my old region, hire two assistants, move the regional office from ninety miles away from my house to two miles away, and move in to our beautiful new home. The demoted manager saw that he was losing his bet and filed a lawsuit against the company.

While this was happening there was a shakeup at the operations center and Jackie, with whom I had formed a great bond, left to become a Regional Manager so we became colleagues as well as friends. My new loan operations counterpart, Larry, was installed and he and I bonded quickly because he also saw that I was his ally and he could come to me with problems that my consultants were causing and I'd get those problems fixed.

Even though the loan consultants had cleaned up their acts, sometimes they would promise to deliver things the underwriters needed like documentation from the customer or Title Company, but they would take their time or deliver the wrong things. That would cause problems on my end and for Larry's group and I had no patience for it. It was reciprocal as well so it made for a great relationship.

In those six weeks we had our first Area Meeting which was a very big deal because we had the executive managers there as well as the Area Manager and all of the Production and Lending Regional Managers. The purpose was to review year-end results, discuss strategies, review and assess policy matters, and deliver our projections. The jury was still out on me because while I was making significant changes at the field level they weren't immediately noticeable at the corporate level in terms of numbers.

As luck would have it, I was the first manager who was selected to speak. Larry was terrified that I was going to have him speak for us, as some of the other managers were planning to do. Larry was one of those guys who got nervous speaking to two people much less an audience of fifty comprised of our colleagues and regional competitors as well as the highest ranking officials of our company.

The objective of the speech was to give a brief overview of our current statistics, our trends and assessments of areas of the greatest concerns along with what we saw as the greatest opportunities. We would wrap up the speech with how we were going to approach those opportunities and measure our success. The thing was, we weren't given any kind of notice about any of that nor did we know the order in which any of us would be speaking. We were handed our packets as we walked into the meeting room, and the executives fully expected us to know our regions or there would be hell to pay considering what they were paying us. By then I was making $150,000 a year in salary plus production overrides, bonuses, and many perks like stock options, great expense accounts and corporate recognition.

I had looked over our packet and saw that our Inland Empire region was dead last in every one of the twelve categories nationally. Larry's face was grim but it soon turned to horror when he heard Linda, our Executive Vice President (EVP) ask us to talk about our region. This was the fourth officer in command of a ten-thousand employee company, and Larry had only been in his position for less than a month. I looked at Linda, thanked her for the opportunity, looked around the room, and began speaking. "Hello everyone, next to me is my partner Larry Smith, and we are the Emperors of the Inland Empire." I paused.

"Before I begin, I want to draw your attention to our performance ranking sheet, and if you all would be so kind as to turn it upside down, then you will see that we are number one in every category." The room went silent.

I knew there was a big risk in taking that approach but took a chance since we all were under tremendous pressure and tensions were high because of the conversions and transitions taking place. I felt that a little levity might help ease some of that tension. I breathed a huge sigh of relief when everyone, including the executive managers, responded with belly laughs. So I went on.

"As you know, Larry and I are fairly new to the region but he and I have developed common goals and are making significant headway toward meeting those goals already. Ours is a region with significant challenges.

I think it would be best to describe our collective group in this way: The staff in our region is kind of like this guy I read about who called a forest ranger in Maine one afternoon with an unusual request. He asked the ranger if his department could move a Deer Crossing Sign from one location to another because there were too many deer getting hit at the sign's current location. You see, he was hoping that if the sign was moved the deer could go to the new location to cross the street and be safer." I waited for a minute while this sank in.

"The staff in our region are much like the caller; doing the wrong things for the right reasons. As a result; Larry and I have begun the process of helping everyone change their perspectives and showing them how the changes are really doing things for the better. We fully expect to show dramatic improvements by the next meeting because we are seeing great results in the field already."

Fortunately for me, the executives had been monitoring the results. They too had seen what we were doing and were impressed. My approach to the meeting had set the tone making it a lot of fun. My colleagues were running with the deer story and were having word plays with one saying he got a brilliant idea while mowing his lawn with a John Deere mower. Another lamented that her operations counterpart had sent her a "Deer John" letter, while yet another had talked about how "enDEERing" it was to have received a letter complimenting him on his loan consultants.

By the next quarterly meeting our numbers had improved dramatically as I had predicted, with us ranking Number 1 and 2 in most of the categories nationwide. Within that time frame, Lori, my Area Manager had shared a recording of an executive briefing following the first month when every one of our consultants had funded one million dollars or more, something that region had never done since its inception. It was Anne, the executive who was the third in command of the bank, reviewing highlights of all the regions with the CEO and the board of directors, but spotlighted our region's success. Anne went on to say, "this is what happens when we put a manager in place who knows what he's doing." It is amazing the kind of motivation that follows hearing something like that being said about your efforts.

Steve, the demoted manager, was doing what he could to bring his suit to trial. The law firm was the same firm that defended us when the prima donna quit and filed suit. The law firm asked me to help them understand a Regional Manager's role and responsibilities, and more specifically where one could commit fraud if he or she desired.

My first response was the Expense Report, at which our attorney handed me one at random. Unfortunately for Steve I remember numbers much better than I remember names and immediately pointed to one expense that was charged to a wrong account number, and commented that it was likely done deliberately. I reviewed the explanation and saw that a significant amount had been expensed to a meeting with Lori, our Area Manager. I looked through a few more and found similar abuses which amounted to serious fraud.

The attorney asked Lori for her calendar and learned that there were no such meetings. When Steve walked in with his attorney expecting to negotiate a settlement, our attorney advised them that we would be filing charges in a separate complaint over the fraud. Steve saw the discovery, walked out, and after dropping his case was never heard from again.

Short-Lived Promotion

Abby, Alex, Andrew, Austin, and I had been settled in our new home for a little over a month when I finally started to relax a little. The house payment was about three times more a month than our previous rent, but I was in good financial shape, earning about twelve or thirteen thousand dollars a month. After the house payment there was plenty left over. However, I was only relaxed for a little while.

One morning I logged on to the executive briefing as I did every morning and learned that our company had agreed to be bought out by Washington Mutual. By then I had only been in my role for a little over three months and starting to see real headway, but I can say my heart sank.

My crew and colleagues and I kept up our professionalism and maintained business as usual, but eight months later I was out of a job. Washington Mutual was a group of arrogant bastards who didn't make a whole lot of room for us . Fortunately because I was an officer of the company, I had a Change in Control agreement, or Golden Parachute, as did my colleagues. Despite being out of a job, I was handed a check for $150,000, some stock, and health insurance for the next eighteen months.

By then my youngest son Austin was eighteen months old so I spent a lot of time with him that I wasn't able to spend with my older boys when they were that age. I also spent a lot of time with them especially through Cub Scouts and other activities which I thoroughly enjoyed since I couldn't before because I was always juggling a really busy work schedule.

Lori, our former Area Manager, was hired on by a large mortgage banking company and brought about half of us with her. It looked like a done deal. While the situation wasn't perfect I was being hired on with quite a bit of money left over from my parachute. I remained an arrogant bastard and made a classic mistake, one that I've never made again. Even though I had completed all of my bachelor course work in my college program and got an A on my bachelor's thesis a few years before, I still had about 15 units of lower division course work to complete. In my mind though, I had completed my degree and that's what I put on my application especially since I was using EzGov to assist my loan consultants after completing the course work.

The company rescinded their offer because I couldn't produce the actual degree. That was a hard lesson because it took over a year of interviewing before I got a good position again. And by the time I did land a job, our money had run out and we almost lost our home.

I had also interviewed for some top lending management positions in the interim and had hoped to land one of them but that proved to be elusive. I interviewed with Chase for a Relationship Manager position and thought I had it, but their main customer didn't like that I lived in Rancho so Chase went with another guy. I was devastated because it was a great position with high earning potential.

Later that year I landed a district manager's job at a mortgage company. That proved to be a disaster because the company was poorly run and over priced at a time when the market was showing signs of dying. The pay was so low that I had to spend what was left of my golden parachute which should have gone to savings had I found work sooner (or not screwed up my previous offer).

Corporate Management

Once I was no longer a loan agent (or loan producer / consultant as we were sometimes called) and hit the executive level, all of my positions were performance based which I liked because the better my team and I performed, the more I made. But when you land with a company that isn't invested in your success then the performance-based pay is a problem because you're not able to do the things necessary to achieve the needed results. That was a big problem with the company I was with. I decided to resign from the company because what they said they would provide was not what they did. I remained on good terms with my boss because my problems were with the company; not with him. We stayed in touch.

Had I chosen to stay, I would have run the risk of them firing me for poor performance, even though I met the terms of my contract by hiring a full team of loan agents to generate loan business as I agreed to do. But the company overpriced our rates while buying a low-priced competitor and keeping their rates low which created direct competition for us within our own company. Our customers would let us do all the work by helping them package their loans, but then they would cancel with us and apply with our corporate owned competitor because the rates and fees were so much lower. The company took no action to prevent it from happening, and by doing that, the company took away our ability to compete and we lost so many loans because of it.

`I tried to file a lawsuit against them but they saw it coming, and by then I had no more money to pay the attorneys. One attorney who had his hand out for a big retainer was trying to convince me to accept a non-financial settlement so I just ended up dropping it.

I was back to being squeezed financially though and didn't have a lot of prospects in sight. The kids were old enough and didn't need as much supervision. A real estate career for Abby, who had a great eye for real estate, would have done wonders for our circumstances. I was able to help out with the kids, and it would have been a flexible schedule for her. Not to mention that the market was actually starting to heat up again and there would have been less pressure on our ability to stay afloat. Even though I met her behind a cosmetics counter, Abby had demonstrated that she had a great eye and grasp of real estate early on and throughout our marriage.

I begged her to go into real estate while I continued to look for a job. I was a mortgage manager and did not have much experience in the real estate sales industry yet so the learning curve would have been too much for me to try and take real estate on as a new career. And since the market was starting to heat up again, that suggested that there might be more job prospects for me.

But by then we were one step away from foreclosure and having our cars repossessed. Back when we were able to afford it, bought a new car for Abby and I paid cash for a Monte Carlo that I bought for myself when things were better, but when things got bad I had to borrow against it at 80 percent interest. Abby promised she would go into real estate but didn't. At the very least if she got her license she could have collected a commission when we sold our house and bought a new one later, but since she didn't it meant that we paid over $60,000 in commissions to someone who didn't even do a good job for us. Those were commissions that could have been Abby's but she kept putting the license off. Any commissions that she would have earned could have been used to augment my earnings and the job would have given her plenty of time to still be with the kids.

I found a start-up position that I wasn't thrilled over because I would be going back in the field and sell loans. It was in my old territory when I started with Home Savings but it would have been straight commission. Unfortunately our budgets and lifestyle was built on salary plus commission and I really didn't have the money available to carry us for the two or three months it was going to take to start earning the commissions. I was pretty depressed about it but I needed something to bring money in so we could survive in our house and put food on the table.

Driving to the bank to deliver all of the completed paperwork to accept the start-up position, the recruiter out of Florida who had placed me in the position I had just resigned from called to ask me if I would be interested in talking with Chase again. He told me they had an entirely new position and I wouldn't have to worry about a client not liking where I lived.

Immediately I agreed and placed the start-up offer on hold. I was very aggressive in the Chase interview because they interviewed me the year before and took almost three months before telling me I didn't get the job. This time I had a bonified offer in my hand and told them I needed an immediate answer. Within two days I had an offer to cover the West Coast while working out of my house at a rate of $110,000 a year plus bonus, commission, and expenses; within a year I was making over $225,000 annually.

It was far from a dream job, but it was a great job. I worked for one of the most talented men I knew in the industry but never had I ever been around such a mean bastard, except for myself of course. From time to time I would see articles in the Wall Street Journal pulling the worst traits from the Top Ten Worst Bosses ever.

Mike was the CEO of our unit, and had every one of those ten traits. We would start our phone conversations very pleasantly but by the time we hung up we would be screaming at each other. The unit was a division of Chase Manhattan Mortgage, and his being the CEO meant he had a lot of pressure on him, but that didn't mean he always had to be so miserable and for a while I thought it was just me who he didn't like.

After a while I realized Mike was like that with everybody. The important thing with him was to be sure of your facts because Mike would always challenge us. That was a trait I didn't mind because it was rare that I would get tripped up and that also served me well throughout my entire career by coming to every boss' meeting fully prepared. I even learned to ask questions they hadn't thought of.

Once I joined Chase, I was actually glad that I had the experience that cost me the job for unintentionally misrepresenting my degree. I modified my resume to show that I completed my thesis but still had some lower division units remaining. This was so important because unlike the other position that I lost, this was a Vice President role in a Fortune 100 company with far more upside potential and it was a bonded position. A bonded position means that there has to be an extensive background check because an insurance company was going to bond me to reimburse the bank in the event I committed fraud or other financial crimes. There was no way they would provide such a bond if my background wasn't clean.

After I was in my role for six months and producing results, I got a call from my corporate office saying that they were unable to validate my high school diploma and I had ten days to correct it otherwise I would be terminated.

I panicked because I was just getting into the job and back into the financial swing of things and yet I was back to looking at a bleak future. I called the school and was relieved to learn that the person doing the research at the school had transposed my social security number which is why they couldn't find my diploma.

I also have to throw out a huge THANK YOU to my sister Suzy because without her efforts I would have been out of that same job. When I left our town of Dover, I left a week before school got out and skipped graduation because I was fed up with school and was anxious to move away. Even though I had completed all of my course work with passing grades, the school wasn't going to give me my diploma because I left early. I remember Suzy telling me how hard she had to fight to get them to give it to me, and while I was genuinely grateful for Suzy's success in getting the diploma for me, the diploma didn't mean all that much to me at the time. It was only when I thought I might lose my job at Chase that I realized what she had done for me.

My job as a Vice President with Chase was to form and manage partnerships between real estate brokerages and Chase on the west coast. The first year, despite the nice income was still a struggle financially because we were playing catch up after just avoiding foreclosure. The stress and the travel were sending me down some unhealthy roads though I was learning to live with it. But there were some days when I just couldn't see an upside.

One night I had to drive to San Diego to join my boss and colleagues to attend a trade show. On the way down Abby called to tell me that our kitchen faucet just sprung a major leak and she couldn't get the water turned off. We figured something out but I remained worried about the cost and the aggravation of having to fix it. It was just another thing to remind me that my life had promise but it wasn't perfect.

I also dreaded seeing Mike because he wasn't my favorite guy and I was expecting that he and I would end up in a fight or he would do something to try and humiliate me. I arrived at that conclusion after being subjected to his wrath on more than one occasion; something that my colleagues told me was a rite of passage when joining Mike's crew.

When I arrived I was genuinely happy to see my colleagues, some of whom had flown in from the east coast and the mid-west, and we had somewhat of a reunion. While we were getting reacquainted with each other, Mike walked up to me and told me I had to meet him after the trade show, and he wasn't looking particularly happy. One of my colleagues, Graham, saw that and looked over at me and said, "Shit bro, I think you're probably a goner. I haven't seen him look like that in a long time. Don't worry about it though; I'm pretty sure I can help you find a new gig."

Graham's comments hit me hard because it seemed as though my life wasn't shitty enough; especially since we were just finally starting to catch up financially. I was angry and upset that I had to work the show with my best professional face and demeanor knowing that I was going to be out of a job in a matter of a couple of hours. Worse, I knew I was losing the job simply because someone didn't like me. I based that on some of the exchanges I had with Mike and some of the staff at the corporate office, and I knew that he had let people go in a similar way before.

The time came for us to meet and as hard as I tried I couldn't muster enough energy to keep an unaffected attitude. Mike asked me what was wrong and I said I assumed I was being let go and it was pretty upsetting to me. I didn't say how I knew I was being let go, but Mike chuckled then muttered under his breath, "Fucking Graham."

Mike went on to tell me that he had handed out everybody's bonuses earlier in the day but didn't have enough time to get mine before the show started. He congratulated me on earning the bonus and in particular on the successes I was having with the partnerships I was forming and managing.

Fucking Graham! I spent a miserable night worrying about losing my job but instead closed the night with an extra $6,500 that went a long way for my family. It ended up being a great night after all!

Things got settled for Abby, the kids and me. Over time my job expanded so that I was covering five western states. I traveled a lot and became an efficient traveler so it wasn't overbearing.

Even though they had a contract with a corporate travel agency, Chase was great about letting us make our own travel arrangements as long as we followed the guidelines. I found it to be more efficient to use the same services when I was traveling to the same locales. I didn't realize how much I was traveling though until the people at different airport counters knew my name once they saw me.

Steady travel had its advantages. I was traveling in Portland and always stayed at the same hotel where I could call and reserve the suite. It was a nice one-bedroom with a fireplace, overlooking a little pond which I found relaxing. This hotel not only knew me, they'd send me holiday cards signed individually by the entire staff. It also came in handy during the 9/11 attack.

On that morning I was due to give a speech in front of two hundred people in Salem and it was about a one to two hour drive to get there from Portland depending on traffic. Since the speech was at 8:00 am, I checked out at 5:00 am, rehearsing my speech on the way down. I found out once I arrived the attack had happened and that airlines were grounded. I was able to call the hotel and get my suite back.

I felt what I had to say was so insignificant compared with the attack and the horror of the day, but my real estate partner,

Byron, was adamant that I should continue the speech even though he couldn't hold back his tears. When I returned to the hotel and checked in again, I got enough information to realize that the best course of action was to drive back to my house, about a 24-hour drive non-stop. I had checked with Hertz and they had no problems at all with my returning the car in California, and only charged the normal day rate without a drop off charge.

I called Abby to tell her of the plan and she had her sister Joanie on the other line. Joanie lived in Los Angeles but was stranded in Seattle where she went for a conference. She had already checked out of her hotel and turned her car in but couldn't find another car or hotel room once she found out air travel was canceled. Seattle is three hours away from Portland so I suggested she grab a train then meet me at my hotel since my suite had two rooms. Amtrak wouldn't book her.

I was already prepared to drive up and get her, but called our Chase Travel Agent first and she was able to book Joanie on a business class seat on Amtrak. Joanie was at the hotel in time for us to get a nice dinner together and map out the route. Even though I normally made my own travel arrangements, this is where the Chase Travel Agency really stepped up to the plate.

Not every travel experience was a bad one, or at least without adventure. Once I was running late for a plane on my way to a very important client in Seattle. This client was the head of a $20 billion organization and I was scheduled to give him a presentation on forming a partnership with us. I was amazed but the plane actually held the door open for me (again, one of the perks of using the same services repeatedly) and I got pushed through security so I could get there in time. The passengers applauded when I boarded the plane knowing that they were able to leave, and I got seated in a group of four, with two facing each other. I was breathing sighs of relief and thanked the stewardess profusely and asked her to thank the captain as well for holding the plane.

After I regained my composure, I was making light chatter with the passengers sitting around me who were sharing their empathy over my having to hold the plane up, but then I was hit with a paralyzing thought.

"Did anyone notice what I did with my briefcase when I came on board?" I asked a little nervously. This was the same briefcase that was carrying my billion dollar partnership presentation with all of the contracts and data.

"Briefcase?" they all asked, "You didn't have one with you when you boarded the plane."

I commented on how lucky they were that we weren't sitting in an exit row because I would have opened the door and jumped. It turned out that in my haste I left the briefcase at the Security Checkpoint, and I was so panicked at the thought of showing up without it.

Not to worry, the stewardess told me. Once we hit cruising altitude she had the captain call the airport and put the briefcase on the next plane where I had it in time for the meeting. Wow, what an experience. That was Southwest Airlines and what a great experience that was.

Business was good, and despite the fact that our particular business unit or division was spread out all over the country, my colleagues and I talked a lot with each other over the phone to build synergy and share what was working and what wasn't. Although there was some competition amongst ourselves, there was far more camaraderie and I think it was because most of us were working alone out of our homes or traveling alone. We were high-paid professionals, but it didn't mean we didn't get stung at times or made to feel inadequate. It wasn't unusual for me to place forty or fifty calls to the same individual over a two- or three-month period before I would get some kind of acknowledgement. I signed a partnership with a broker but only after placing over one hundred and thirty calls to her over a nine-month period.

It wasn't that I was harassing anyone; it was simply because the principals or owners of the businesses I was soliciting at one time or another told me during one of our meetings that they wanted to explore a business venture with my company. Once they said that, I would call them until we formed that venture or until they told me no. Highly paid or not, that environment is not for anyone who is insecure because it would drive them to drink. Unreturned calls are a form of rejection, and it's not hard to feel rejected when you spend five or six hours calling people you've called forty, fifty, or sixty times without them calling back even once.

There were also times when we got to play a little, especially when traveling to conventions or group meetings. My best memory was a group meeting in Winter Park, Colorado where our entire unit met to share our marketing strategies and projections, year-to-date results, concerns and management outlines for our partnerships, and best practices. There were eight of us plus Mike, and each of these presentations would be about two to four hours depending on the depths of the partnerships being managed.

Winter Park was actually a central location because of where we all were scattered across the country; and it turns out because Mike was a skier and so was three-quarters of the group including me. I used to be a hot-dog skier but hadn't skied since my kids were born and by then I was as fat as a house, over 300 pounds. I didn't have any ski clothes and at that time I was still too broke to afford any because I was still new to the company and playing catch up with our finances. But I didn't care; I kept hearing the slopes calling my name.

Say what you will about team building at offsite meetings, but I can tell you that when they are done right they work very well. This was where I got to see an entirely different side of Mike and it changed our relationship for the better, at least for the most part though we still had our outbursts. We had three days there at Winter Park, two of the days were for presentations and one for fun in the snow. Instead, all of us pounced on Mike and convinced him to let us do the presentations on the first day so we could play the following two. Amazingly, Mike let us do it and that's when I encountered the worst kind of torture, listening to and analyzing management strategies from 8 am to 12 am, and mine was the last.

We hit the slopes the next day. It had been about fifteen years since I had skied but I knew it was much like riding a bike. My colleagues poked fun at me showing up in some old Khakis and boat shoes to go skiing in 14 degree weather. I had my Alpine ski jacket, some great gloves, and I picked some mid-range rental skis knowing I was going to have to re-learn a few moves. That too raised a few chuckles among my colleagues who had already been planning to watch me roll down the mountain side and turn in to a big fat snow ball.

I rode up in the chair with Harlan, one of my colleagues, who was particularly gleeful at what he thought would befall me while fancying himself to be an experienced skier. He fell off the chair as we were dismounting. Stopping to help him up I realized that he wasn't as experienced as he thought he was, so I went ahead but skied backwards for a little while to give him tips so he could make his way down. If that wasn't enough to make him eat his words, once he told me he was comfortable I did a couple of 360's then flew down the hill leaving him in the powder.

Graham and I found some track gates left up from some slalom races that were held earlier in the day and we used them. Track gates are the flags that line the ski lanes that the competing skiers have to stay within while racing. Graham won each time we went down but that was alright with me, my time improved each time we went down and he wasn't beating me by much. He had spent the year before skiing somewhere like in the Swiss Alps, so I didn't mind losing to that kind of competition especially since that was my first time skiing after fifteen years.

Although I kept most of my skill, falling down then getting up when you're over 300 pounds is no piece of cake, so I made it a point to ski very aggressively without falling down. My colleagues appreciated the fact that I suckered them into believing I was some kind of bumpkin and that made the day all the more fun. The next day we did some more skiing but then went tubing and drinking after and had a total blast. Unfortunately there weren't any more outings like that but that one was indeed memorable.

Over time I was getting really well settled but became a little disturbed when we all heard there were going to be upcoming changes in the structures of a few corporate units including the one I worked for. Although concerned with the changes, I wasn't concerned enough to make a move but was setting my sights on doubling my income for the following year and was contemplating how I was going to go about it. I was earning $225,000 plus bonus and commissions but was looking for about $400,000 or more a year. One of the reasons for doing it was because high paying jobs tend to create comfort zones where you can stagnate and roll backwards, or where you become a liability if you get too comfortable and stop moving forward.

I knew from experience and observation that for one to progress they had to leave their comfort zones and take reasonable risks. I just didn't know where to begin. Around that time, I was getting calls from a manager from Wells Fargo to see if I wanted to meet with him. Ironically this was Patrick, a manager whom I had tried to reach many times for an interview when Home Savings was sold, but he never would return my calls so I wasn't eager to return his.

My friend Charley who had just left Chase put Patrick in touch with me and told me I should meet with him because of the opportunity, so I did. After six months of getting to know each other and then seeing what an offer would look like, I told Patrick I would think about it for a while. The opportunity was a good one indeed, but a lot of changes were going to have to be made.

I wouldn't be working out of my house anymore, and we would have to move from our home in Rancho to Orange County where the cost of living and housing was so much more expensive. The job was going to be very stressful because Wells had a team of high producing loan agents who had gone without a manager for over a year and were planning to leave if they didn't get a manager. The base salary was going to be $75,000 a year plus bonus and commission; they would pay for my moving expenses plus pay me another $50,000 in a signing bonus. My earnings by then were at $250,000 and climbing and I worked out of my house, and my partnerships were seasoning so I could do a lot of the managing by phone instead of traveling so much.

It was a tough decision but I knew the kind of money Charley was making even though I was already doing ok financially with some decent future prospects. The thought of needing to leave my comfort zone was nagging at me though because of my desire to be making so much more.

One day while those thoughts were still fresh in my mind, Mike called me and we got into a screaming match because he blamed me for doing something I never did. His direct reports had screwed up royally on one of my new partnerships and rather than own up to it they convinced Mike that I was the one who screwed it up. That wasn't the first time it happened, but it was the last. Even though I managed to show Mike that they were the ones in error, I was pissed. I called Patrick right after I hung up with him. We talked and shortly after we inked a deal.

Within six months after joining Patrick's group at Wells Fargo, I had saved $100,000 for a down payment on a custom home we bought in Orange County. The house was customized by the builder we bought it from, and was going to work out great for us. Since Abby didn't get her real estate license as promised, one of our friends made just under $70,000 in commissions by the time everything was settled. The house we decided on was beautiful, a 5-bedroom, 4.5-bath house with a walk-in attic, office, upstairs laundry, fireplaces in the master bedroom and living room, and the master bath had a marble tile shower and Jacuzzi tub. The first night Austin got in it he aimed the jets to shoot right out of the tub and managed to soak me and the entire bathroom.

The lot was small but it backed up to a wooded common area that made it feel like we owned acres of land. We were free to plant things and landscape it, we just couldn't build on it. The kids and I hiked and biked on the horse trails that were just up on the ridge, and although we never did we could have gone a full thirty five miles on those ridges if we chose to.

The neighborhood was part of the location where the show 'The Real Housewives of Orange County' originated in Coto de Caza; I did business and was friends with one of the original cast members. We lived in an area called the Village and of course we referred to ourselves as the Village People. Though our houses were in the $800k to $1.5 million range we jokingly referred to the Village as the Coto Ghetto because the houses in the sections nearby would go from $8 million to $15 million plus.

It was a park like setting complete with all sorts of wildlife like rattlesnakes, owls, deer, bobcats, and mountain lions. The little road leading up to our house crossed a stream surrounded by pine trees and gave it the feel of being at a mountain or lake resort. At the end of the street was a little general store where the kids would go for ice cream and snacks. We joined a country club that had a restaurant and a pool where we could go and order food and drinks that waiters brought to us poolside and simply charge it to my tab. It used to just drive me nuts to hear my kids complain about being bored and never wanting to go to the pool even though there were many teenage girls and teenage boys there all the time. It wasn't only a pool with food and drinks, there was a weight room and tennis courts too.

The job itself was a challenge and before buying and moving in to our custom home, I commuted for eight months and slept at a hotel for a couple of nights each week. I was pretty stupid at the time because the hotel was costing me $1200 a month, I should have just rented an apartment or gotten a shared room during that time.

The team of loan agents and I hit it off well, and instead of them leaving the company as they had been planning, we all made a hell of a lot of money. I made over $500,000 that year and the Orange County branch (my branch, which is the Wells' equivalent of a region or territory) made the company over $4 million in net profit which they would not have made had the team left. By the following year four of my agents were listed in a national trade magazine in the Top 200 loan originators among all lenders in the country. Two of them were in the

Top 10, and one other was named the magazine's Rookie of the Year.

I made Leader's Club with Wells Fargo, a top designation for branches because of profitability and because of it got a big fat bonus. My branch was constantly winning production awards for volume, and we were shining. My income had climbed to over $600,000 a year; a couple of my agents were making about $1,000,000. Since some of my peers, fellow Branch Managers / Assistant Vice Presidents were already making over $1,000,000 a year so I was setting my sights on it as well and for a while it looked like I was going to do it. But things changed, and the stress had become unbearable.

Each week I would have at least one loan agent in my office either in tears or screaming at how they wanted to kill themselves because the stress was more than they could take. Imagine making $500,000 or more a year but wanting to kill yourself because of stress? I knew what they felt like because I was right there with them, not only from the stress of the job but from stress at home too.

My days consisted of at least a hundred and fifty emails with all sorts of urgency, and in the time I'd gone for lunch there would be thirty new phone calls. After a while, it was getting harder to take and my home life was taking its toll. The company was going through major policy changes on the heels of some critical audits by the federal regulators and it was affecting how we did business. Any audit by a federal regulator is critical because they could shut a bank of any size down, but they could also require a bank to change its policies which was what was happening to our division at Wells. The market was also changing so the company was making significant cutbacks while one of our biggest competitors was building a private group and making significant plays for the top members of my team.

After about a year and a half of non-stop stress at work and at home, things got to a point where some nights I would go to bed wishing I would just die in my sleep. My health took a nose dive and I had some severe chest pains at different intervals which led to some heart attack scares. My team got raided and went to a company I'd predicted would go out of business and two years later the company did fail, but the damage to my group was already done. The team left in part because of my health scares but mainly due to the policy changes our company was implementing. The company they went to didn't impose those rules and for a while the team made a lot of money until the company was forced to shut down.

Wells consolidated the branches which eliminated my position, leaving me as a loan producer where I was once again making my living by originating loans. In four of the first six months I hit the Top 10 for production out of 8,000 producers nationwide, but my heart wasn't in it. It was hard to go back to being a regular loan agent after reaching the levels I had reached. Some of it was ego, but it was also my having to go back to being on straight commission especially while the market was beginning to go through changes that were affecting my livelihood; meaning it was getting harder and harder to get loans approved. And the only way I got paid was when loans got approved and then funded.

I went through that for about five or six months but then started looking for a management position that would still allow me to do my own loan production too. I was a good producer but I was also a good mentor and coach for loan agents who were willing to do what it took to be successful, so I felt that management was what I was best suited for.

I went through a number of interviews as part of the process and really hit it off with a senior manager for one of the largest banks in the country which will remain unnamed. After a series of meetings and business plan submissions, it was clear to them that I knew my way around the loan business and could give them the help they needed for their region as a manager. The last phase of interviewing was a psychological test conducted by the Gallup Company, the same that does the Gallup polls.

I was familiar with it because I had taken one when I interviewed with Home Savings and scored just fine, and I didn't really have any major concerns but maybe I should have. During the test, I emphasized that I wasn't willing to compromise my ethics especially if it was just to be number one. At that time, mortgage fraud was pretty rampant because business was so hard to get, so I wanted to be adamant that I was going to be on guard for unethical and illegal behavior.

Surprisingly the bank saw that as a huge negative and decided not to make an offer. As disappointing as it was at the time, I'm sure I wouldn't have lasted long there because I have no patience for that kind of compromise.

Even while that was going on I was working with a recruiter who indicated Citi group was interested in me for their 28 San Diego lending offices as an Area Manager, and we were able to ink a deal. The agreement was for a one year contract and ended with a conflict that ended with mutual satisfaction, but I'm not at liberty to discuss anything beyond that, other than to say that I was very surprised to see a company that was so big hire such inexperienced managers.

I was shocked to hear a senior manager in charge of lending for the state stand up in front of a group of loan officers and say that he had never taken a loan application. HUH? How in the world was this person going to manage a lending group if he had no idea what it took to get a loan through?

One of the conditions of my hiring was for me to be allowed to originate and submit loans, something that I had done as a manager with every company I was with. I didn't do it to compete with my loan agents; I did it so I could understand every aspect of what they had to go through while they were funding loans. It was not only a way for me to coach, but it also helped me understand whether or not what was being asked from them was reasonable.

There were times when I would take the operations managers out in the field so they could understand what the loan agents had to deal with from a customer's end, and those trips often helped bridge conflicts that naturally developed between operations and production.

The experience at Citi soured me though and the continual drop in the market caused me to seek other career possibilities away from the lending business. Once the bottom fell out, people with mortgage and real estate backgrounds were considered pariahs so I had to find a way to reinvent myself if that was possible. Toward the end of my contract with Citi I got my real estate broker's license and later got my insurance license and formed my own agency. For a while it showed promise because I was booking deals that if closed would have given me about $100,000 in commissions but those too became casualties of the mortgage market.

I did earn some money from it and I continued to apply for work. The fact that I was working at my own agency also helped on my resume to show that I was still somewhat gainfully employed.

I did get a few offers from companies but they kept going out of business before I could actually report to work. After submitting over 1,200 resumes I finally landed a position with the FDIC. There were a lot of reasons that this hiring was significant, of course not least of which was it gave me an income with health insurance and opportunities for advancement.

This was my first experience with working in the public sector and was a big step for me to get experience outside of lending and real estate. And since the FDIC is in fact an insurance group it gave me some experience in the insurance business as well on the claims side. The experience was a great one overall, and I made some good friends there. It also gave me the boost I needed and it wasn't long before I was embroiled in everything I needed to know.

It was a contract position for two years with an option for two more years depending upon the need and my performance. After about a year and three months I was offered a significant promotion that required me to move to the Chicago area which I did. That was a good move both financially and for the experience. They needed me as much as I needed them and I got put to work right away in helping everybody in the group get up to speed.

I landed a few awards and got corporate recognition for a variety of things that I brought to the table, and even landed an interim Section Chief appointment. But I mainly got those awards because of the great managers I worked under who took the time to show their appreciation, something for which I'll always be grateful.

The bad side of the job was the politics that existed especially when dealing with the seasoned employees who weren't on contract. The politics of it all went against my grain and that was part of why I didn't get selected for positions for which I was extremely well qualified. I remained outspoken and held people accountable, including myself but that often produced animosity since it was considered politically incorrect. Regardless, it was an experience that I badly needed and for the most part I did what I thought was right despite making a few colossal screw ups. Like my screw up that cost me a job offer, the screw ups I had at the FDIC taught me some extremely valuable lessons.

Even though the promotion got me an extended contract, our entire Chicago office was closed after about two and a half years of my getting there. The Irvine office I started in had already closed nine months before. There were other positions that I could have applied for and likely would have been selected, either in Dallas or Jacksonville, but by then Austin had approached me a number of times throughout the year before the office closed and told me it would help him if I moved back.

He had had a rough go with my being gone after the divorce, even though he was very much a part of the decision before I accepted the promotion. Sure, I wanted to keep with the job which was great in terms of earnings, recognition, and travel perks, but the fact that my son asked me was so much more important.

There was no way I could have refused it or ignored his request. The job market was bleak especially in California, and moving back would mean that I would have to interact with Abby, but with Austin hanging in the balance it was an easy choice.

I moved back and started my real estate and insurance agency all over again, and went to work in the newest job dynamic which was contracting. It was a far cry from being high up as a Fortune 100 officer and manager, but by then I had a different motivation.

Coming back and starting over put me in an interesting place. I was in essence, having to market myself all over again with a whole new dynamic.

The job market changed dramatically thanks to Obamacare, corporations found it too expensive to hire full time so they went to contract work in order to avoid the mandates. I was up against that plus I was old and overqualified, and despite having a track record for managing multimillion dollar divisions for major international corporations, nobody was interested.

The good news for me was that I'm a survivor and based on early results I hadn't lost my customer relationship skills. Once I knew the dynamic and the landscape, meaning what and who were my competition, where was my skill set most needed, and where could I make the most money, then I could start to focus on doing what I needed to do to find success.

It will be a while before I can make $500,000 a year again, but it's a focus I needed to have for quite a while. At this point, I was so far down, I had nowhere to go but up, and up is exactly where I planned to be. I just had to get back on the road to recovery, and given my state of both physical and financial health, that was going to be much easier said than done.

SIX

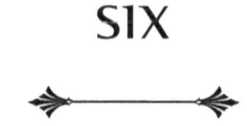

The Unhealthy Years

It has been said that if you put a frog into a pot of boiling water, it will leap out right away. But, if you put a frog in a kettle filled with cool water then slowly boil it; the frog will stay there until he boils to death...

    I was that proverbial frog and it took me what seemed like forever to figure out that I was hanging on to circumstances that were slowly killing me. As I said before, as a bachelor I kept myself healthy and in shape, and when I separated from my first marriage to Rachel I went back to being healthy by resuming a workout routine while sticking to a good diet and getting plenty of rest. The routine and diet also led to some great sleeping habits which helped me lose the weight I had gained during that marriage.

    When I married Abby I tried to incorporate exercise with things that I had to do every day, like riding my bike to school or walking places whenever I could. For a while it worked but working two jobs seven days a week and going to school full-time was too much especially when being married to a prima donna who felt she was entitled. I wasn't getting enough sleep so my energy levels were way down. After marrying Abby, my life was solely focused on doing whatever I had to do to bring my family out of poverty and build a life for us but that unfortunately led me to take my health for granted.

    Surprisingly I was able to physically endure the stresses of work, school, and the marriage complete with two new babies for the first six or seven years. I had put on about twenty or twenty-five pounds but my heart was sound and my blood pressure stayed in check. I had a few scares and went into the doctor's office thinking I was having a heart attack but was found to be just fine. I really didn't start getting unhealthy until I got the Assistant Regional Manager position at Home Savings.

Once I got that job I started traveling a lot and my diet started going down the tubes. As I traveled to each of the offices I would take doughnuts or candy and nibble on them without even thinking about it. Then I started skipping a healthy breakfast to save time; instead grabbing a scone and a coffee on my way to work. Then I would eat doughnuts when I got there.

Over time, I would skip eating anything for breakfast altogether and would be starving by the time I got lunch which often wasn't until two or three in the afternoon. At lunch I would eat appetizers with big salads doused in double or triple dressings, then dessert. Even though I would be stuffed I would go home three or four hours later and eat a big meal which I would wash down with a few beers or glasses of wine.

It never occurred to me the damage I was doing to myself, but I started putting on weight fast. My home life was pretty much the same as it had been in terms of stress, meaning Abby was herself and had no qualms about leaving any significant problem for me to resolve. But the stress of the new job, especially after getting the Vice President position then losing it was tough. I had worked very hard to shape up a floundering sales team while dealing with dramatic policy changes. The successes were equally as dramatic but I only got to enjoy them for a short time before the company was taken over. The routines I had built before I got married had completely disappeared and though I tried a few times to build new ones I could never get my head around it.

Austin was born a few months before I got promoted to Vice President at Home Savings, and what a blessing he was and still is, except for the fact that he just wouldn't sleep at night and that went on for two and a half years. I still did what I had done with the other boys which was to go get him in the middle of the night and change him then bring him to Abby to nurse.

Once I got into a deep sleep for more than twenty minutes I would be wide awake for hours if I woke up. That used to be a great asset because I would power nap before meetings and I would go into those meetings supercharged with energy. In this case, I'd fall asleep at about 11:00 pm then I would be woken up at 1:30 am by Austin for his feeding. After that I'd be up for the rest of the night until it was time to go to work.

So instead of building workout and diet routines like I had done in the past, I was building a very bad combination of poor diet, no exercise, and not enough sleep. The sleep part really became problematic because I would go for three or four days that way, sometimes five days before I'd collapse from exhaustion and get at least one night of eight hours. But when I wasn't getting the rest I needed, I wasn't performing at my very best either.

The lack of sleep made me very irritable and I yelled a lot at work and at home. It also made me goofy at times, meaning that it would take me a while to grasp a concept because my mind would keep drawing blanks.[6]

Warning Signs – A-fib and Pre-diabetic

Over time and not long after my promotion I started noticing a change in myself. By then I was about 280 pounds and growing, and I started waking up in the middle of the night because my heart would be beating so fast and hard it would shake me. This was the other problem I had with sleeping; if it wasn't Austin waking me up, it was shortness of breath and my heavy, rapid heartbeats doing it. Abby's reaction to my telling her that I was having these rapid heartbeats was to say that I was just looking for attention, even though I was thinking it was something more serious but I never did anything about it. I also started noticing that when I would be lifting heavy things or exerting myself I would have these rushes and black out momentarily but like a fool I never listened to what my body was telling me.

I tried some workout routines but they didn't stick. I was sexually frustrated though I can't blame Abby for not wanting to have sex with me when I looked like that. It made me angry though because I

---

[6] I had about ninety people on a conference call and I was setting new expectations when I realized that I was dozing off in the middle of the discussion. It really sunk in once I heard people on the line saying things like: "What did he say?", "Wait, that didn't make sense" and so on. My assistant clued me in that I started talking gibberish so I promptly ended the call then went home and went to bed.

realized that I became that way by not paying attention to what was happening to me. That realization started to keep me up at night.

Hell I was the one controlling my destiny and I should have recognized the impact that my getting unhealthy would have on all of us not only Abby and me but the kids as well. However, I also had to look at something else. While I didn't acknowledge it then, I know looking back that I had a wife who had no interest in being my partner nor did she ever. I looked at our friends and saw how they had all teamed up and shared the burdens and each chipped in while supporting each other. Ours was the one-way relationship of give and take; I kept giving and she kept taking.

Once our financial stress eased I traded the stress of simply surviving for a different kind of stress after joining Home Savings. Not only was I being held accountable for some lofty production goals, I also had to manage a hostile and mercurial group of producers. I replaced Steve, a well-liked regional manager who was demoted and had to work under me as a producer. My management style was vastly different than his. Mine was direct and firm, his was vague and accommodating, especially if you were his friend. For a while I rubbed my new team the wrong way until they saw themselves becoming more successful. By forcing them to do things more efficiently I helped them find greater success with a lighter workload and no more customer complaints.

Ironically, I helped my crew become less stressed while I took on much more stress. The more stressed I became, the more depressed I got and I poured myself into escapes like drinking, eating, and television. I don't manage exercise or diet regimens well when I'm under stress. I've since learned to do better, but there's still plenty of room to improve. Like with almost everything I do, I have to focus and block out other things so whatever it is I'm focused on can be a bigger priority. What I saw as my most important role was to make and keep my family secure. Anything else, including my personal well-being was a lesser priority. I see now what a mistake that was, not only for my sake but for theirs too because over time I couldn't sustain my energy levels and got too sick to move ahead.

I kept growing heavier because of my eating and drinking as a means of escaping depression. Because I could well afford it I kept buying new clothes as I put on more weight, outgrowing my wardrobe instead of breaking my bad habits and keeping the weight off. It wasn't long before I was a very fat guy with nice new clothes.

My excessive weight caused me to reach a point where I accepted how heavy I had become and even resigned myself to it. Before I married Rachel when I was working out all the time, I used to think that 250 pounds was really, really fat but here I was blowing right past it to over 300 pounds. Even though I recognized what was happening I still didn't put any effort into fixing myself by working out or eating right. There were too many other things occupying my mind like looking for work and the challenges at the jobs I did find.

By the time the bank was sold I was over 300 pounds and still climbing, but even then I just considered myself overweight and thought I could fix it by getting serious with a workout and diet routine. There was so much more to factor in but I continued to ignore it.

After Home Savings was sold to Washington Mutual I got my large severance check which was nice so I took some time to relax. I spent a lot of time with Austin who was nearly eighteen months by then, and because we had only moved into the new house we bought about six months earlier I worked around the house and painted rooms that we wanted painted. The house was a repo that was in good shape but needed cosmetic work which I did while I was off from work.

I also tried some running and biking for a week or two but none of it stuck as a regimen because I just didn't see the value of it. I didn't see any value in myself as a person. As time went on and the money supply kept dwindling, along with the rejections at the job interviews, I started to get depressed and started with negative self-talk. Subconsciously I was punishing myself for not finding work sooner and kept letting myself get fatter and more unhealthy. Consequently, I was keeping myself in a deep depression.[7]

First Health Crisis

Following a very dark period of financial strain and depression because we had to spend my payout money, I eventually landed my new job as Vice President with Chase. I had a really tough boss named Mike and a very heavy travel schedule since I covered the

---

[7] Many people don't realize that exercise stimulates the chemicals needed to combat depression. Being sedentary bars those chemicals from coming out, but once a person gets active the adrenaline takes over and leads to a clearer and generally more positive outlook.

West Coast for them. Within a year of working there I had my first real health scare.

It started because I decided it was time to lose weight so I went to a weight clinic for help. As part of their pre-analysis, the clinic staff did an EKG and the technician was visibly freaked out. When she rushed out of the room I thought maybe something was wrong with the machine. The doctor looked at the readings and he wanted me go to the emergency room; I told him I wasn't going. First, I really didn't believe there was anything wrong with me other than being overly tired and full from having eaten a big meal with coffee and dessert. Second, I had a business trip planned for the next morning to meet with my potential partner so there was no way I was going to cancel.

The doctor told me I was crazy so I agreed that I would come back to see him when I returned from my business trip; if the symptoms were still there then I would check myself in. He continued to advise me against it; after learning where I was going, he gave me the name and phone number of a doctor in the area. He told me that I could be walking down the street and could have a stroke or a heart attack without any notice. If something like that happened I was to give the paramedics the name of the recommended doctor for help. He said he would let the doctor know what was wrong with me.

Even though I was a little shaken after that conversation, I didn't dwell on it and moved on. When I returned from the trip I went back to the doctor as agreed. The symptoms were still present so I went to the hospital as I said I would. It turns out this doctor probably saved my life.

After waiting a while in the emergency room, a triage nurse came over and asked what was wrong. I told her nothing was wrong, I was only there because the clinic told me I needed to go in. When she listened to my heart I watched as her face paled. She jumped up and burst through the double doors of the emergency unit yelling that she needed a heavy bed for a patient "stat!"

While they were prepping the bed the triage nurse walked me over to the admitting clerk and told her to just get my driver's license and take my basic information. The clerk got right on it and handed me a sheet to sign agreeing to release my organs upon death. Having never been in that situation before, I looked down at the paper, then up at her and said, "I'm not leaving here, am I?"

She didn't respond so I just went along. It was all so strange to me because I didn't feel anything different about myself in terms of physical problems, other than being a big fat hombre. I had to do a series of special testing over the three days that I was in the hospital, during which was the first time that I heard myself referred to as obese. Until then I thought of myself as heavy compared with other people whom I deemed fat or obese. My obesity was underscored when the testing was delayed until the doctors could locate a testing table strong enough to hold me which meant that I had to be transported to another hospital.

The tests were not fun, especially the one where they injected me with something that stressed my heart out and made me feel like I was going to die. They were eliminating things like leaky valves and blockages. In one test they injected me with radioactive die and I watched the isotope course through my blood stream. The test that made me feel the worst was an injection that constricted my vessels and the pressure on my chest was unbearable, like a semi-truck parking on it. The doctor was watching me closely and asked how I was feeling but I could barely answer him. "Like I'm dying," I could barely squeak out.

"Good, good," he said pre-occupied. "That's how you're supposed to feel." It turned out that I had Arrhythmia and was in Atrial Fibrillation, or A-fib. A-fib is a condition affecting many people on different levels but no one seems to be sure why.

In simple terms, it is an irregular heartbeat that can often cause your heart to beat very rapidly. Mine has gone to over 260 beats per minute (BPM) while sitting, but I have known others who have had over 300 BPM, versus the normal 72 BPM. Due to the irregular beat which is like a thump...thump-thump...thump...blood doesn't clear the heart valves as it should and can cause blood clots if the blood stays in there too long. A blood clot can lead to a stroke or even death over something as simple as getting up from your chair too fast or something more intense like strenuous exercise.

I had been planning to play football starting that week for the following six weeks on teams formed by local churches. I had done it in previous years and had a great time, but this time I had to skip it. Based on what he saw, my doctor predicted I would die on the field.

Over the next few weeks I assimilated to a new lifestyle of managing my medical condition which included injecting myself six times a day with a very expensive medicine to thin my blood. Since my new job with Chase had taken the stress off us financially

I was able to join a diet clinic, hire a trainer, and buy a treadmill. Over the next eight months or so I lost sixty pounds by avoiding carbohydrates, riding my bike about twenty miles a day on the weekends, working out with my trainer in the early mornings, and using my treadmill after dinner while watching TV in the garage.

I went through four cardio-versions at different times. A cardio-version is when you are hooked up to a defibrillator and then shocked until your heart stops. The doctors wait to see if your heart will start up on its own in hopefully a normal beat rhythm of 72 BPM or less. The first time I was to have it done I told a friend about it. He was really concerned about my heart stopping and told me to wear sunglasses so I wouldn't be tempted to follow the light if I saw it.

One time the anesthesia wore off and I woke up in the middle of being shocked. I could feel the jolts of electricity going through my chest. I remember screaming at the doctor about how painful it was; he just pushed my head back down and told me it was supposed to feel that way. I passed out right away but when I woke was in tremendous pain and felt worse after finding out the procedure hadn't worked.

Eventually I self-converted so my heart began to beat normally at below 70 BPM and I felt really good. I realized that I had been feeling bad for so long that I didn't know what it was like to feel good anymore. Intimacy with Abby improved and we were active sexually, and my stress levels were diminishing. In fact the depression that caused me to use various escapes like too much TV, excessive drinking and poor diet had pretty much disappeared. A lot of things changed for the better: we had money again, our sex life was regular and good, and we were very active socially. We were having fun. My bike rides were getting longer and my body was beginning to show muscle tone.

My routines were sound, I managed to incorporate healthy eating and workouts on my travel schedule and I stuck with my routines when I wasn't traveling. I had to get smaller clothes and was looking better in jeans. Life was pretty good, but it changed once I decided to leave my comfort zone to pursue more money by going to work for Wells in their private group.

Once I joined Wells Fargo all of the routines I had set in place went out the window and it wasn't long before the stress of the new job and the interruption of my workout routine took its toll again. In order for the kids to finish out their school year before moving to a new county, I commuted for eight months and started getting back into bad eating habits again, eating beef jerky and orange juice for snacks over the mountain road I commuted on. In order to lessen some of the stress of the commute, I stayed in a hotel in my office complex but I was too tired to do anything because of the long days. I never slept well while I was away from home, so it wasn't long before I was back to not sleeping and my energy levels were dropping once again.

I tried to duplicate my earlier weight loss success while I had been with Chase, so I joined a nice gym across from my office and hired a new trainer but I never showed up because something else always got in the way. I still didn't realize how badly I needed an active routine to keep my mental and emotional health in top condition and to keep my body fit.

In time, I went back to my old habits of skipping breakfast or drinking coffee and eating sweet rolls or scones on the fly and being starved by three o'clock in the afternoon. In no time at all, I was back up to weighing over 300 pounds and once again my attitude toward life and intimacy with my wife were impacted. She played games with my need for her and withheld sex as a way to frustrate me because she no longer concealed her hatred for me. The fact that I became obese again made it so much easier for her to ignore my advances.

Our home life was miserable to say the least. As a result of the stress at work combined with the stress at home, I had no avenues for relief anywhere and I was unbearable to be around. I should have focused on using exercise as a way to relieve my stress but the stop-and-start routines I had in the past just added more frustration. My lack of sleep kept me from having the energy to establish good workout regimens.

Alex and Andrew had reached their teen years and started experimenting with marijuana and alcohol. Alex in particular decided he hated me[8] and everything I stood for and his mother was right in there with him, helping Alex to find reasons he hadn't thought of.

I was paying about $25,000 a year for private school tuition for all three boys and I was supposed to be happy with Ds and Fs on

---

[8] He and I continued to have problems for a while, but being the incredible kid that he is he found ways to help both of us build bridges to allow us to become close again as we still are today.

their report cards. I had a basic philosophy that Abby either couldn't or didn't want to grasp mainly because she always took the easy way out in life and never wanted to aspire to or accomplish anything. This particular trait in her was always a point of contention with her family members and mine because all of them and I accomplished a lot in our lives while she never bothered to try.

I didn't want my boys adopting her parasitic ways, and my approach was a simple philosophy really. If the subject was so hard that the best grade they could get was a D after trying their hardest, like getting help from me, the teacher or a tutor, then we would celebrate that D because it was the best they could get and there was no shame in it. But if they were turning in poor grades because they weren't trying at all, then those were unacceptable grades.

I heard every excuse in the book and it usually boiled down to two reasons both Alex and Andrew were giving me; the teacher was bad, or I had to stop telling them how smart they were and simply accept that they were too dumb and unable to understand the subjects.

Abby was perfectly content to accept both assertions since she never attempted anything that would shine any light on her inabilities and lack of ambition. She couldn't and wouldn't face the possibility of failure, mainly because it meant that she would have to actually try to succeed at something which would have meant work in the form of trial and error.

In terms of the boys, I wouldn't accept it because I knew differently. I would talk with their teachers, observe their study habits, and get really pissed off when they would be screaming that the subjects were impossible and the information they needed wasn't available, yet when I'd open their books the information they needed was usually in the first few pages of the chapter.

I'm not sure who said it since the quote is attributed to at least two sources, but there is a saying: "a mind is like a parachute, it only works when it's open". And I'd like to take it a step further by adding that "the person in control of the parachute needs to make the effort to open it".

Needless to say I didn't back down and often times it was the three of them against me telling me what a bad person I was. Although Austin wasn't subject to any of the frustrations I was having with his brothers, he joined in with them for a show of support. It was ugly, especially as I was coming to the realization that I had sacrificed so much for my family yet it seemed like nothing was good enough.

Abby pummeled me over the last five years or so of our marriage with claims that I was ruining the boys' lives. In her view my expectations of them achieving grades higher than Ds and Fs were unreasonable.[9] She also chose to ignore that I placed far higher expectations on myself to take care of their needs while never once expecting her to do the same. Never mind that she had everything she needed at her disposal to find success on her own, but in her eyes her job was to stay on the sidelines and criticize rather than try and form a partnership where we could have capitalized on and expanded the things we had. Had we been able to find common ground and work together as partners, I am fully confident that we could have retired very young and had a nice life together.

I was worried about what my kids were turning into. They had all forgotten what it was like to be poor and it went to their heads without ever stopping to consider what it took to generate and maintain the lifestyle we had. I joined the Club for them, so they had full use of a pool with poolside service like food and drinks except they never wanted to use it. We had fun Jet Skis and after I got the better jobs I bought a new Cadillac for me, and a new Suburban for Abby and the boys which was fully pimped and complete with a DVD player.

Each time we went to a hotel on vacation the kids had their own room separate from us, yet each vacation was always beset with problems. Alex made it a point to criticize every aspect of our outings and made sure each day would start with a major argument, and Abby was his coach and mentor.

That might have been Alex's job as a teenager, but she decided to take sides in front of all of the kids because of her hatred for me which she no longer chose to hide. That only empowered them to scream and throw out insults at me whenever it suited them, which was usually when they were caught lying and didn't want to own up to it. Ultimately everything became my fault in their eyes.

Deepening Stress

I stopped sleeping at night because the stress at home and at work was so intense. I would often go to work having had only two

---

[9] Not so ironically, both Alex and Andrew understood why I had expectations of them when they had to work side-by-side with poor achievers after having joined the military. Over time they volunteered their appreciation of what I had been trying to do.

hours of sleep or sometimes none at all. My productivity suffered and the fact that I was beginning to perform poorly added even greater stress. I went to a hypnotist for a while to try and calm down but it didn't have any lasting effects for me.

My doctor prescribed an anti-depressant but I never took it. I come from a family with extremely addictive personalities and I can't tell the difference between taking prescription drugs, non-prescription, illegal drugs or alcohol to escape my problems.[10] In my view, because I was so vulnerable, taking anything for it would have been my escape and an easy addiction to develop. I've seen too many lives ruined by people turning to drugs and alcohol to ease their problems, exactly what I had done in my early teen years so there was no way I was going to put myself in that position if I could help it.

Over time the housing market took a nose dive and I lost not one but two jobs in the course of about a year and a half, and there seemed to be no hope in sight. My job with Wells was gone due to the raid on my staff and the company consolidation, and the same for my job with Citi.

As a career mortgage lender I was one of thousands looking for work as banks and mortgage companies were going under. My age and appearance didn't help; I surmised that one or two interviews did not go well specifically because I was so old and so fat. After we exhausted our savings and investments which were over $250,000 at the time, I did what I could to bring some money in by getting a real estate broker's license and insurance license in hopes of landing a job because of them but times had never been as dark as they were then and there were no jobs out there.

I continued to develop feelings of self-loathing and worthlessness; I abandoned what little self-control I had and was secretly and intentionally trying to kill myself through poor health. Despite having plenty of time on my hands since I didn't have a job to show up for every day, my state of mind was so congested with all that self-hatred that I couldn't find a routine to help myself, nor did I want one. In my eyes, I just wasn't worth it and it wasn't the first time I felt that way.

---

[10] It turns out that I did the right thing by not taking it because a year later the drug was found to cause death by heart attacks and the company was hit with a major class action suit.

Everything I touched, every investment I had made had gone downhill and we had to liquidate everything just to survive and eventually could no longer pay our mortgage which was over $1 million. There were days again when I didn't know how we would put food on the table and keep the utilities on that I needed in order to look for jobs while working on real estate and insurance deals. I worked real estate for about a year and a half and was able to collect some income but not much. Abby was still in denial and it was a few years before she finally figured out that we needed her to try and sell real estate.

I had to help her get her license by helping her study and coaching her through her tests, but unfortunately I no longer had the funds to invest in her business nor did I have the contacts. She eventually made more money than I did one year and that's when she stopped selling real estate for some reason. I think laziness may have had something to do with it, but I think a bigger part was that she had been telling everybody that our entire financial ruin was my fault. Her early success in real estate contradicted that notion, especially since she seemed to leave out the part that six years before she promised she would start her real estate career to help us out.

If Abby had done what she promised, we could have stockpiled her commissions and saved ourselves from our financial ruin. At one time we had over $400,000 in equity in our house and we could have sold it and paid cash for a smaller house and she could have collected the commissions on both transactions which would have amounted to about sixty to eighty thousand dollars.

We argued a number of times because I kept telling her that even though I was making so much money I was extremely vulnerable because of the volatility of market conditions, and because my income largely was based upon the production of a few talented sales people. If those people were to be recruited away, we would be sunk.

The days I predicted finally materialized and we were facing the prospects of being broke. I worked hard trying to find a job while desperately trying to figure a way for me to bring some income in until I found one. Unlike my separation from Home Savings, there was no golden parachute. I had savings, investments and equity in the house but those were dwindling pretty fast. Around the time my job with Wells ended I worked on seeing what I could do for us to become self-employed. I worked on my licenses and. I built an online business that had promise and was showing early signs of success, and it was run out of the house so it was a great after-school job for our sons.

Once it was up and running it was generating some decent cash flow. The business plan was formed around a product that was going to be short-lived because of a pending lawsuit so I wrote a second plan to expand the business while eliminating the use of that product. We would have been able to expand it on the cash flow it was already generating.

I hoped the business could generate enough income for me to work it as a sole means of income but it didn't. I didn't stop looking for work and finally found a job through a recruiter and went to work with Citi. Though Abby enjoyed the limelight that the business was bringing she wanted nothing to do with helping it grow. Worse, Abby made it a point to tell me that our sons and some of their friends' parents were talking about how they thought it was stupid, yet for a few hours of work a day we were generating a net of three thousand dollars a month after only six months in the business. One of the kids slipped one time and told me that Abby was a big part of talking about it with the parents behind my back, an item she conveniently left out.

Instead of embracing the business plans and working with me, Abby didn't want to work to help grow the business and let the boys complain about having to work after school. The job was pretty easy since it was a mail order DVD business something like Netflix only the movies were like the ones you see on an airplane with the sex scenes and foul language removed. All they had to do was pick up the mail every day and process the DVDs that came in and then ship the ones on order. It was all out of our garage and the working conditions were pretty cool since they could watch movies or play music while doing it.

But they followed their mother's lead of not wanting to do anything and in a short time began doing a poor job at customer service. In six months I had built it to where we were shipping all over the country and Australia while picking up new customers every day. My business plan included keeping the business completely family oriented and I had begun negotiations with a book distributor that would give us access to 120,000 titles that we could sell on our site while adding more to the business. But in the time I went to work on the contract job with Citi Group, Abby decided she wouldn't participate at all and let the business die, even though each time we would set goals and talk about plans to expand and move it forward she always pretended to be supportive.

In hindsight though, what we could have and should have been doing around that time was to buy houses and fixing them up for resale while I still had the cash and credit to do it. That was my fault directly but it was influenced a lot by Abby's attitude and her unwillingness to partner. I started a real estate brokerage after I got my real estate broker license and my contract with Citi Group ended.

I got into doing property valuations called Broker Price Opinions or BPOs for major banks that had foreclosed on properties or were about to. Back then the values of the properties were very low because of the condition they were in, and I could have used some of our cash to start buying them and fixing them up to rent or resell. I had enough experience in rehabilitating houses and I had two hale and hardy sons who could have helped me with the work.

Abby could have also used her real estate license to sell the properties. But by then I was losing my fight. I was tired of taking the blame for everything, whether things were going right or wrong, especially from the people I cared about the most who saw me as a target for their dissatisfaction. Over time, Abby had seen what I'd accomplished from the time we were married right up until things were taking a turn for the worse, but in all those years she would not work with me as my partner despite all of my attempts to get her to do so. She just wanted to have me do it all and take the blame for whenever things didn't go right.

But once I started looking at how our world was crumbling, I knew I couldn't do it the way I had done in the past. I didn't want to carry her dead weight anymore; I was not the man I once was because of the stress and burnout. Gone was that cocky kid who thought nothing of hitchhiking in downtown NYC at 1:00 a.m. And gone was the arrogant bastard who welcomed battles of wits while climbing the corporate ladder. There was nothing left inside of me that was worth anything, and so I succumbed to all the noise around me. I continued to try to kill myself through poor health and just kept getting worse.

The money ran out, and I lived in terror of being forced on to the street while doing what I could to keep my family insulated from those same feelings of terror. They still had a comfort in knowing that I wasn't going to stop trying to make things better, but in reality there were no job prospects and the real estate market was getting worse. Right up until I got my job with the FDIC, I kept hitting walls very hard and losing hope every single day. No job prospects, too many clients that I couldn't qualify and later on fewer clients every day.

The FDIC

I was offered a job with the FDIC on January 20, 2009. Because of my financial hardship I couldn't start until March 16, 2009 when I was fully vetted and it was deemed that I wasn't able to prevent the financial ruin that had occurred. Less than a month after I got the job it was confirmed that our house had been foreclosed on and we would have to move. That was one of the worst experiences of my life and I understood why people in my situations were killing themselves. I also was finally able to look past it a little, and saw that we had indeed hit bottom which meant that it was time to try to start climbing back up.

Abby found us a tiny house near the beach and the bank gave us money to move, in part so we didn't tear the house apart to sell the expensive items. I wouldn't have done that anyway but the funds were helpful just the same.

The job paid me enough to pay the rent and food and gave us healthcare, and Abby set out to try and earn money from real estate. Up until that point, she had no interest until she saw what I predicted could happen actually materialize. Once she came to that conclusion, she briefly stepped up to the plate though once she saw herself becoming successful at it she realized that she could have done a lot to help us avoid ruin.

It didn't take long for me to realize though that she didn't consider what she was earning as ours. In her eyes it was hers and she was using it on things like eye tucks, face peels, and refurbishing her car. People say that the worst times can either bring out the best or the worst in a person and I've known that to be true. The remarkable thing here though was she hadn't changed, the bad times weren't bringing out the best or the worst, I simply had begun to see her for who she really was.

Despite the new images I had of her, I was still committed to making our marriage work and was willing to do what I needed to do to get us there and that included losing weight and getting healthy. However I was no longer willing to shoulder all of the burdens because I decided I didn't want to die from the stress it caused, and frankly much of it was from her. Even though the boys had settled in and were actually enjoying their new home, my relationship with Abby got progressively worse. In an effort to start to get myself healthy I was riding my bike regularly, walking, watching what I ate, and. I also started going back to the gym. At the same time, Abby's hatred for me grew worse and she no longer made any attempt to conceal it and our home life was deteriorating. But she was targeting some of her hatred on things she was imagining.

For example, I was getting ready to go out the door to get on my bicycle with barely enough time to catch the train so I could get to work. I kept my gym shoes I used to ride near the door. When I went to get them I found they weren't there and got angry knowing one of the boys had taken them and didn't put them back. Abby launched into a diatribe about how I accused the boys of everything when it was my fault. I ended up driving to work that day because I used all my ride time looking for the shoes.

Andrew admitted later that he took the shoes for Alex to use at the gym and never put them back. I pointed out to Abby how these tirades and her accusations of me targeting the boys were the same accusations in the six blowups we had in the previous two months, all ending with the boys copping to their guilt. Yet she wouldn't admit that her hatred of me was clouding her judgment nor did she stop with her accusations despite them being groundless.

Another time she heard me whispering to the two oldest boys then came in and started screaming at me for trying to turn them against her. What I had done was give them money and got their commitment to make sure that they were going to do something nice for her on Mother's Day that weekend. By her rants though she exposed herself because it slipped that she had actually been trying to poison the boys against me and thought I was trying to turn the tables.

I started writing around that time and would write in the morning before anybody woke up. I'd also do research but I didn't tell anyone what I was doing. She would come down in the morning and see me at the computer and launch into this rant of insults. I slept on the couch often and it was clear we were falling apart.

The Divorce

One of those mornings after sleeping on the couch I woke up with numbness in my left arm and couldn't shake it. I drove myself to the hospital where they admitted me for several days. They determined that a pinched nerve had caused the numbness, but also discovered that I had diabetes and had it for at least a year.

Abby didn't come to see me until the last day of my hospital stay and she didn't bring the kids, nor did they come to see me on their own. She had the boys convinced I was completely to blame for being there, for contracting the disease, and was hospitalized in large part because I ate a lot of mayonnaise. Her disdain was pervasive and when I got home I saw that she had been in the phone books looking up divorce attorneys.

Not long after she announced that she was leaving me. I wasn't surprised that I dismissed her fairly easily which I think bothered her. I moved into a cheap extended stay hotel and gave her a large part of my salary even though we hadn't gone to court. Once Abby realized that being away from my kids was tearing me up she did everything she possibly could to stand in the way of my being with them.

My concern was for Austin who was traumatized by our split and I was trying to help him stabilize, so I wasn't going to put him in the middle of a custody fight. Alex and Andrew were already of legal age and could go where they wanted but Abby and Austin moved in with Susan and John rent free. John is an attorney and his office prepared separation papers that deprived me completely of my rights to Austin. John's comment was that if Abby was going to have physical custody then she would need legal custody in case of a medical emergency. I didn't sign the papers and told Abby exactly what I thought of her crap. She had announced to everyone that she was going to work on finding a new man; no doubt to find somebody to marry and she wanted to make sure I had no rights to my kid. There was no way I was going to let that happen; Austin needed me as much as I needed him.

The medical emergency was a serious issue that had to be addressed and the possibility that our custody agreement might require both parents to authorize treatment for Austin if something bad happened to him. By her having both legal and physical custody, that meant that Abby could act on Austin's behalf if he needed it. But by my giving up legal custody, then she would be free to keep him away from me, something she tried to do a few times through her applications to the court.

Even though I'm not an attorney, I came up with a simple remedy to the emergency; I executed a medical release and kept joint legal custody. The reason I didn't push for joint physical custody right away was because he wasn't of legal age and he would have been forced to come live with me for six months out of the year. His life had already been turned upside down by the separation and I was living in substandard conditions in order to provide support payments for them that I was paying on my own.

Abby also chose not to work or sell real estate and she spent money faster than I could send it. I was giving Abby anywhere from $3,000 to $5,400 a month on my salary at the FDIC which had grown to about $80,000 a year but she kept complaining that it wasn't enough. My payments to her became a sore spot with me years later because when we did go to court neither child services nor the courts gave me a dime of credit for all the years I paid her without a court order even though I proved it by showing each transfer from my account to hers.

I had gotten a promotion with the FDIC and moved to Chicago and had begun to focus on a targeted plan for getting healthy. And it was working. I began to drop weight, was dating and starting to enjoy myself a little.

Once I had gone to work at the FDIC my life had stabilized somewhat because of the steady income, and though it was low I began traveling a lot for bank closings and that gave me opportunities for overtime and per diem reimbursements. It was good because the money was steady and the overtime was substantial but bad because the hours were often long and usually interrupted any routines I had established.

A Busy Lifestyle at Work

Working at the FDIC was quite a bit different than what I had done before. It is different from what most people are familiar with which is why I'll digress a little in order to give you a better perspective of the work and how it impacted my daily living.

At the FDIC some of us were hired for both day jobs and weekend closings in the field. My day job as a Resolution and Receivership Specialist was processing claims against banks after they were closed. A lot of people don't realize that the FDIC examines banks and reports the findings to a regulator like the Office of the Comptroller of the Currency or various state regulators which are the actual agencies that regulate the banks and decide if they are to be closed or not. If the regulator decides to close a bank, then they usually appoint the FDIC to be the receiver of the bank and then task it with taking care of the customers while disposing of the failed bank.

Once a regulator told us at the FDIC that a bank would be closing some of us would get assigned field work in different functions which would entail creating and submitting closing strategies for the bank then traveling to whichever city and state the failed bank was located. My functions in the field were usually as a Subject Matter Expert or Claims-Agent-in-Charge.

We would work our day jobs during the week; then on Friday night at 6:00 pm, the regulator would close the bank operations and would appoint the FDIC as the receiver. So we had from 6:00 pm in the evening on Friday to 8:00 am on Monday morning to receive the bank and transform the rest of it then hand it over to the bank that bought it.

This happened about ninety-seven percent of the time, the other three percent of the time was often more difficult and lengthy because we couldn't find a buyer for the banks we were closing in those instances. If we found a buyer for the closed bank, then we would work over the weekend and reopen it as part of the bank that bought it so the customers never really knew the difference. But if we couldn't find a buyer, then the bank would close and customers would be left stranded which is something we desperately tried to avoid.

On occasion, people would be in the middle of buying groceries or paying for dinner in a restaurant but have their cards rejected because their bank was no longer operating. And when we couldn't find a buyer, it also meant we had to deal directly with depositors, some of whom were losing money which would not have been the case if there would have been a purchasing bank. At times it became stressful because customers became scared and angry, especially if they lost money due to the closure.

I enjoyed going out on closings which meant travelling all over the country to where the failed banks were closing. One week I'd be in Seattle and the next I'd be in Baltimore. I enjoyed it because of the extra money and because I was good at it. When we'd close a bank we would take over their offices and put the former employees to work for us over the weekend to do what was necessary according to federal law to dispose of the bank.

But the process was often scary for the employees of the bank being closed, so we would do what we could to allay their fears but were careful not to give anyone false hope. We were just the receiver, the old bank was closed by the regulator and whether or not an employee had a future with the new bank was entirely up to the new bank's management. And while there were many success stories, there were also sad ones.

The way the FDIC structures the teams to close and transform a bank is nothing short of amazing, and it is something that any company or major corporation should learn. As a former corporate manager who went through two significant mergers and one takeover attempt I know something about how slowly most groups move. But the FDIC has a structure in place that has proven successful time after time and has merged banks with net worth's in the tens of billions or more.

Regulators such as the Office of the Comptroller of the Currency (OCC), or what used to be the Office of Thrift Supervision (OTS), or individual states would be the ones to make the final closing decisions. The FDIC would analyze and examine the banks, and once the regulator put the bank on the watch list the FDIC would go to work on marketing the bank to potential buyers. While that was happening, a Receiver-in-Charge (RIC) and Closing Manager (CM) would be assigned, and the bank would be given a code name so as not to be divulged to the public and risk causing a bank run. A bank run is when customers get in a panic and rush to the bank to withdraw their money.

The RIC would then begin assembling the team which consisted of approximately fourteen field managers each responsible for a specific area of the closing. Those areas included setting up all the equipment, organizing hotels and meeting areas, others were accounting, real estate, investigations, public relations and taking care of depositors. My typical assignments dealt with the analysis of depositors and deposit insurance. Once the managers were assigned, then each would be assigned support teams for the respective areas and each manager was then tasked with doing the analysis then completing their individual Strategic Resolution Plans (SRP) to submit to the RIC by a certain date.

All of us assigned to field teams were still required to perform our day jobs without interruption, so it was important that we organized our time properly and remained efficient because as a general rule overtime wasn't allowed in the preparation or post-closing functions. It was only allowed on the actual events. There would often be meetings during the day to review the plans and report updates until the actual moment of the closing.

On the day of the closing, we would meet at the bank to wait for the signal that the bank was closed and the appointment was met, then we would assume our roles and do our jobs, ensuring that on Monday morning we turned over the keys to the new buyers. What was and still remains so remarkable is that each of the functional managers doesn't necessarily know what the other is doing beyond a general scope. And that is true of the RIC and the CM, meaning that we all know what needs to be done, but for anyone to take on another's role would be extremely difficult. Yet we all performed within the expectations and timelines that we set, and each night we would review our progress with the RIC and CM among our peers and we'd get the job done.

Most of the days were twelve to fourteen hours though some teams as well as my own have had to put in as much as twenty hours in a single day depending upon the urgency and complexity of the closing. The projects were stressful for various reasons so we were encouraged to go out to dinner together to blow off steam and unwind. The greater value those times had was the bonding and information sharing among ourselves.

These teams were assembled from offices all over the country and the experience levels of some of these individuals were very high. At times we might never see each other again but interact on the phone, or other times we would be on multiple closings together and those outings would often set the tone for trust building and smoother closings.

I did my best to maintain a diet and workout routine especially after moving to Chicago, but it was hard and about the best I could do was recover from each trip and resume my routines enough to where I didn't put on weight while traveling. There was one period where I worked thirty-three straight days in a row. The overtime was great but the weekends included travel in some cases and fourteen hour days with dining and drinking in between. By the time I moved to Chicago, I had settled into some routines that kept me losing weight though I had made some new friends and would often go out partying which caused me some setbacks.

I was extremely lonely from being away from my sons. Austin would call me on weekends sometimes when he was lonely and bored, but it was about nine months before I was able to see him again. Even though we talked and Skyped, it wasn't the same. I had pretty much written Abby off, she was someone I didn't care to be around. I took off my wedding ring and was setting my sights on new horizons, very glad to be away from her. The fact that at times I was living in squalor just to ensure that I was supporting her and Austin while she lived in luxury rent-free made it easy to despise her, especially since I was supporting them on my own and without a court order.

But for her it wasn't enough. Abby would complain that I wasn't giving her enough money and apparently convinced her family and friends that I wasn't giving her anything at all. The two older boys told me later that their mom had begun parading guys she found on the internet in and out of her life. Abby had a habit of leaving Austin alone so she could go out. I saw very little of it firsthand but our sons observed it, though no surprise that she denied everything when it came up in conversation but I no longer had any reasons to believe anything she said.

In less than a year after being separated, Abby starting calling me and began making gestures toward reconciling. Once I understood how much of our past relationship contributed to the stress that caused me to get so sick, I wasn't interested in going back to a vacuum with someone who had no interest in sharing the burden. My focus was on getting healthy again and I didn't want any kind of relationship where I couldn't keep that as my primary focus.

I would rather have no one at all. I asked her point blank what she would be willing to do to start a new relationship. Would she be willing to seek independence and bring in some income? Would she be willing to step in my shoes to see what carrying the family for twenty plus years was like? Would she be willing to take a twenty mile bike ride so she could celebrate with me when I crossed the 50, 75 and 100 mile marks, knowing what she had to do to achieve twenty miles? And would she be willing to acknowledge her responsibility in what went wrong in our previous relationship and accept those areas where she could have partnered with me to save us from our demise? Of course the answer was no to all of the above.

Abby moved out of John and Susan's and took over her mother's luxury condo since her mother was placed in a home. The condo was owned free and clear and she lived there rent free even though she put that she was paying $2000 a month in rent on her court documents. After moving in there, she went on the prowl and trolled the internet for any guy who would respond. But she wasn't happy with the guys who were accepting her invitations and according to my boys they were losers in their eyes.

I never asked them about her nor did I want any details about her escapades, I simply wanted to move on. Except Abby would call me at all hours of the night to try and wear me down, ignoring my specific pleas for her to stop because it was breaking my sleep pattern which I fought so hard to maintain. Of course everything was all about her so Abby didn't stop and my sleep patterns broke. It would be three more years before I came close to getting them back because of my work load and because of her. I couldn't turn my phone off because Austin or his brothers would often call me in the middle of the night and I didn't want to risk missing their calls.

Austin confided to me that he wished his mom and I would get back together. He also confided that Abby told him that the break up was my fault and I wouldn't get together with her no matter what. She painted such a dark picture of me that I knew I was going to have to swallow my pride and let her back in so he could see that I was willing to do it for his sake. But I knew then that I was going to go through hell before it was over.

I responded to her gestures, and for the next year Abby put me through an emotional roller coaster because it had become her favorite sport. She pulled all of her strings together and got me to fall in love with her again to a point where I almost put my wedding ring back on. Abby would call me and text me telling me how much I was her rock and how much she loved me, and when she got me to say it back she added a different twist.

Abby would tell me how much she loved me on one night and beg me to call her the next day because of how much she needed me. Then she would leave me voice mails saying she had met someone who expressed an interest in her and didn't need me anymore. She'd call me a week or two later begging forgiveness and asking me to build her up.

What I found out over time was that she had latched on to a complete loser who would put her down, and she would call me so I could give her some emotional boosts, and then do it all over again. This went on for nearly a year and it was tearing Austin up only I didn't know it. Abby kept telling me that his problems were all my doing because I had moved away. Not surprisingly she left out the part about how what she was doing was actually causing Austin to be so stressed.

Abby brought her new guy Ralph[11] into Austin's life as a substitute for me but forbid Austin to tell me anything about it. They'd have BBQs and go out to dinner, while at the same time she

---

[11] Abby met another Ralph later on who is referred to as Ralph2.

was calling me at night telling me how she wished I was there with her and how much she needed me in her life. It got uglier and uglier, especially for Austin who had developed some intense anger issues. Abby blamed everything on me because I wasn't there and ignored the impact her garbage was having on Austin.

I didn't know about the boyfriend until one of my sons told me about him nine months after Abby had made her overtures to try and reconcile. Abby's real game was to keep me sending her money so she could go out and play with Ralph1. One of my sons saw the impact trying to reconcile was having on me, and told me about Ralph1 and how they were playing me.

At one point Abby admitted the relationship to me, told me it was over, and confided in me that she was afraid of what the guy might do. I expressed my concerns about the guy based on what she told me and I told Abby I wanted to put a restraining order on him to keep him away from Austin, especially since I couldn't be there to protect him. She assured me it was over and she wouldn't let him back where he could be a problem to Austin, so I accepted that for the time being. It came out later that Ralph1 had been a full part of the family gatherings while she was pretending to reconcile, but when the relationship was over she felt a need to announce to everyone in her family that it was over between them.

Several weeks after she told me and everyone else that it was over with the loser I got a call from Austin at about three in the morning my time, one o'clock a.m. his time. He was in a panic worrying that Abby had been killed. Abby told Austin that she was meeting with a new guy whom she'd met online and was expecting to be home around midnight. Austin was alone and didn't like it; he started calling and texting her around 12:30 when she hadn't returned. Since he didn't get any call backs or return messages Austin went into a panic.

I tried calling and texting her, and her sister Susan did as well but got no response so I called the sheriff's department to ask about reporting a missing person which they said we could do right away. I held off but had Austin call Susan who agreed to come pick him up and take him home with her. I stayed on the line with Austin to calm him while waiting for Susan to pick him up.

While on the phone with me Austin went through an entire litany of things about Abby and his observations about how she was throwing herself at anyone who looked at her. This was not a conversation I wanted to have, especially since I was still coming down from the emotional roller coaster she had put me on, but she was his mother and it was impacting him really hard so I had to listen.

It wasn't the kind of thing a thirteen-year-old should have to see his mother doing either, but he is an observant kid and noted all of it. After having listened to this for much longer than I wanted, Susan finally arrived just as Abby returned Austin's call. It was the usual excuse, that her phone wasn't working but she totally ignored the question about why she didn't call him from another phone to say she was going to be late. She knew that Austin always stayed up late waiting for her.

Shortly after that scare, Austin told me it was time to stop trying to reconcile because he knew it would never happen. I was sad for him, but relieved for myself because I wanted to be as far from her as possible.

Once Austin turned fourteen he came of age in California and I wanted to make good on my promise to put his life in his control by requesting joint physical custody. Abby refused, not because it would be in his best interest but because she didn't want her child support to be cut. I told her in an email I would continue to give her full payments even if the courts lowered it and I would give it to her in writing, but she refused. When Austin asked Abby why she wasn't giving me joint custody she told him I only wanted to do it so that I wouldn't have to pay for child support.

She left out the part on how I was willing to keep giving her full payments. By then I had learned to do everything with her in writing so I was able to show him several emails that I sent to her saying that very thing and ones that she responded to so he could see that she had received them.

That wasn't anything that I wanted him to be involved in but she was constantly trying to wear him down and turn him against me, and he and his brothers were and are the most important thing to me in the whole world.

Ironically it was Ralph1 who inadvertently helped me gain joint physical custody through an email. I did file a restraining order after Austin told me that Ralph1 had put him in a headlock and after intercepting some messages to Austin where Ralph1 was trying to get Austin involved in a fight he was having with Abby. Ralph1 sent me an email to try and buddy up to me prior to the court date and, he opened up all the stops.

Ralph1 wrote about how she would leave Austin alone at all hours of the night so she could have sex with him and smoke pot, and how she was having sex with him anytime during the day instead of looking for work like she told me, the courts, and her family she was doing.

While she was doing that she was playing me and sharing our intimate conversations with Ralph1 so they could have a good laugh. Ralph1 also admitted that he was monitoring her emails. Based on what he was monitoring he claimed that he knew she was playing around with at least four other guys while she was shacking up with him.

He offered to share his files with me but I was pretty clear in my reply to him that I wasn't interested in anything he was doing with Abby. But I did tell him that I was interested in anything that he felt was putting Austin in harm's way.

I also told Ralph1 that if he was continuing to play his games with me that he was fucking with the wrong guy. I took a copy of my response to the restraining order judge as did Ralph1. I had no problems showing the judge my disdain for this loser. This idiot thought he could present it as some kind of threat that I made to him, but I was simply making a statement about who he was dealing with. I had his address and could have just as easily gone over to his house and put him in the hospital for having touched my son, but I preferred the court system so that I didn't have to see my son from behind bars.

Through Ralph1's revelations I was able to give Abby a simple option, sign over joint physical custody or I would drag her to court. I planned to use Ralph1 as a witness to show the judge that she wasn't providing a safe environment for Austin then demand full physical and legal custody because of her actions. Abby realized I was serious and signed it over; Austin was very grateful that I had done it.

By then Ralph1 had begun stalking her and unbelievably she called to ask me to beat him up for her. I told her exactly what I thought of her and made it clear that I didn't care what Ralph1 did with her or to her as long as he didn't go near Austin. Anything she got from that guy was her doing.

For Austin's sake though I did offer to appear as a witness in court if she wanted to put a restraining order on him, but she apparently was worried about what Ralph1 had in his files that might show up in court so she never took me up on her offer. Interesting to me was how much she had lowered herself to be with a dead-end guy who had nothing to offer except for a high opinion of himself.

What pissed me off about all this beyond the devastating impact it had on Austin was despite how much of this I showed to the family court and child services, they continued to treat her like she was some kind of queen and did her bidding to make sure that I had no access to my son. Worse, she knew that by keeping me under stress and through lack of funds she was keeping me from getting healthcare and medication. That meant there was a very good chance that I could succumb to the diseases and become disabled or die, which was something Ralph1 said she hoped would happen.

I moved back to California because I promised Austin I would when he asked at a time he needed me most. But in order to fulfill that promise I had to stop looking for work in other states and even passed on some opportunities to work with the FDIC in Florida. I also knew that I was going to have trouble finding steady work once I got back to California because I had been looking for work for more than a year and a half and only landed a couple of interviews.

Once I arrived, I had no income, no job, and the court and child services were helping to make sure that I had no access to my son and no access to medication which was put into motion through Abby's deception. Her fraud on me empowered the Court and Child Services to take away what little money I set aside to start a real estate and insurance business while continuing to look for work. It was hardly a way to embark on a path to getting healthy.

This was quite a change from the first time I arrived in California, and it wasn't a good one. What I did get out of it though was a chance to see the change in Austin's outlook and behavior once I got back, proving to me that it was and still is worth what I've had to go through. I just wish that would have been the end of it, but as you will soon see that wasn't to be the case for some time to come.

SEVEN

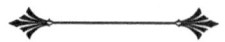

The Road to Recovery

"We cannot change our past... we cannot change the fact that people will act in a certain way. We cannot change the inevitable. The only thing we can do is play on the one string we have, and that is our attitude. I am convinced that life is 10% what happens to me and 90% of how I react to it. And so it is with you... we are in charge of our Attitudes."

- Charles R. Swindoll

I spent a tremendous amount of time focusing on becoming successful while battling the pressures of being married to Abby. She saddled me with the responsibility of making her happy yet was unwilling to find out for herself what happiness meant. Unfortunately the time I spent doing that led to the undoing of what used to be solid workout regimens and a genuine desire for good health. It took its toll in a very big way.

Over time I looked in the mirror and didn't recognize myself. Not only was I a big fat guy, I was an emotional basket case and could no longer find the confidence to pull myself up and move forward. In the past I could never see the obstacles and instead could only see the target, but at that moment I couldn't see anything but the obstacles and every single mistake I made since the day I was born. I blamed myself for everything and often thought things would have been so much better had I never been alive.

I suppose those thoughts are something most of us think when we're faced with what we perceive as a disaster in our lives, and I recognized that but it didn't stop me from wishing I was dead. My view was that my wife and kids would have been so much better off if they didn't have me around, and so for about two or three years and at first without realizing it, I was deliberately trying to kill myself through poor health. I stopped taking my heart and blood pressure medications, and I didn't care about what I ate or drank.

Little by little though, things were starting to turn around for the better. There were only small things at first but enough to give me some hope so by the time I learned I had diabetes and realized that it wasn't only death that I could be facing, I decided I wanted to live and knew I had to start figuring out exactly how I could go about doing it. But that was far easier said than done.

Throughout my entire life I had learned how to visualize targets to get me from where I was to where I wanted to be, and once I fixated myself on those goals there was no stopping me. Each time I achieved a goal I became more and more confident and that just propelled me even further.

What I never did learn to do was to cope with a colossal failure since failure was an option I never considered. Once I saw the failure that I had become, I lost all confidence and with it went my ability to visualize targets that I could use to get myself out of it. But if I was going to be able to move forward, I had to find a starting point and what better place than at the bottom of the barrel which was my life in ruins?

I assessed where I was when I began what I call my recovery journey, and it took more than six years including a more than four year divorce period before I could finally start to find some peace of mind. I know, to a lot of you reading this, you might think it was an exceptionally long period so it might help if I give this illustration so that you know what kind of person I was dealing with.

When Alex was about fifteen years old he went through a very tough period where it seemed as though he challenged me at every step through our relationship. Abby jumped in and encouraged him as often as she could; not because of anything I was doing to him but because of how much she hated me. Shortly after Alex turned fifteen, a friend of mine gave us a cockatiel that was a lot of fun. The kids played with it, the dog and the bird played, and it took showers with us on a perch and acted as though it was bathing in a rainstorm.

In the daytime we would put the bird's cage with the bird in it out on the back patio so it could get fresh air, but we always felt it was important to bring it in before dark since it got really cold at night. One day before going out on some appointments, I asked Alex to take the responsibility of bringing the bird in since I wouldn't be back in time and he said he would. When I got home that night I asked him if he had taken the bird in and he panicked while saying he didn't, so we both went outside and found the bird dead in its cage.

I was obviously upset and started chastising him and he felt genuinely sad because he is an animal lover and he felt responsible. Abby immediately intervened and cautioned me to let it go and leave it alone, and because I felt he and I both had said enough I did leave it alone and never held it against him from that point on. In fact, I never even thought about it again until it came up many years later after Alex and I moved in together as roommates following his discharge from the Army.

Alex brought the issue up out of nowhere because he had recently spoken with his mother who told him that she poisoned the bird. I'm not sure how the conversation with her came about nor did I pursue it with him because he was very upset. The two things that upset him the most were how she killed the bird but more importantly how she let him think he had done it for all those years.

Alex and I had a chance to talk it through so that he felt better about it, but it gave light to a much darker side of someone I already had learned was a real monster. Abby apparently took up after her father who told me one time that he poisoned the little dog who belonged to a four year old neighbor boy because Abby's father didn't like the noise the dog made. So at the beginning of my journey toward recovering I didn't know exactly what Abby was capable of but I did know that she was someone who had never tried to succeed at anything except at bringing people down.

And for more than the six years or so that followed our separation and divorce, Abby made sure to put up road blocks at every crossroad I came to and using every willing accomplice she could find. Abby was relentless and recruited her family and boyfriends; she had no qualms lying to anybody including the court and Child Services in order to get them to do her bidding. She had also exploited my greatest weakness, my kids. Because Abby can be such a persuasive liar I lived in fear for a long time that I might lose my kids and I just couldn't bear it.

It took a few years, but once my kids figured Abby out they went out of their way to make sure I knew how much they loved me and I gradually became more secure. When her attempts at turning them against me didn't work, she used the court system to make sure that I had as much trouble as possible finding a home so that Austin couldn't come to live with me at least fifty percent of the time. She blocked me by lying to me about a document and getting Child Services and the courts to take the funds I had set aside to build a real estate and insurance business so I could generate money to live on while I looked for permanent work.

When our divorce was finalized the court set up the alimony and child support based upon my nine thousand dollar a month income that I earned as part of my promotion at the FDIC in Chicago. At the same time I presented the court with the formal announcement that the FDIC office was closing and I would be out of a job in a year, and pointed out the difficulty I'd been having in finding work in light of the announcement. The court simply said to come back in a year for a review.

During that year I began to assess what lay ahead and started to act on it. I made the choice to move back to California and that was by far one of the best decisions I've ever made since I got to see Austin's outlook improve. I also knew that the California job market was very bad so I wrote a business plan to re-form my real estate and insurance agency and set fifteen thousand dollars aside in the event I couldn't find work. I had already finished my business plan, and out of that fifteen thousand I budgeted about five thousand for real estate board fees and dues, licensing, and errors and omission insurance.

The rest was to help me with gas expense for presentations and showing properties, phone and office expense, and some marketing. I was also going to have to use some of it to live on while I built up clientele. The market was pretty hot at the time, and since I used to be a top producer with great customer service scores, I had a pretty reasonable expectation that I would be able to sell commercial and residential real estate as well as life, health, and property insurance. I was covering a lot of bases which could have opened some doors to a pretty good living once I was able to get to work.

I couldn't access my funds for a minimum of forty five days, and during that time I filed some documents with the courts to show that I not only lost my job, but I would be getting about fifteen hundred a month in unemployment. This was what I attempted to tell the courts a year earlier when I gave them the formal announcement that my contract was ending, and I was hoping to get relief once I filed the updated document.

I actually went without collecting anything from unemployment for at least ten weeks for reasons I won't bore you with here, but I barely had enough money to live on much less afford an attorney to help me with the filings. I had to borrow money against my Suburban at a 50 percent interest rate and sell the trailer I hauled my things with in order to have money to live on for over three months before I actually started receiving money.

Within hours after I crossed the California state line I got a call from Child Services. Almost exactly a year after we were in court for divorce proceedings, Abby enlisted her thugs at Child Services to come after me with every bit of the same hatred toward me that she had. At least that's how it seemed based on their actions and condescension toward me, and through her telling me that they laughed their asses off when they got my submission in response to her opening a case against me.

I filed my new income statement but ended up doing it incorrectly, and had I been able to afford an attorney it would have been filed correctly and probably would have stopped me from what I was about to do next. Presenting what appeared to be an original form from our divorce a year earlier, Abby claimed her previous attorneys didn't complete the paperwork correctly and told me I needed to sign it.

According to Abby, the incomplete paperwork caused us to still be married. She said she needed it done because she was going to be marrying a guy she had been shacking up with for a while but couldn't because technically we were still married. In reality she had been shacking up with other guys while we were still married but asked me to lie to her family for her to say that we were already divorced. I wasn't about to lie at all, but fortunately for her the topic never came up so I never had a reason to comment on it.

The fact that she would be getting remarried had a lot of appeal to me because it would relieve me of a lifetime of having to pay her alimony. Because of my action with the courts to gain joint physical as well as joint legal custody, Austin could choose to live where he wanted since he was fourteen and of age in California, so I wasn't worried that he would be stuck with them if he didn't want to be. I fell for it as Abby figured I would.

I told Abby that I wanted to try and find a lawyer to review the document. She was persistent, hitting all the right buttons; and I couldn't see anything that indicated she wasn't telling the truth. She even recruited her sister Jackie to put pressure on me to sign while I was staying with her son Hank who was Abby's nephew. Broke and facing the prospect that there was indeed some idiot who was actually going to marry this ugly person and free me of alimony, I signed.

The legal aid people told me months later that, in language that was couched so as to avoid potential liability, I had been tricked into signing what I thought was an original document clarifying our divorce but was instead a document that caused me tremendous harm. The document stated that I was agreeing to continue to pay the alimony and support of $3,200.00 a month, and after I found out about it and confronted Abby with it, it was clear that she had known about it all along. She was just surprised that the lawyers at the family law center told me about it.

Intentional Harm

It was my mistake for thinking Abby would be telling the truth about anything. For the two months that I didn't receive any income except for unemployment[12] and in the subsequent months when I was earning less than forty percent of what I earned when the court first ordered payments; I went into arrears and they had me listed as a deadbeat. This is exactly what I tried to avoid when I gave everybody the notice about my job ending a year before.

Since Abby and her thugs took away everything I had set aside to start the business up, I took any work I could find which was to do contract mortgage underwriting and later contract insurance sales. And when that happened, she also made sure that every one of my contract checks were attached to pay her so that I barely had anything left to survive on, thanks to her and her thugs at Child Services.

It just keeps getting better. When I landed my first contract job it paid about four thousand dollars a month and Child Services kept coming after me for the thirty-two hundred a month. Forget that because of the distance I had to travel it cost me four hundred dollars a month just in gas to get to work, plus whatever I needed to live on. The thugs garnished my wages and left me with nothing to live on so

---

[12] Which I received more than ten weeks after applying for it.

that I continually had to pawn things like my bike and a few coins I had collected just so I could eat. Had I not been tricked, I could have worked on the contract job and sold real estate and insurance while doing it and that could have helped me get financially stable.

I couldn't afford to get my own place where Austin could stay with me for fifty percent of the time, so I was only able to rent a small room from Abby's nephew Hank. I would have to scrape everything I could just to see Austin when he did come and barely had enough to buy groceries for us without borrowing or going without.

The cost of the gas to go pick Austin up was twenty dollars round trip and though I always found a way to make it happen, I could barely get there for any other times like for school outings or maybe to have dinner with him during the week because it would mean that I may not be able to afford to get to work. Abby was well aware that I couldn't afford to see him more than I did and she always refused to drop him off where I lived.[13] When we were in child court reviewing support payments Abby told them that I never saw Austin more than just a few days a month even though I now lived in the area. This caused them to charge me more for child support as she knew it would, and true to form neither the Court nor the Child Services lawyer let me clarify the circumstances. They just weren't interested.

Abby never bothered to tell the court that she and Child Services were the reasons I couldn't see Austin more. When I tried to bring it up in court her Child Services attorney told me to be quiet because what I had to say was irrelevant and the judge sustained it. I wrote a letter to the director of Child Services describing how they treated me and how they were helping Abby keep me from my son but of course I never got any response. I also pointed out that they were keeping me from getting any kind of healthcare and the stress they were causing me could harm me enough to kill me, but they never bothered to respond to that either.

Not only did Abby misrepresent my relationship with Austin, she lied on her income and expense statement by claiming she had to pay two thousand dollars a month in rent while she was living in her mother's condo. She wasn't paying rent at all because Susan

---

[13] Abby's nephew Hank made it a point to not take sides and took some heat for my living there. I paid rent but I couldn't always do it on time so I did what I could to compensate. We had a great relationship, and still do.

and John were paying her way out of her mother's trust which was also paying for the lease on a brand new car which was a very gas efficient Prius. I don't think she disclosed the gas allowance she was getting while working for John, yet each time I brought it up the court and Child Services were adamant that they weren't interested. Abby also told Austin that she couldn't wait for me to find a permanent job so she could sue me for more money.

I finally got some relief through the courts by getting reductions in child support and alimony after they paid attention to the proof of my lack of income, but the thugs at Child Services never bothered to update their computers and they instructed the state to pull my real estate license not long after I was finally able to activate it. When I say the people at Child Services are thugs, I mean it. They can pull any license issued by the state if they feel like it and they did just to make my life miserable. And even though they were wrong the first time they did it and it was reinstated when I showed Child Services and the state license bureau the correct documentation, I still had to pay the state $100 as a fee for the license getting pulled. I was penalized by $100 that I didn't have for their mistake.

Child Services was showing me in arrears even though I had been compliant after having caught up. Of course I never got any credit at all for the tens of thousands I had paid Abby voluntarily in the years before a court order while she was trolling for dates on the internet and shacking up with various men before and after we were divorced instead of looking for work. My motivation had always been to try and keep Austin in a somewhat stable environment, and the payments I was making to her before the court order were one of the ways I tried to do it.

About nine months or so after this happened; a real estate investor friend approached me because his wife had recently died. In addition to losing his life-long friend and partner, she was his real estate broker and her death left him exposed on a few of many properties he owned. Larry needed help with two important real estate transactions and knowing my circumstances he lent me the money to pay the board fees I needed to get started. I was able to start working with two listings and two offers, and the commissions provided me with some living expenses and seed money to get my real estate and insurance business going after all. I was starting to see some light, and I had been hoping that the unemployment extension would come through to help me have money to live on until the transactions closed.

But the transactions weren't closing in time for me to start making a living on them. If that weren't enough I faced losing my Suburban because I couldn't afford to make the payment on the 50 percent interest loan I had taken out on it. When my contract job ended I went back on unemployment insurance until it ran out leaving me a week short and once again without money. The license issue came up again but with far more serious consequences while illustrating just what a vile person Abby is.

I closed a real estate transaction at the same time I had to find a new place because of Hank's new girlfriend, plus it was time for me to go anyway and find a place of my own because I had lived there long enough. Around that time, Alex had been living with Abby and Austin and worked with Abby at John's law office. According to Abby, Alex was becoming verbally abusive to her and somewhat unruly and she had concerns. Even though I have no trust in anything Abby has to say I have to concede that Alex does have the capacity to be that way, and because of his size and military training he can be a very imposing figure.

Abby and her new boyfriend also named Ralph[14] kicked Alex out about the same time that I was starting to look for a place to live. I was behind in my support payments due to no job and no money, and I hadn't made my support payment out of my commission yet because I didn't know what I was going to have to pay to get into a place.

While that was going on, Alex found a room to rent for about seven hundred and sixty bucks a month but he couldn't use the shower or kitchen facilities, and he had to walk three miles to the train station each way so he could get to work. Alex was showering at the gym very early in the morning before going to work, but wasn't able to every day.

After about a month of Alex renting this room, Abby called me and appealed to me to find an apartment with him. Her concern was genuine as was mine. Alex and I ended up finding an old place not far from the beach that was perfect for us. I ended up having to advance Alex $2600 to help him move in, so it took everything I had put aside leaving me with only two hundred dollars to live on for

---

[14] This Ralph is Ralph2, who is different from Ralph1.

the month until I could either close a transaction or find some work.

Alex and I moved into our new place in the beginning of the second month following my real estate closing, and because of my insurance license I was fortunate enough to land a two and a half month contract job set to begin about three months after we moved in which would pay me an hourly wage plus bonus on my sales.

Abby was well aware of my circumstances and while I was barely affording enough to eat, she was basking in the glow of her substantial inheritance plus the twenty-eight thousand dollar commission that she got in July for closing the sale of her mother's condo. The condo was one-quarter hers from the inheritance so for the month of July she made about $175,000 from her share of the sale proceeds plus the commission for selling it. It's easy to see why she kept telling everyone how poor she was.

I was planning to get caught up on some of the support payments in October once I had money since nothing else had closed, but in early September Child Services had my insurance and real estate licenses deactivated so that I couldn't work on my contract job. When I had first learned of what they were planning to do I appealed to Abby to drop the case so that I could work, not solely because of me but because of Alex whose name was also on the lease and who would be heavily impacted if I couldn't work for that two and a half months.

Alex had stabilized emotionally and was finally feeling like he had a home once again. Money was tight for both of us, but we were learning to make do. I had no resources, and if I couldn't work for those months while still trying to close my real estate deals and trying to find permanent work I would be in breach of my lease contract and out in the street. Alex would be stuck covering the rent and would have to find a new roommate so that he wouldn't be in breach as well. I laid that out for Abby and she initially didn't respond much less drop the case.[15]

---

[15] My phone and internet got cut off during that time as well, no doubt a high point for Abby and her thugs. Alex being the great guy that he is stepped up to the plate by paying me more than normal payment toward what he owed me for the $2600 advance. Abby sent me an email accusing me of leeching off Alex and calling me a big, fat disgrace. She ignored the fact that Alex was still paying off the rent and deposit that I advanced him in July and September. She also ignored that she never bothered to help him despite the windfalls from her inheritance and the $175k she made in July.

I screamed at the case workers asking them how they slept at night knowing they were going to keep me from a job over a lack of payment because I had no job. I couldn't believe that they would pull the licenses but they did, and to her true character Abby had a good laugh over it. She was having so much fun with it she even hired Alex to clean her house once a week for $50 just so she could rub my nose deep in it. She still had the thugs at Child Services convinced that she was the poor, innocent victim, even though I showed the case officers proof of what she was making compared to what I was earning.

I managed to find a way to get temporary relief, but this goes to illustrate the hatred that drives a soulless individual not because of any way I may have mistreated her or left her wanting, but because of how I had exposed her for who she really is. That was the unpardonable sin that I committed, which was to show how her only successes come at the expense of someone else, such as her mother dying or tricking desperate boyfriends into paying her way with false promises that she'll bring them happiness. Or she would badger family members to do her bidding like giving her work and rent-free accommodations, just like she did with me for more than twenty years of being married to her.

By her keeping me down, it perpetuated the lie that she told about everything being my fault. She pointed to my lack of ability to move forward as proof that I was the one responsible for everything going bad, while leaving out the parts of how her deception and vile behavior were the biggest parts of what caused me to stay down as long as I did.

Had my kids not been at stake I could have easily moved on even though I still loved her in the early stages of our separation. But in looking back into the early years of our brief courtship I'm confident that I would never have dated Abby beyond a year much less married her if she hadn't been pregnant. Instead of moving on though, I had to learn to bide my time because through the bits and pieces that my kids would let slip occasionally, she was playing the innocent victim and portraying herself as someone who could never be capable of causing the damage she had caused me over and over. Had I ignored Austin's pleas to move back to California, I would have been fine because I would have likely secured a new contract.

I could have taken a job in Florida at the FDIC satellite there so I would have had an income and making the payments wouldn't have been a problem. But I might have lost my son because of what she was putting him through while having her fun. At the time he asked me to move back he was still talking about suicide and there was no way I was going to ignore him even though Abby kept calling him a drama queen each time he talked about killing himself. I can overcome an evil person and lack of money, but I can never replace one of my kids.

Trying To Get Ahead

Around the time these things started happening Andrew was also getting married. Because my financial straits were so bad at the time, I wasn't able to contribute to the rehearsal dinner, but I was still able to attend and could have at least paid my own way. Abby made it a point to make sure that not only was I being excluded from the rehearsal dinner but she and some members of her family were actually rubbing it in. I could have forced the issue and found a way to go in, but she would have created a terrible scene and I would likely have lost my temper which would have ruined Andrew's and Renee's night.

The heartbreak was almost unbearable knowing that no one stood up for me. A few months after he got married though, Andrew came by to have a beer and without my asking told me he and his mother had a huge argument over it and she won because he couldn't ruin Renee's night. He said he was sorry and he meant it, and I told him just how happy I was to hear that he stood up for me.

Twenty-three years earlier when Abby and I found out that she was pregnant with Andrew her family had put pressure on Abby to have him aborted because of our terrible financial situation at the time. These were some of the same participants who had attended the rehearsal dinner and were claiming him as their own. At the time they were putting pressure on Abby to have him aborted, they didn't have the guts to pressure me about it but it didn't matter because my position was clear. I didn't care if I had to work fifteen jobs to support my family; there was no way that I was going to let Andrew get aborted simply because his being born would have been inconvenient for us.

According to Abby, that was the route that one of her sisters had taken for herself before I met Abby, for convenience and because her sister couldn't face their parents with being pregnant out of wedlock. But that wasn't who I was. I didn't care what anyone thought of me for getting Abby pregnant, I was in love with her when it happened and I fully accepted the responsibility of my children. After knowing who the young men Alex and Andrew grew up and turned out to be showed me that I had indeed made the right choices.

Abby was a part of the choice, of course, but she told me she had already had one abortion before I met her and had I not been adamant about keeping the babies when we found out she was pregnant with both of them, she would have very likely given in and had Alex and Andrew aborted because that's who she is. During the time I had to deal with all of that garbage involving licenses, no job, and the emotional ups and downs being meted out by Abby and her complicit thugs, I spiraled down once again into a deep depression.

Before it all started happening, I was breathing fine, sleeping fine, starting to work out three to four times a week with some pretty good intensity, and I was eating a much better diet with minimal alcohol intake. It was strange that I didn't see the depression creeping in, but after a while I could tell by the changes in my habits and how I was feeling. My patterns changed all over again. I stopped working out, began eating a poor diet including desserts, started drinking more (Wal-Mart had wine at $1.97 a bottle), was again having trouble breathing, and found myself falling asleep on the couch and waking up after only a few hours of sleep instead of going to bed. I watched yet again as my successes in the battle against this disease began to give way to the additional stress and the bad lifestyle.

I don't need the researchers to tell me why diabetics who are depressed end up dying; I began living everyday wondering if I'd even make it through the next year. My good friend Vince had four strokes while sleeping because of his stress, and he was healthy up until the strokes. I have heart disease, high blood pressure, and diabetes, how in the world was I going to survive with all of this hitting me without any sort of relief especially when I kept falling into depression due to a vicious ex-wife's evil pastime?

Despite that ugly prospect, I still held firm in my commitment to not only live, but to exact the best revenge possible which is to live well. I had a vision and that meant I was going to finally be able to move on.

Finding The Right Road

Once I had decided that I wanted to live and to find a way to live well, I realized I just didn't know where to start. I assessed the circumstances and had to find a way to look past the ruins. I knew I needed to develop some routines so I could eat better, get plenty of rest, and exercise. I also needed to see a doctor to help me stabilize. If I chose to focus on the obstacles, there was no way that I would have survived.

Over time, some of the pain and confusion began to subside and I began to see a path. The most important thing I could do was to learn how to grow that vision once again. There is a fine line between wishing for something versus knowing where you want to end up. Wishing is pure fantasy, and although wishing is a good place to start when you are trying to follow a vision, it can also be a waiting place from which you never want to leave. Wishing gives you a happy place, like wishing you had a million dollars and imagining what your life would be like. This makes for a fantastic escape mechanism to ease the drudgery of everyday living, but it can be very wasteful if you stay there too long.

A vision on the other hand can form the beginning of an actionable plan well beyond a fantasy. A vision is bringing your fantasy into a reachable place and then taking steps to achieve the goals that will take you to that place for real. A visionary who wants to make a million dollars won't wish for it, but might break it down into bite size pieces so that he focuses first on improving his circumstance like finding a job that pays between $60,000 and $100,000 a year with growth potential.

Then if the employer doesn't offer opportunities to accumulate wealth through advancement, investment or downright purchase of the company, then the next focus might be to get $500,000 through investments and seek out opportunities to double the investment at each juncture. The point is the million dollars is an end goal while the interim actions are designed to improve the present then ultimately working toward that goal of accumulating wealth that might lead to a million dollars.

My goal has always been to accumulate at least five million dollars but I've been doing it so long I need to adjust it to today's dollars and set my sights on ten or fifteen million dollars to be more realistic. I realize if I said that out loud anybody looking at me or my circumstances would brand me as an absolute idiot and they might be right, but it doesn't mean I'm going to stop trying simply because they don't think I can do it. It's likely they don't think I can do it because they don't think they can do it. But what others think is hardly anything I lose sleep over. What does matter is whether or not I'm heading in a direction that could bring me opportunities that can help me achieve those goals.

Despite how broke I am, I have managed to hang onto two licenses in professions where someone in my age group can make a million dollars a year or more depending upon how hard and how smart they want to work. Now that I'm practicing in both I'm able to see that I haven't lost the qualities that have made me successful in the past. I've also had a chance to sit with people who have been very successful and have been able to learn from them.

It came time for me to redevelop my style and approach, and to find cash flow to keep me current and fluid enough to act on opportunities as they appear. But first a quick look back at how I got to this point. Learning how to develop and act upon visions is a lot like building routines for health and exercise. You have to start small and celebrate the small successes then expanding your reach.

Embarking On A Targeted Journey

I was still living in Chicago when I told my buddy Mick that I was going to attempt my first fifty mile bike ride, he offered me these sage words of advice, "Gerard, what you need to do if you want to make it all the way is to get behind a nice looking blond and keep her ass in focus."

We both had a great laugh about it, but then the day of the ride came and I was a little apprehensive about whether or not I could go the distance. I wasn't sure if my body would hold up, and I wasn't sure if I would be up for it mentally. I told my kids and a few friends that I would be doing it so I didn't want to face the embarrassment of coming up short.

The ride was for a charity sponsored by the Evanston Bike Club and the route went in and out of some beautiful neighborhoods overlooking Lake Michigan. There were about sixteen hundred riders who had signed up for any of the five distance options, 25, 50, 62, 75, or 100 miles. The ride was marked and very well organized, and it was a beautiful day.

I started about 7:00 am and since the farthest I had gone before was forty-one and a half miles comfortably, I decided to pace myself at about fourteen to fifteen miles an hour to ensure that I had enough energy to make my goal, even though both my body, at two hundred and ninety-three pounds, and my bike were capable of a faster ride.

After a few miles though I started to get a little concerned that boredom might do me in before I actually ran out of steam. Just then four riders passed me and one of them was a very attractive blond with a, as you might have guessed, nice ass. Mick's words echoed in my head.

"To hell with it", I said to myself, "I really don't have much to lose, and if I run out of steam at least it will have been an enjoyable ride." For the next twenty-five miles I paced behind this beauty's behind at about eighteen to twenty miles an hour in order to keep up. I had no intention of catching her of course. After all in my shape I really had nothing to offer this attractive woman, but it was a fun adventure just the same. I followed her at that pace until the first rest stop when I lost her in the crowd. Energized and motivated, I kept the pace between sixteen and twenty miles an hour for the remainder of the ride, and my total mileage was 51.4 miles.

A year before passing the fifty mile mark, two friends at work who saw that I had an interest in bicycling encouraged me and gave me important tips. One of them, John, a large fellow like me; but an avid rider in the ten to twenty mile range gave me a lot of very useful tips, probably the most beneficial of which was his telling me to get Kevlar tires. Before I did I was getting a flat a week, but once I got Kevlar I had no more flats.

One day John asked me if I wanted to meet him early on a Saturday to go for a seventeen mile ride. I told him that it was too long of a distance and I would need more time to work up to it, so I asked him to invite me on the next ride. He said no problem but then shamed me by telling me that our colleague Sally was going on the ride with him. Sally was not only older than me and had never gone beyond ten miles either but that didn't stop her from jumping on his invitation. We left at 7:00 am on that Saturday and immediately started up some very long hills but the good news is that we went downhill too, making for an exciting ride. At the sixteen mile mark, Sally and I stopped at the top of a particularly steep hill to catch our breaths while looking at the even steeper hill ahead of us. John took his break across the street. Sally and I were feeling a sense of accomplishment thinking that John's house was just around the corner.

"Hey John," I could barely squeak out due to lack of oxygen, "how much further?"

He answered with the same matter-of-fact tone of a doctor who proclaims the procedure will "be slightly uncomfortable" as he proceeds to torture you in the most painful way possible.

"Oh, not bad," he said while pointing straight up that very long and steep hill, "right about a mile and half."

I would have belted him right in the kisser had I been able to drag myself across the street.

Well we made it, and I for one was better off having done so. Not only had I nearly doubled my distances but I did it on hilly terrain. The fact that I had done it and felt good about it gave me new targets to visualize. It became much easier to take on bigger hills and longer distances because I could already see myself having done it.

There is a big lesson here, and it's one that no journey should be without. Whether you are trying to improve your professional success, launch a new venture, or like me, trying to reinvent yourself, each segment is a journey and each journey requires a visual target that you must follow if you are ever going to succeed. Sometimes you need others to help you get jump started.

Setting Action Plans And Achieving Milestones

Both Mick's and John's philosophies underscore some critical points not only for a targeted journey but for a life journey. The first place to start is to know where you want to go, but sometimes you have to let someone else lead the way. Go along for the ride; see yourself in new places, then find a target to follow that will take you even further than you've ever been.

Visualization is truly one of the cornerstones of success. Every time I hit a new high, I saw it in my mind first and I never lost sight of it. When I went through the darkest moments of my life, I lost my ability to see any positive outcomes, and not surprisingly only found life's negativity. I still fall prey to that at times but the cycle I was on eventually started to break apart and I began to see more positives. Once I did my approach to other things changed too because my attitude was more positive and even though I was still prone to bouts of depression, those bouts didn't last as long and they were less impactful.

My routines continued to be intermittent since having started my move to heal myself, I not only needed to recover from what the sickness did to me I needed to change my life in a way that I dealt with things differently so that I didn't give in to stress and depression. For a short while I had worked my way up to running

1.5 miles non-stop and the results were showing. That's not much of an achievement for the average person, but to a guy weighing over 300 pounds it's a major challenge.

Every part of me was affected, especially my back and joints because of the pounding they had to take every time I ran. I kept trying and as I did I dropped more weight, my stomach started to get a little flatter, and about an inch came off my girth. That might not seem like much but every bit helps. My heavy travel schedule kept interrupting my routines. I'd go on extended work trips for the FDIC and that took its toll, in part because of the long work hours also in part because of the drinking and partying. I also took trips to each coast to see my sons on weekends following my work trips, and even though I struggled I managed to get some workouts in, which consisted of some long walks or 10 mile bike rides, or half-mile runs.

The travel was hard though, and I was more exhausted than anything. Most times I had neither the energy nor the place to sit still or lay down to visualize what I needed to do. Each time I went home after my trips it took me about two or three days of just sleeping and resting before I even was able to go back to my workout routines. I would restart my workouts slowly then build them up, like with a short run or a five to ten mile bike ride, and after a while the workouts would grow into something more significant.

There were always new barriers to contend with each time I'd try to build a routine, both mentally and physically. I moved to a new apartment with a couple of friends from work and started a new routine by taking advantage of a path around a little lake outside my building. It was about a mile around and I started running on the path early in the morning. My biggest problem then was getting a full night's sleep. I would fall asleep about 10:00 p.m., wake around 1:00 or 2:00 a.m. and was unable to get back to sleep.

This was a big problem on a few levels, especially being diabetic. The lack of sleep totally sapped my energy and it was very hard for me to follow a routine. It also made me emotionally unstable at a time when I still struggled to find reasons to live when I'd hit my lowest points through the years of that journey, and I had a hard time staying focused on my visual targets.

I'm one of those guys who has to visualize in detail over and over again, and at times I squander the time that I could be acting upon achieving a goal. My visual targets can often be wishful thinking and they stay that way until I actually begin to take action. That is and has been one of my greatest obstacles to overcome, and it is a constant battle. One of the reasons it happens though is because I'm so negatively impacted by any kind of stress.

Most of us know there is good stress and bad stress, but my life over the past ten years had been just a constant barrage of bad stress and it affected everything about me so much that I didn't know how to relax and unwind. As I started out to achieve my goals it took about a year of re- learning how to go to some great places in my mind and to find things that relaxed me.

Even though I had lost my ability to visualize due to all of the stress and failure that had become my life, I eventually gained it back. Over time, I slowly managed to overcome the obstacles, one at a time, and with each event I found new confidence. Each time I hit an interim weight goal, cleared a debt, or completed a chapter, I found the achievement gave way to a feeling of accomplishment and boosted my confidence. From there I began to see a new life ahead.

Looking Beyond The Negatives

Before I was able to see a new life ahead, I looked in the ruins as my whole world crumbled before me and I came to realize that I could very likely die because of what I was doing to myself. It's one thing to toy with the notion of doing something bad but it's quite another to see the bad things in action and what they can do. How do you walk through ruins to see what can be salvaged or even if you want to salvage anything? My custom mansion had been foreclosed upon, my family was torn apart; I was one paycheck from being homeless, was fat as a house and riddled with disease. If the diabetes didn't kill me, my high blood pressure could, and if that didn't do it my heart could likely give out, or if not I had a very good chance of having a stroke.

When you work for the federal government, especially in a position of public trust like I was in, you have to go through some very serious background checking about every two years. If the investigators find that you or something you did are the causes of the problems in your life like financial hardship or DUIs then you will get terminated on the spot; and if caught lying you face prison time. I had already been through this once before when I first got hired on but it was required that I go through it again, so I was on my second one and it was grueling. Most of my friends and colleagues got through their interviews in about twenty minutes to cover their previous ten years; my first one took two and a half months, and the second one went on for nearly four hours because of everything that kept coming up.

Through the course of the discussion, all I could do was describe the events as they happened and show their impacts on my circumstances. This was important because two weeks after the interview Abby filed a false charge against me to keep me from filing a restraining order against her boyfriend Ralph1 over what he had done to Austin. She later dropped it because it was a bogus charge but had she filed it before my interview instead of two weeks after I would have been fired whether it was a false charge or not. That just showed the kind of idiot Abby is especially when she realized that she nearly cost herself her livelihood by doing it which she admitted during the court appearance when she dropped the charge.[16]

The investigator had started my interview as a tough, rigid guy but after listening to the explanations his stance softened and he became quite different.

"I've been in my job for over twenty five years," he said before starting to wrap it up. "Most of it went pretty smoothly over that time. I don't know if I could have survived half of what you've gone through, but the fact that you are able to smile and look ahead is a real inspiration."

He was a good guy, but I was still sweating the outcome until six months later the office let me know that I had once again been cleared.

The investigators parting comments caused me to reflect on why I wanted to move forward, and the answer ended up being pretty simple. My kids were and are too important for me to ever want to give up. I wanted to show them that no matter how hard things got, there was always a way out if you just persevered. Now understand that it took me a long time before I was able to say that with any conviction, and you can see that I'm filled with doubts a lot of the time; doubts in myself and doubts about my future.

---

[16] She wanted to drop the charge without going to court but I wouldn't agree to it because it was a completely bogus charge and I had all the documentation and witnesses to prove it was a false charge. Both Austin and Alex offered to testify on my behalf once they knew what the charges were and because Austin was a witness to the entire event. She dropped it before I had a chance to show the fraud and the case was dismissed, but unfortunately the fact that she filed it still stays on my public record.

Perseverance is about having faith and pressing on even when you can't see the end of the line. I can tell you though; if my kids would have believed Abby and abandoned me as she hoped they would, I'm not sure that I could have gone on.

Every once in a while I reflect on the past when the boys were little and life seemed simpler. I used to have a refrigerator magnet that had a picture of a little rowboat on a lake with a fishing pole sticking out of it. The caption read "if money is your only problem, then you don't have a problem." I used to look at it every day before hitting the streets to face the day, realizing that I didn't have a single problem. Back then, my family was healthy and secure, and I had three little guys whose worst worry of the day was whether or not they would have to wear a shirt that was a color that they didn't like. Even though I was scrambling to make ends meet, that magnet reminded me that life could have been so much worse. Breaking it down that way helped me to focus on what I needed to do to succeed without whining about what I didn't have.

My focus from that point was to earn more money so we could live comfortably. And back when I was a new lending manager while they were still little, I always made it a point to start early and finish late. Since I was a producing manager, meaning that I had to generate my own deals while managing the branch, it was important for me to lead by example and as such was always the first one in and usually the last to leave.

One day I came in a little later than normal but still pretty far ahead of when we were due to open, and I found that one of my agents was already there. Walter made the comment that he was paying attention to what I was doing and said he appreciated the example I was setting. I responded almost apologetically that I had come in later than normal but I had been playing with my oldest son Alex who was about five at the time. I said that I couldn't bring myself to leave him before he was ready to let me go.

Walter, who was a new father-to-be looked at me and said, "You know, I've never heard of anyone who, as they lay dying, said they wished they had more time to spend in the office." He drove home a point that day that has never left me.

As I looked at my life in ruins, I realized that it wasn't a total loss and far from it depending upon what factors are used to measure. I had three sons to whom I devoted my entire life; strong, handsome, and sound young men who had and have very bright futures ahead of them. That in itself could be marked as a source of pride, and the fact that they still loved me proved that I was indeed blessed.

On the night before leaving for Chicago to relocate for my new job through the promotion with the FDIC, I took Alex and Austin out for our version of a night on the town, Andrew was already at boot camp in the Marines so he wasn't able to join us. Our rocking night was dinner, movies, bowling and dessert, and I treasured every last second of it. When it came time to say goodbye, I hugged Austin who was thirteen then, long and deep because I didn't want to spend a minute away from him if I could have helped it. As I started to pull away, he was holding back tears and couldn't let me go. He didn't see my tears, but once out of his sight I don't think I stopped crying until I was out of California.

Laying The Foundations

After leaving Austin I started to ponder what lay ahead. I knew that after working that hard and that long for the past twenty plus years, I was having to start all over again, only things had changed and really not a single one of them for the better. .

Then I had to look at what I had to work with because a lot had changed with that too. I was an experienced executive with a Fortune 100 manager background, and that helped me be one of the 275 people hired out of the 6500 applicants who applied for the same jobs offered by the FDIC.

The other parts though were that health-wise, I was a walking time bomb and had I not gotten focused on understanding what I needed to do to survive, the stress and strain of the job and the divorce probably would have killed me.

Ralph1 sent me an email before I met him in court to get a restraining order on him to keep him from touching Austin. In it he said Abby told him that she hoped the disease was putting me in a lot of pain, and she didn't care what happened to me because of it.

Clearly I couldn't control what she and her loser boyfriends were going to do, so all I could do was brace myself for the worst and do what I could do to get through it. What I knew was that before I could even start to fix my financial problems and get past an ugly, vindictive ex-wife and her parade of losers, I had to first fix myself, physically, mentally, and emotionally and to do that I had to learn about what it was that was wrong with me.

At first it seemed like an overwhelming task, and indeed it was. So I approached it in the same way I would if I had to eat an elephant and in fact I was eating an elephant, that elephant was me. The way to do it is to eat it one bite at a time, and if it is still too big of a task then you turn it into a banquet and invite your family and friends to a feast.

I started learning about my health problems and talked to my doctors so that I could understand the risks I was facing and what I needed to do for maintenance and ultimately if there was anything I could plan to do to cure them. This helped me create boundaries and parameters so that I knew which lines I couldn't cross but what framework I could use to reshape my life. Changing my life and knowing what to change about it was exactly what I needed to do to start to get my life back.

Emotionally I was strung out and had been for about the past four or five years, and it got so much worse before it ever got better. Austin held out hope for almost two years that Abby and I would reconcile and build a new life together, and I did what I could to try and make that happen for him but it was he who saw the hopelessness of it over time and finally told me it was okay with him for me to move on.

Despite the wreck I was, I managed to have a couple of cute girlfriends and that went a long way toward helping me boost my confidence. It helped me realize that I probably wasn't going to be lonely the rest of my life if I didn't choose to.

My mental condition was the other hard part. For so many years I listened to my negative self-talk, and it seemed like it was so many years since I had any achievements to point to. All I could see were failures. The images of the blob I had become emasculated me into a weakling. I used to make this joke about being a fragile flower, but in truth that's exactly what I had become. I knew at that point that I needed professional help. The stress of my son Andrew being in harm's way in Afghanistan and being away from my other two boys was delivering some pretty crushing blows. Add to that my ex-wife trying to make it so I couldn't see my youngest on top of her other games and you might see why I was back to losing hope every single day.

At that point and once I started paying attention to what I had become, I began going through some different changes as I pressed ahead bit by bit. It wasn't long before I wasn't the fragile flower anymore. I was pretty friendly most of the time, but I started hanging out in biker bars more and more and it got to where people made it a point not to piss me off because they couldn't be certain of what the consequences would be. I wasn't looking for fights or anything like that, but that part of me that used to be there started coming out in conversations and in actions so it was pretty clear that if somebody wanted to start trouble with me I planned to finish it.

I was still in Chicago when all of this was happening, and even though these new outlets seemed to help my overall outlook, I knew I needed professional help before doing something really stupid. This realization came to me after a night of drinking when I woke up in my car and had no idea where I was or how I got there.[17] After getting a referral through the Employee Assistance Program (EAP) at work I was fortunate to meet Dr. Deidre Alexander around the same time that I was forming a long-distance relationship with a lovely woman named Deanna whom I had met on a plane during one of my trips from Texas to California.

Deidre helped me put it all in perspective and into those bite-sized pieces I'd been looking for, like the divorce, the separation from my kids and my efforts to rebuild myself. She also walked me through what I was trying to process so I could distinguish between what was real and what was imagined. There is no way that I could have moved ahead the way I did, virtually unscathed, had it not been for her guidance.

Deanna helped me in a far different way. She was fun and beautiful and totally high maintenance, and it wasn't long before I had fallen madly in love with her. We met on a plane while I was flying on a first class ticket given to me as a gift by my sister Iris. The seats reclined and I spent most of the trip with Deanna's German Shepard lying under my feet. Although I didn't start the trip being talkative, eventually Deanna and I started talking and hit it off. We traded names during the flight and a few weeks later I contacted her and to my surprise she contacted me back. It wasn't long before she and I started spending hours on the phone with each other, and each time we did I couldn't wait until the next time we'd get to talk or see each other.

---

[17] I had an upcoming court appearance to confront Abby after she filed court documents to try to ban me from seeing Austin. I caught her in lie after lie on the documents prepared by John's office but she still tricked me into thinking she was postponing the court date. In reality what she had done was to make it appear that I wasn't interested in appearing so the court would rule for her in my absence. I figured it out in the nick of time and managed to book a flight, but the idea that I almost lost rights to my son left me numb and I lost myself in too many drinks.

This is probably the best way to sum her up: A high class, big-breasted beauty from Texas who was a teacher and occasional model. She drove a convertible sports car, smoked cigars, drank vodka from the bottle, and owned a .38 that she most certainly knew how to use. And she got a Ph.D from USC under some really tough circumstances. What's not to love? I was hooked but alas, it was destined not to work out I'm sad to say. But the time I spent with her was exactly what I needed, like it was with Deidre because both relationships went a long way to helping me recoup my sanity and my confidence.

Deanna helped me regain my confidence and helped me realize that I could have a relationship that I could look forward to while Deidre taught me to break down the barriers and obstacles in my life into manageable pieces.

So what did those bite-sized pieces look like? The first thing I came to realize was that I had to work on things that I could probably control best; diet, exercise, and sleep. I had originally worried that by moving to Chicago I might have had to stop my bike riding, because I never envisioned that Chicago was a bike-friendly place. I was very pleasantly surprised to find out that I couldn't have been more wrong. Illinois in general is a very bike-friendly state. The humidity knocked about ten miles off my rides at first, but I was able to adapt and move past that in a relatively short amount of time.

I joined a couple of gyms and started following some routines but my sleep problems and travel schedule caused me to fall into a series of start-stop-start patterns. To me, the fact that I would keep falling off a schedule didn't sway me as long as I stayed focused on my objective which was to get exercise however I could and as often as I could. And I had to stop the negative talk about the futility of what I was doing; otherwise I would never get the benefit of what I was doing. After two hours of sweating then stepping on a scale the read my weight range of 297 to 303, it was disheartening at best.

So I worked on learning to master the start-stop cycles to ensure that I was getting enough exercise. I biked, cross-country skied, took long walks, ran, took Zumba classes, worked out at the gym, and used the treadmill as alternates to help get me the movement and exercise I needed.

At the same time I was learning healthier ways to eat, and focused on looking for foods that not only were diabetic friendly but could help me lose weight while staying energized and could help me build muscle. There was some trial and error while trying to find the right diet, and there are still some times when I fall off the wagon so to speak, especially when travelling. Still, I didn't always want to be so confined because I knew I would want and need to cut loose once in a while, so I developed some lifestyle offsets to help me manage that.

There was a village about four miles away from where I lived in a Chicago suburb, and on those nights when I needed to cut loose, I'd walk the four miles (sometimes in 100 degree heat with 98% humidity) and hit the Chinese-Sushi buffet, then take in a movie, and walk four miles back. That helped me accomplish a couple of things. It gave me a little freedom so I could mix in exercise with 'porking' out. I always kept the pace at about four to four and a half miles per hour to burn off the bad stuff I had just eaten.

While I wasn't doing the best things for my body, I wasn't doing the worst either. It kept me from putting weight on during those times, and my blood sugar was at okay levels because I had meds. It also helped me get my body back to being accustomed to waking up some muscles that weren't getting much use. I bought some excellent New Balance cross-training shoes but even with those it was often hard to walk the next morning because the heavy weight over the long miles was really hard on my feet. I would sometimes trip and fall during those walks and get banged up, three hundred pounds falling at four miles an hour can cause a lot more damage than one might think. The good news was that I was the airbag to help protect my bones from major damage.

I would also get big blisters and bursitis in my heels. Anyone who has gotten bursitis knows how severe the pain can be for months on end. Yet I really didn't have a choice, the only way to get past the pain was to keep getting up and working at it until things got easier.

I would share some exercise milestones with my sons and Renee, then my future daughter-in-law, and some family members and a few close friends. The milestones were like when I passed the nine mile mark when walking or when I would do forty, fifty, or sixty mile rides. I'd share it with them so they'd know I was working on getting myself fixed, and they in turn would cheer me on.

Instead of looking at the start-stop-start patterns as a problem, my pattern actually was my focus on developing new, good habits to replace old, bad habits. And I came to understand that I had to take each exercise event one at a time in recognition of the fact that

I didn't get fat and unhealthy overnight, I did it over a long period of time. So it stood to reason that I wasn't going to get trim and healthy overnight either, but I could take comfort in knowing that I would be able to get fixed in much less time than it took me to get that way. I needed to let that sink in so that I didn't get impatient and depress myself even more. Yes, I still have issues with it, but it doesn't stay with me for too long as I have learned to adapt and attack the problem when it arises.

The sleep problem was a much harder one to deal with. Not only were my health issues causing me to lose sleep, so were the frustration and loneliness which would often hit me very hard. I'm a pretty social guy and not afraid to venture out so I would hit clubs and make new friends. I also had a few good friends from work and that helped me a lot, at least as a cure for the loneliness, and it would lessen my frustration by giving me brief escapes from it. The downside was that I would stay up late drinking with my friends and that wasn't good from a health perspective.

In time, I learned to manage that as well so I kept the staying out late to a minimum, and I tried a few methods to help me get to sleep. My sleep problems were a combination of not falling asleep quickly enough, and once asleep for one or two hours I would wake up and take another three to four hours to fall back to sleep. So on average, I was getting at best two to three hours of sleep each night.

I drank alcohol, took Melatonin and Nyquil on a regular basis because of how well it worked. I found in one of my diabetes diet books that red wine was good on occasion so I would drink a couple of glasses a night but that would lead to drinking the whole bottle each night. It seemed like Nyquil was a good way to go but then I read the warnings on overdoing it because of the acetaminophen, too much can be bad on the liver and I already knew that my organs were at risk because of my diabetes. There is also a warning for diabetics to let the doctor know when you are taking it because it can impact blood sugar levels.

Eventually Vick's came out with 'Zzzquil' which worked great for me, and Walmart came out with a comparable product under its Equate brand, which is probably made by Vicks. Overall it is listed as safe, and seems to work fine for me, but WebMd.com lists precautions for people with any of my conditions (as opposed to all of my conditions). I would really like to reach the point where I don't have to use any sleep aids, but for now I'm glad that I'm getting the new habit of sleeping through the night and the energy that results from a good night's sleep.

So my bite sized pieces seemed simple to achieve on the surface, but like many things was much easier said than done. Getting a handle on things meant that I had to first identify why I even wanted to do it, why did I want to live and get fixed? After all, if you don't have the right motivation there's a pretty good chance you aren't going to succeed.

Once I knew why, then I had to assess what needed to be done while isolating those things that I could change immediately so I could start right away. And while that was happening, I had to start planning my approach to changing the things I had less control over. There was no way that I was going to change my ex-wife or her vicious antics, but I could work on dealing with it until I could remove the emotional impact while keeping my son in focus. I couldn't change my travel schedule, but I could continue to focus on making better choices while I was traveling and sticking to routines when I got back.

And I could persevere; I found new faith in my ability to persevere by identifying goals I hoped to achieve, and that helped me to get past the rough stuff, and it still does.

I heard a great saying by former newscaster David Brinkley, "A successful man is one who can lay a firm foundation with the bricks others have thrown at him."

I realized after hearing it that I've been trying to do just that without even knowing it, and after each time I revisit where I've come from I can see the foundation that is being laid. It's getting more solid every day.

EIGHT

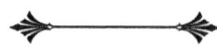

How Diabetes Got Me on the Right Road

Your life does not get better by chance, it gets better by change.

- Jim Rohn

I've learned that nutrition, exercise, and blood monitoring are probably the most important parts of coping with diabetes. I am lucky that I have type 2 diabetes instead of type 1 because I am able to keep it under control mostly using diet and exercise. That said, I'm not without risk by any means whether I'm on medication or not. But reversing the disease is my ultimate goal instead of simply trying to keep it under control.

Easier said than done for some of us though, right? First thing I had to look at was how I got to be so fat and stressed out in the first place. Eating and drinking too much were high on the list. So was being under heavy stress, lots of travel, eating all the wrong things. Sound like you? Changing all of that for me wasn't just simply finding the right diet plan. Diet and exercise plans for me often added more stress by having to follow rigid guidelines or impractical routines, and because of my lifestyle and fluctuating work schedules I would have a very hard time succeeding.

The best way for me was to incorporate diet and exercise into my normal, everyday routines. At different times I rode my bike or took my bike on the train to work, then rode longer on the way home, sometimes twenty miles to get home on bike. Or I walked to work at times when I lived close enough to the office, like less than five miles away.

When I was traveling I usually picked hotels that had refrigerators and kitchenettes in the room, then I shopped at a local grocery store to get the foods that best fit my personal needs. The Hyatt House chain was one of my favorites since it was like living in a one bedroom apartment at very affordable rates. This gave me the chance to eat healthy and cut down on the nights out partying with my colleagues. Going out and interacting with my colleagues and new coworkers was very good and helpful most of the time, but more than twice in a week took its toll on me.

When I wasn't working long hours I used the treadmill or exercise bike at the hotel gym, or walked in the city instead of taking the train or a cab. If I was in a place for more than a week, I'd rent a bicycle and map out a bike route and ride. I got a great ride along the Potomac on the Mount Vernon trail which goes from the Virginia side of Washington DC and ends at Mount Vernon where George Washington once lived. I went for a few hikes there too, and I'd highly recommend it to anyone out there.

When I would go to LA to visit Austin, I rented a room in a trailer near a beach trail so I could save money by skipping hotels. It was far from ideal because I couldn't have Austin with me, but I was able to leave clothes and one of my bikes there so I could ride to the beach or run on the trail on my trips out. Problems with that arrangement though were the bed and the travel conditions. My personal travel was focused on finding the cheapest rates rather than something convenient, so the flights were often cramped red eyes. A lot of times my back would be in so much pain that I often had trouble walking for a few hours after getting up, but I learned that I could eventually walk the pain out or at least dull it enough so I could get some exercising in.

Because I didn't have cooking privileges there, I had to eat out and it usually wasn't the best menu options. Mostly it was McDonalds or other fast food joints and not very healthy, but it was about a six mile roundtrip hike so I would walk there to get my breakfast which offset the high fat calories. So despite the obstacles I was facing, it helped me a lot by simply incorporating exercise into my daily living.

There were a lot of stop and starts while I was trying to develop exercise and diet routines, and at first it slowed my progress. But once I realized that interruptions were part of my daily life, I focused on getting exercise and staying active rather than the exercise routines themselves. In other words, instead of trying to commit to getting to the gym for a set workout every day, I knew my schedules often wouldn't allow it. So I would focus on maybe taking a really long walk at the end of the day or doing some exercises in my hotel room.

Parts of my other problems were the bad habits I had developed in the past, so I really needed to get some new, good habits to replace them. One bad habit was to get a frozen yogurt almost every night. I'd trick myself into thinking that it wasn't ice cream so it was healthier, discounting the fact that the portions and the toppings actually had a lot more calories than the ice cream I would have eaten instead. Once I realized what it was doing to me, I stopped altogether, and later went to letting myself have a dessert at the end of the week to avoid developing cravings.

Another habit was portion sizes in general and meal seconds. Reducing the sizes and eliminating the seconds actually became easier once I learned the damage I had been doing to myself by starving myself early in the day and then stuffing myself later. The body is remarkable in that it adapts to the environment in order to try and save it, but in my case I was tricking it. By skipping meals, I was causing my body to think it was in a starvation environment, so instead of processing the food like normal to use as fuel, it was storing it as fat to use later since it technically wasn't sure when the next meal was going to come.

By overloading my body with food once I did eat, I piled on the weight quickly and put my metabolism under a lot of strain. I can remember being so full sometimes after starving all day that my heart would beat really, really fast and I'd have trouble breathing. I also had a lot of trouble breathing when I'd lie down to sleep at night because my weight seemed to be crushing my lungs and I couldn't get deep breaths. More importantly though, was the constant overloading of my system which taxed my metabolism in ways that caused a lot of damage and contributed to my diabetes.

Bit by bit I knocked those things off, letting myself go off the wagon periodically at the end of the week, but inserting some exercise habits like walking and biking in the same day to offset the temporary indulgences. Over time and as I continued to lose weight, one of the first things I began to notice was my inability to breathe, something I thought would have gotten better after getting thinner. To me there is nothing as scary as not being able to take a deep breath.

I learned later that it was my heart that would cause me to not be able to breathe right. Stress and too much sugar are major contributing factors, but my atrial fibrillation and high heart beat rates were causing the shortness of breath.

It was a long while before I was able to mitigate the stress, but the diet, exercise and subsequent weight losses definitely had positive effects overall. I'd still indulge in a mushroom burger with fries and a diet coke, but I'd often do that and workout shortly after. Or sometimes I'd have a low-cal meal consisting of a six-inch Subway tuna sub with double meat, no cheese or dressings on whole wheat bread, with a bag of chips and a diet coke. From a calorie perspective that was a pretty good meal, especially if I ate it right before or during a bike ride.

As part of my routine, I used the Sparkpeople.com 'Nutrition Tracker', which I found to be an excellent resource. It did a great job helping me know how many calories I was consuming, how many I was burning during exercises, and helped me to track my eating habits. It also exposed some red flags which helped me make changes for the better.

The red flags were the nutritional values or lack thereof. On one of the days that I chose to eat a Swiss mushroom burger for lunch and a tuna sub for dinner, I offset the meals with a twenty-five mile bike ride at about eighteen miles an hour so calorie wise I thought I did ok. But when I was pluggin g in the menu in my nutrition tracker food diary, I went down to the bottom of the page and flipped out. I never noticed it before, but they have a weekly progress report that shows the nutrient composition. The nutrients were what really started to stand out.

Below is a series of tables (Tables 1-8) which I created with the help of the nutrition tracker to show one day's diet when I thought I was eating right. I then compared to another day's diet after I learned otherwise and you'll see the differences are significant. I started out by watching calories and fat, but realized later on how important it was to focus on nutrition just as much. Like anything, menu planning and execution require learning and adapting to what is at hand. I traveled a lot, sometimes was without money, and until I started paying closer attention, I usually ate meals that were low in calories thinking they were healthy, but it turned out those meals were actually bad for me because they were so high in sodium and often lacked important nutrients.

TABLE 1: Low Calorie Breakfast

FOOD	CALORIES	FAT	CARBS	PROTEIN
Omelet	233	8	11	6
Pork Sausage - 3 patties	299	25	1	16
Whole Wheat Tortilla	130	3	22	4
Swiss Cheese - 2 slices	213	16	2	16
Totals	875	52	36	42

This was my typical breakfast which focused on low calories and low fat. In retrospect, this is still higher in calories and fat than what I eat now on a regular basis, but quite a drop compared with the 1,500 calorie breakfasts I was eating before. These tables don't show the sodium counts because I wasn't monitoring them at the time but you will see them in **Table 8**. This is to illustrate how I came to think what I was eating was okay.

TABLE 2: Low Calorie Lunch

FOOD	CALORIES	FAT	CARBS	PROTEIN
Mushroom Swiss Burger	820	46	60	48
Fries	396	15	62	6
Diet Coke	0	0	0	0
Totals	1216	61	122	54

This was actually an occasional lunch in which I would indulge myself if I was planning a long bike ride or other intense workout. My typical lunch is more like 500 to 700 calories.

TABLE 3: Low Calorie Dinner

FOOD	CALORIES	FAT	CARBS	PROTEIN
Subway Tuna	663	39	55	28
BBQ Chips	150	10	15	2
Totals	813	49	70	30

This was a standard dinner though not always sandwiches but usually meat and cheese with crackers or fish and rice.

TABLE 4: Healthy Breakfast

FOOD	CALORIES	FAT	CARBS	PROTEIN
Turkey Cheeseburger (2)	713	55	6	50
Coffee w/2% Milk	54	1	8	0
1/4 PB&J	58	8	0	2
Fried Egg	35	2	1	3
Totals	860	66	15	55

This is a typical breakfast before a bike ride but focused as much on nutrients as well as calories. **Table 8** shows the significant difference in sodium compared with my previous diet regimen.

TABLE 5: Healthy Snack

FOOD	CALORIES	FAT	CARBS	PROTEIN
Green Iced Tea	8	0	0	0
Peeled Cucumber	8	0	1	0
Totals	15	1	1	0

This was enough to take the edge off of my hunger, and it was healthy.

TABLE 6: Healthy Lunch

FOOD	CALORIES	FAT	CARBS	PROTEIN
Oil/Vinegar	8	9	0	0
Peeled Cucumber	8	0	1	0
Jalapeño Pepper	4	1	0	0
Tomato	35	0	7	11
Thin-cut Beef Steak (3)	519	45	0	28
Totals	574	55	8	39

I was amazed at how filling this meal was and how much energy I got from it.

TABLE 7: Healthy Dinner

FOOD	CALORIES	FAT	CARBS	PROTEIN
Chicken Tandori - Organic chicken thigh (boneless/skinless) (2)	187	4	7	11
Green Iced Tea	8	0	0	0
Totals	195	4	7	11

I have found that discipline is a much needed piece to managing a healthy regimen. There is no way that I would have considered a couple of chicken thighs to be an adequate meal in the past before I knew I had diabetes, yet this meal was very satisfying.

TABLE 8: Low Calorie vs. Nutritional Meals

TYPE	GOAL PER DAY	HEALTHY FARE	LOW CAL
calories	2600-2990	1779	3154
fat	80-100	115	181
carbohydrates	330-374	32	257
protein	132-150	115	140
potassium	4500-6000	1034	2179
calcium	120-200	60	144
sodium	< 2300	1832	5393
magnesium	80-175	9	34
folate	100-250	7	26
cholesterol	0-300	22	869

Originally when I focused on low calories and low fat I felt pretty good at largely meeting those targets until I saw my sodium intake while I was looking deeper into the Sparkpeople.com tables at the end of the week, something I had never paid much attention to before even though I set the targets when I first set up the tracker. Notice in the Healthy Fare row, the sodium count for the day is at 1,832 and well below my target of less than 2300 mg, because of my high blood pressure. In the Low Calorie row when I ate the Swiss Burger and the Tuna Sub my sodium for the day was over 5000 mg. The burger was approximately 3,200 mg of sodium and the tuna sub was about 1,600 mg. That sodium reading explained why I was feeling flushed, having rapid heartbeats and had trouble sleeping. I had no idea I was eating more than three times the amount of sodium recommended for diabetics with high blood pressure.

I used that information and started looking at everything I was eating. While I thought I was eating a pretty healthy diet I learned that just the opposite was true. A normal breakfast was a couple of hard boiled eggs, about a half to full cup of cottage cheese, and some fruit or peanut butter toast if I was going out to exercise. Lunch a lot of times was the tuna sub from Subway, and dinner was salad or deli turkey, Swiss cheese and crackers like Wheat Thins or Triscuits. From a calorie standpoint I was doing pretty well, but the sodium count was still extremely high according to the Tracker. The eggs and cottage cheese combined were over 800 mg, the tuna sub was a whopping 1,600 mg, and the deli meats and cheese combined were over a 1,000 mg. What I thought was fairly healthy was over 3,400 mg of sodium a day.

I quickly changed my diet by eliminating a lot from it like deli meats and cheese, eggs and cottage cheese, and substituting naturally low sodium foods like fruits, vegetables and lean meats. I still eat eggs and cheese at times but sparingly and I use olive oil to cook with. A good rule of thumb is that processed foods are often high in sodium, so I have learned to limit portions to offset it like when I have a hankering for Costco potato salad which is very tasty but high in sodium.

In comparison, look at the differences now. Turkey burgers with a fried egg for breakfast is not a normal meal (Table 4) but every once in a while I do it to break up the meal boredom or when I'm planning on a long bike ride. My normal breakfast is low carb granola and one slice of peanut butter toast; and that knocks off about 400 mg of sodium from the 1,893 mg for the day.

Although I focus primarily on calories, carbs, fats, and sodium, I still look at the others like cholesterol and potassium. My potassium reading in Table 8 shows that it is still very low, but for reasons I discuss in other chapters I consult a doctor before taking steps on my own to correct. Potassium is listed as an essential mineral that benefits the heart and helps to lower high blood pressure, but it is hard to find a general range of recommendations for diabetics online because the wrong amount can be problematic and can result in doses that are either too high or too low. Most of the websites defer to your doctor or healthcare professional because the dosages are based on your individual circumstances.

Also note the cholesterol levels once I changed my eating habits (Table 8). When I indulged myself with the mushroom burgers once in a while and eggs frequently, my cholesterol was way over target. After I converted to a healthier fare it dropped considerably.

Once I realized I was eating bad foods while thinking I was eating right, I added food research to the list of things that needed attention. I ran across these five foods as bad foods from the Trim-Down Club www.info.trimdownclub.com. This site, like Sparkpeople.com, has many helpful features including apps for food planning tools and journals. The list was a little surprising to me in terms of what I needed to know about food and it was reinforced by what I had seen on other sites.

> *Five bad foods:*
> *1)Concentrated fruit juices*
> *Fiber removed = sugar water that goes to fat storage*
> *2)Margarine – (trans fats), butter can be a better alternative because saturated fats can be burned*
> *3)Whole wheat bread is a high carb food despite being heralded as healthy*
> *4)Processed soy (tofu, soy milk) vs. edamame*
> *5)Corn that has been genetically modified, instead of farm fresh*

The offset is to focus on nutrient dense foods and the need to balance carbs with protein meals. Here's an example:

Low carb foods include beans and nuts while high carb foods include breads, pasta, and beer. High carb foods quickly convert to glucose, but since diabetics have trouble using the glucose in their system, we need to balance our carb intake to help our bodies process them better. If you're a stress eater seeking out comfort foods, you're asking for more trouble. Cortisol induced by stress increases appetite and heightens cravings for carbs. Experts say that high stress eating is a quick way to gain weight and eventually contract diabetes. That is exactly what happened to me.

I've said before that having a strict meal plan didn't necessarily work for me because my work and travel schedules didn't allow much room to comply with a strict plan. But I know the food groups I need to watch out for and how to balance my food intake so I can adapt to what I might be stuck with for food choices. I have friends who have been on strict plans and have reaped tremendous rewards by getting a healthier diet and a change in their lifestyles.

As I've mentioned before but worth repeating, there are quite a few offerings online for recipes, trackers, and monitors like Sparkpeople.com and WebMd.com. There are also health retreats like the Joslin Diabetes Center, Whitaker Institute, and Duke University.

Whitaker, Duke, The Mayo Clinic and many others also have published diet plan books which are life-saving guides. One of my favorite books on nutrition is 'How to Prevent and Treat Diabetes with Natural Medicine' (Lyon, 2004). It is a compelling book that guides the reader through the how, why, and what to eat if you want to cure your diabetes. It is a detailed guide for both Type1 and Type 2 though the authors do not give hope of a cure for Type 1. Type 1diabetes happens because the body is not producing insulin or not enough so a cure can't be found simply through diet and exercise.

Type 2 on the other hand is due to the body not processing what it is producing or consuming and those can be altered or reversed through diet and exercise. One item that struck me was how the authors had a similar notion about the disease being a good one for people who have a genuine desire to get healthy. This truly is a disease that makes getting healthy a life or death choice.

After going through various books, nutrition guides, and diabetic cookbooks, I began to develop a better sense of the right and wrong things to eat. Processed foods, sub sandwiches and restaurant burgers were all problems for me because of the sodium, but there was nothing wrong with a double-meat Tuna Salad at Subway instead since the tuna is natural and not processed. I can still indulge myself with a bag of chips if I want. Lots of vegetables, fish and chicken are far better for me and that's what I now gravitate toward so that I can shop and eat without having to overthink it, but still focus on getting healthy.

In addition to covering my diabetes concerns, I also needed to find ways of eating that reduced the risks of the associated ailments like heart disease and stroke. I found that there were a wide variety of foods available including vegetables, whole grains, fruits, non-fat dairy products, beans, lean meats, poultry, and fish. In simple terms, anyone with health problems like obesity, heart disease or high blood pressure should eat as though they were diabetics. They'll get to eat great stuff that will be really good for them.

I'm not so keen on the non-dairy stuff like soy milk or tofu as substitutes for dairy, but I also limit my intake of dairy to begin with so in general I don't have much of a problem in that area.. In my research I have seen Mediterranean diets heralded more and more as great diets for diabetics because they are comprised of lighter fares heavy on the fish, fruits and vegetables along with lots of olive oil.

So I have been working on getting recipes, finding stores that sell the foods, and locating Mediterranean restaurants because I happen to really like the food.

It's important to note that there isn't a perfect food for diabetics which is actually good news because it lets us enjoy a variety of different foods. The critical element here is to watch portion sizes and make sure that you are picking natural foods rich in vitamins, minerals and fiber over those that are processed.

Diabetics can also eat what their peers or families are eating, but if the family chooses to adapt to eating more like you as a diabetic then they will definitely benefit from the healthy choices. For some with the disease, especially those with type 1 diabetes, it takes advanced planning but favorite foods can definitely fit into a meal plan while paying attention to glucose, blood pressure, and cholesterol levels.

The National Diabetes Information Clearinghouse (NDIC) is a great resource for getting a start on understanding portion controls, good and bad foods and a whole slew of information to benefit people with the disease. The first time I talked to a nutritionist she summed it up pretty easily for me: try to eat five or six meals a day about the size of your balled up fist. **Table 9** is helpful to gain perspective of what lands on your plan and portion sizes.

While each portion below may seem small, remember that these portions combine to form a full meal. Think of a chicken thigh with a small salad and mashed potatoes; even for a guy my size I find that to be very satisfying and doesn't leave me feeling stuffed.

TABLE 9: A Guide to Sensible Serving Sizes

THIS MUCH	IS THE SAME SIZE AS
(open palm)	**3 ounces:** 1 serving of meat, chicken, turkey, or fish
(fist)	**1 cup:** 1 serving of cooked vegetables, salads, casseroles or stews, such as chili withbeans, milk
(thumb)	**1/2 cup:** 1 serving of fruit or fruit juice, starchy vegetables, such as potatoes or corn, pinto beans and other dried beans, rice or noodles, cereal
(cupped hand)	**1 ounce:** 1 serving of snack food, cheese (1 slice)
(thumb tip)	**1 tablespoon:** 1 serving of salad dressing, cream cheese
(fingertip)	**???:** mayonnaise

Source: U.S. DEPARTMENT OF HEALTH AND HUMAN SERVICES, National Diabetes Information. Clearinghouse (NDIC) - *What I need to know about Eating and Diabetes (08-5043, 2007)*

Once I became aware of how my diet affected my overall well-being, I started paying attention to food labels and bought the foods according to what was going to give me the best results. As I indicated earlier, eggs are naturally high in sodium so I cut down on those and looked at cereal as an alternative. Then I paid attention to the calories and carb counts, and found Bear Naked natural granola worked for me. Most cereal has 36 to 48 g of carbs, Bear Naked has 18 to 25 g, and it's delicious and filling. I also was going with peanut butter toast because the peanut butter was a healthy fat that helped keep me from getting hungry, but I was adding extra carbs and sodium with the bread, so I went with a tablespoon to a tablespoon and a half of peanut butter without the bread.

There are other important things to look for when reading the labels. Look for heart-healthy stuff like whole-wheat flour and oats. Also watch the fats and try to stick to things like olive, canola or peanut oils because they're better than butter and promote heart health. The American Heart Association is a great resource to help identify heart healthy foods. Although butter is listed as a healthier food earlier in the chapter, it is less healthy when it is compared with the oils listed here which are natural vegetable fats vs. animal fats. Try to stay away from hydrogenated or partially hydrogenated oils whenever you can. In fact, you really should stay away from those altogether because they're trans-fats and will cause your cholesterol levels to rise.

Fiber is very important for diabetics and I get mine from a variety of fiber-rich foods like baked beans, brown rice or bran, and psyllium, which, admittedly, doesn't taste all that great but does a great job at ensuring you're getting the fiber you need. Something else to be careful about are sugar-free or no-sugar-added foods, at least read the ingredients so you can tell if the product is high in carbs even though it says sugar free. There is a difference since carbs will convert to sugar, so don't be fooled if you're objective is keeping your sugar intake low.

I don't know if this can still happen because of the labeling laws, but one mother I knew was bragging that she was watching out for how much sugar her kids were eating and pointed out on the label on the drink she was giving them wasn't sweetened with sugar. It was sweetened with high fructose corn syrup instead. I guess you could give her an A for effort, but she needed to dig a little deeper. Had she done so she would have learned that she was trading sugar for more heavily processed sugar; any time you see the "oses", fructose, sucrose, dextrose, and of course glucose, then you should know these are sugars and your body treats them that way. The other ones you have to look for are sugar alcohols like sorbitol, xylitol and mannitol. These aren't always low in carbohydrates or calories either.

By now though it should be getting pretty clear that anything processed is what you have to be looking hard at. If it's natural, you mainly need to know what you're eating so you will know how it impacts you, but you don't have to worry about Mother Nature sticking in some other ingredients then calling them by different names.

Diabetes, while now a fairly common disease is still based on the individual who has it, therefore not everyone is going to have the same goals. Some are going to focus on counting and cutting calories while others are going to need to watch fat and salt. Still others may need to have more fiber. I have set an aggressive target and need to lose another forty-five pounds as quickly I can while doing it and staying healthy so I'm focused on watching calories, fat, and salt and making sure I'm getting regular exercise.

If you eat out a lot, the American Diabetes Association has some helpful tips on how to order at restaurants, whether fast food or sit down venues at www.diabetes.org. If you are able, order only what you need and want, like if you are getting a simple bacon and eggs breakfast with an order of toast, go with one egg and one slice of toast if that's all you need. Be sure to know how to make changes in your meal plan in case the restaurant doesn't have just what you want.

Here are a few tips:

» Just because the restaurant serves you a bigger portion doesn't mean you have to eat it all. Put the extra food in a container to go or share it with your partner.
» If you're going to order a baked potato, put the toppings on yourself and control what and how much you put on.
» Get sauces and dressings served on the side, dip instead of pour.
» Stay away from fried foods.
» Don't forget to ask for substitutes like extra vegetables instead of potatoes. Most restaurants are aware of individual tastes and needs and will probably accommodate you.
» Remember, just because they end up serving you some food you want like rolls or breadsticks it doesn't mean you have to eat it.

Find a restaurant or restaurants that are health and calorie conscious so you can relax a little about your diet. Seasons 52 is a great restaurant chain that not only serves great food in a relaxing atmosphere, it guarantees that nothing on its menu is over four hundred and seventy-five calories. I've eaten there quite a few times and found it to be a very enjoyable experience.

Knowing about the foods you eat in terms of nutrients, calories, carbs, sodium and cholesterol is probably the best defense when having to eat on the fly. If I'm with my son who is a committed high-school athlete and health nut, we often eat out but try to visit healthy venues like Daphne's, Flame Broiler or Subway. Austin orders what he likes best, and I order what I like as well as what is good for me. If we wind up in a not-so-health-friendly joint, I look for fish or places that serve non-fried foods as part of the menu. If it's burgers then I eat them without the bun, or I make up for it later by intensifying my workout to offset the higher calories This is also where food diaries or the Sparkpeople.com Nutrition Tracker can be big help because they let you keep track of how you're doing overall.

More on eating on the fly, especially for fast food:

» On average, fast-food meals can be one-thousand calories or more and are high in fat.
» If you have to eat a fast-food meal, offset it by eating healthy on the others and working out.
» Stick to broiled, baked, or grilled, and stay away from fried. Fish and chicken are good choices.
» Some places will let you substitute sides with extra vegetables; this is an option that works great.

There's a whole lot more to be said about fast food, and buffets for that matter but at some point you're going to have to inject some common sense. A good rule of thumb that will apply no matter what the circumstance is this: everything in moderation. We diabetics have to learn right off the bat that portion control is one of our biggest worries, right along with processed versus natural.

Fast food and buffets are usually very unhealthy combinations of both processed and natural. Just because their portions are big or the food is lying out there for the taking doesn't mean you have to eat it. One-half of a Big Mac is about the same as a regular burger, so take the other half home for another meal. Hold the mayo, and grab a side salad instead of fries. Know your proteins and your carbs so you can offset them on the fly.

> » Medium Fries = calories + carbs + fat
> (380 cal., 48g carbs, 19g fat)
> vs.
> Side salad w/oil & vinegar = low calories + low carbs + low fat (90 cal., 4g carbs, 8g fat)

Buffets are real problems for anyone who seeks comfort in eating. We get up there and start eating like the world is about to end; and it is rare that anyone at an all-you-can-eat buffet sits down with less than two plates then goes up for seconds. When the seconds are gone, then there is the dessert buffet.

One of the things that got me looking long and hard at buffets is the average weight of the people eating there; many of them were obese. Still, I had a bit of a weakness for a sushi/Chinese buffet but as I mentioned earlier I learned to offset it and I did so by doing an eight mile roundtrip walk to get there and back whenever I had the urge.

But more often than not, when we are eating at buffets and fast food joints, we are just adding fat and pounds and blocking ourselves from developing good eating habits.

Preventing or controlling diabetes really boils down to one thing, lifestyle. Everything else falls inside of that. We can make a huge difference by changing the lifestyle that got us in trouble in the first place, and losing weight is the most important thing to get in check. The good news is that you don't have to lose it all overnight to start seeing results. Many experts say losing a small percentage, five or ten percent, will help you lower your blood sugar levels significantly. Ten percent of my weight was about thirty-two pounds, and the experts were right, I began to see a lot of changes. I don't know if anyone else would take comfort in this, but I was very relieved to know that I had some control over this disease that could otherwise hurt or kill me. By making some positive lifestyle changes I have been able to keep that lion in its cage.

Obesity is by far the greatest risk factor for developing diabetes, but it's important to know details about the type of fat you're carrying and how it is distributed. Muffin top or spare tire shapes, where weight is stored in the abdomen, are at greater risk than people whose fat is distributed more evenly. A pear-shaped person has less risk than an apple-shaped person. The difference between the two is the pear-shaped person has most of their fat stored closely below the skin whereas the apple-shaped individuals have their fat surrounding their organs, like their livers. According to a number of studies, this type of fat storage is tied in closely to diabetes and insulin resistance. Studies also show that the size of a person's waist is a better indicator of whether or not they'll get diabetes than their body-mass index (BMI).

Men whose waists are forty inches or greater and women with waists thirty-five inches or more have higher risks of developing diabetes than those whose waists are smaller. Foods and drinks sweetened with fructose or high fructose corn syrup will likely cause you to store fat in the belly, so it's important to know what kinds of foods and drinks these are.

Doughnuts, cereal, granola bars, candy and muffins are big offenders, as well as energy drinks, sport drinks, coffee drinks and of course non-diet soda, so choose carefully and read the labels. As I researched the disease and the best places to immediately act on to help gain control, I quickly learned to go natural, reduce portions, and to balance my diet. The objective was and is to spread eating out so as to avoid being hungry or full. Even though I'm not a hardcore body-builder I learned during the process that food was indeed fuel for my body so I needed to be sure that I was using a quality fuel.

One of the first things I learned was the difference between good carbs and bad carbs, and also how to balance carbs. Good carbs consist of whole grain foods, fruits, vegetables and legumes. Bad carbs are sugar and anything refined like sweets and desserts. Natural vs. processed is a major factor when developing a diet plan for diabetics, but even if it is a natural food you still have to consider what it is you're eating. Natural fruit, especially if it is ripe can be high in sugar like bananas or peaches, so you may have to eat less or balance it with protein. A great snack is an apple with a piece of cheese.

Once you know what to eat, it's important that you know how to eat meaning that food is fuel and needs to be on a regular intake. I was able to validate this in an interesting way. Once when I was starting to focus on increasing my bike riding distances, I was shooting for thirty miles for the first time. Weather wise it was a great day. I was a little over three hundred pounds at the time and determined to make the changes

I needed to make. I ate a filling breakfast to make sure I had enough energy for the ride, and balanced it with protein, some fat, and good carbs and I made sure I had plenty of water at breakfast and to carry with me on the ride. It started out as a great ride with minimal wind, so I was averaging about sixteen to eighteen miles an hour and feeling good. But by mile fourteen, I was starting to drag and could feel my energy levels dropping way down. I was upset that I might not be able to make my goal for the day, but reached into my pocket and pulled out a peanut butter granola bar and ate it while I continued to ride. It was amazing but I could actually feel my energy levels rise as I ate it. I ate a second one shortly after and without stopping finished my ride with a half mile over my goal.

Had I not been paying attention and getting a good understanding about how food works in diabetics, I'm not so sure I would have made my goals that day. There is a great resource at Helpguide.org, with a great web article called 'Diabetes Diet & Food Tips'. They offer some great suggestions about the best ways to deal with the disease and do it in a simple, easy to understand format.

Glycemic Index

Something else that's important to know is the glycemic index (GI), a measure of how a carb impacts blood sugar, and it ranks the food on a scale of low to high. A food with a high GI could cause blood sugar levels to spike more than a low or medium one.

When you develop a diet plan making note of the GI is important but it shouldn't necessarily be the governing factor as some diets seem to do. Simply put, simple carbs rank high on the GI while complex carbs are medium to low, so it is a good way to get an understanding of which foods you should eat more or less of. Meats and fats are not on the list because they're not carbs, but that doesn't mean you should ignore them. Fish and skinless chicken are good ways to go, and so are lean meats.

A rule of thumb is that processed foods usually rank higher on the scale, as do foods with higher fat or fiber content, but that isn't always the case. Age and ripeness of fruit and vegetables can cause it to rank higher on the GI scale because the sugar content can increase in certain ones if they ripen on the vine. Fat and fiber can lower the

GI of a food, so you could have a food very high in fat that could look great on the GI scale if you're not careful. A good rule of thumb is the more cooked or processed a food, the higher the GI, while foods high in fat can look good on the GI scale but not be good for you.

There are many Glycemic Index Charts available through a web search, including GI Calculators for anyone who is interested. I constructed a simple table using information gathered by a few random charts to illustrate how such a chart can be used.

In the table below, the 100 ranking means pure sugar or pure glucose, so everything else is based on how much sugar is contained in a particular food. This table illustrates some basics about certain foods. The scale is 70 and above = High, 55 to 69 = Medium, and 55 and below = Low.

The Glycemic load is based on the amount of carbohydrate in the food, meaning that the food has other things like fat and protein in some cases. So at first glance these all look pretty good on a GI scale, but how does it impact the rest of your diet? It depends on where you're getting the cake from and how it was made. The typical banana cake has a calorie range of 98 to a whopping 463 calories per slice, and a fat range of 6g to 18g. That is a big difference and could impact your other goals.

TABLE 10: A Sample GI Chart

BREADS and CAKES

FOOD	Glycemic index (glucose =100)	Serving size (grams)	Glycemic load per serving
Banana cake, made with sugar	55	60	14
Banana cake, made without sugar	47	60	12
Sponge cake, plain	46	63	17
Vanilla cake made from packet mix with vanilla frosting (Betty Crocker)	42	111	24

The Mayo Clinic offers some great suggestions on how to properly use the GI rankings and offers a few suggestions and cautions in a web article titled Glycemic Index Diet: What's Behind the Claims (Mayo Clinic Staff, 2014). Remember that the index is a guide and not necessarily a good way to plan a diet. Rather than building a diet around the index, focus more on your individual needs based upon how your body processes what you eat and what you need for balance. For myself I don't eat any of the items in the table so it wouldn't do me any good to build my diet on it.

I avoid processed foods and cakes, and what I do eat like chips, granola cereal, yams, and so forth fall in to the low scale on the GI and I achieved that by focusing on natural foods and balancing what I eat when I fall off the wagon. I'm a firm believer that you can develop unconscious habits so that eating right becomes second nature. I had some cheesecake the other night which was the first time in at least a year. It was tasty but I felt uncomfortable eating it because it wasn't part of my new habit. I was going through some pretty intense stress which caused me to fall back in to an older routine which was to eat (and drink) to forget.

I ate a very health conscious meal like normal, but had one beer with it then strawberry cheesecake with whipped cream for dessert. I also had two glasses of red wine later in the evening. That was me going off the deep edge but in a new way. My blood sugar after all that was 130 mg/dl, without any meds. When I compare this menu to what I used to do to myself, I realized I wasn't doing anywhere near the damage I had in the past.

A note about alcohol when it comes to diet, we all tend to forget or underestimate the number of calories in alcoholic drinks, especially if the drinks are mixed with juice or soda. There can be a lot of sugar so if you are going to enjoy a few drinks, plan ahead and try not to overdo it, especially if you are on medication. Diet and sugar-free mixers can work well, and dry wine if you like wine. I cut down on my drinking quite a bit. I was having a couple of glasses a night and partying on the weekends a few years back, I'm now down to maybe a couple of glasses every couple of weeks on average. I pretty much stay with dry red wine though on occasion I might mix it with diet Seven-Up which makes a poor man's Wine Spritzer. Or I might have a couple of fingers of whiskey. I noticed a while back that alcohol seemed to keep me from dropping weight plus I had overall concerns about adding complications to the disease, so I've learned to be more cautious.

Finally, and before moving on to exercise habits, I found that keeping a food diary is an important way to get your eating under control and to develop new eating habits. Making big changes such as daily living means that you have to know what you are doing on a day-to-day basis so you can start to identify what you need to change. It also helps you identify the things that are easiest to change, because like anything else making changes requires practice and determination.

If you are making changes on your own, it's best to start small and build from there. Small changes will show results that will encourage you. You're not going to lose twenty pounds in your first week, but eliminating a food that causes you to feel bloated or raises your heartbeat will give you an immediate sense of satisfaction. Once you see your blood sugar levels getting under control because of the changes you're making, you will have a real sense of achievement even though you may have only lost a pound or two. Any of us who are obese and have diabetes because of it can never lose sight of taking the weight off and keeping it off.

It's also important to develop an eating schedule so your body can adapt. Our bodies are remarkable things and will help us thrive if we help them by not overloading them. A regular eating schedule will help eliminate the hunger/full peaks and valleys as well as the glucose spikes caused by carb overloads.

Psychologically, if you avoid letting yourself get hungry by eating healthy snacks and small meals, you can resist temptations much more easily. When I travelled a lot for work, I used to keep some healthy, low-carb/high-protein snack bars along with a bag of raw almonds in my computer bag. I ate those at a moderate pace so it kept me from starving by the time I was able to eat a meal. When I did get to sit down to eat, I was able to manage my portions better. I'd like to say that I always ate sensibly but there were a lot of times when I didn't have that luxury because I often worked under intense deadlines and had to grab whatever was handy.

The Importance Of Exercise To Burn Food As Fuel

Just as important as diet is exercise, for a whole lot of reasons. One of those reasons, and it's a big one, is weight loss but there is also evidence that exercise can help you increase insulin sensitivity which is needed to process glucose levels.

I talked earlier about the struggles I've had with establishing routines, but I always kept my focus on getting some kind of exercise whenever possible and that has helped me tremendously. The beauty of this is you don't have to start out big you simply just need to start and work your way up, just like when trying to adapt to a new diet.

Some suggestions are to try walking for thirty minutes five times a week, and if that works for you that is a great place to start. I worked exercise into things that I had to do because I couldn't always commit to something like walking five times a week. While I lived in Chicago, my room was about a mile and a half from some stores where I shopped with a paved trail leading to them. With a short list to fill, I'd walk there instead of driving so I'd get some supplies while walking a total of three miles at a brisk pace.

I also would alternate between walking and bike riding. I'd try to get at least ten miles in at between sixteen to eighteen mph, but I kept reaching for longer distances. The idea of exercise is muscle movement that causes you to work up a sweat. House work and yard work count.

The first thing I noticed was an indirect benefit as it related to diabetes. Exercise has a tremendous impact on warding off depression and releasing adrenaline to keep you sharp and alert.

There is so much more that exercise does for you especially if you have type 2 diabetes, some benefits are obvious and some are not. Some of the obvious ones are burning off excess body fat to help you drop weight while improving muscle strength and tone. Most will increase your energy levels and help you relax by reducing stress and tension. I usually take a mini DVD player with me to the gym and watch some exciting shows while I spend up to an hour on the exercise bike. I do that because the gym I use only has TV on it and what plays on it is stuff I hate watching. Having my own DVD helps pass the time and keeps me from getting bored when I'm doing it, especially if it's a good show.

Not-so-obvious benefits are lowering blood pressure, increasing bone density, and improving blood circulation, and helps lower bad cholesterol. In short, exercise is good for you whether you have diabetes or not, but if you do have it exercise can help save your life.

A funny thing about exercise and blood sugar levels; when I've tested my blood sugar after various workouts I saw that my levels actually went up and that first gave me some cause for concern. Shouldn't exercise help you lower blood sugar? As a general rule that's true, especially if the workout is easy to moderate. But the more intense it is the more likely that it will go up temporarily because your body treats exercise as a form of stress and your liver releases more glucose to help fuel your muscles.

This is why you will often see cautions to talk to your doctor about the kinds of exercising you should be doing, because there is such a thing as your blood sugar being too high for exercise. When that happens the results could be fatal. Ketoacidosis can happen when your body is burning fat for energy instead of glucose. Fat burning produces ketones, and too much in your blood can cause a diabetic coma or in some cases death.

Some of the best exercises for diabetics are strength training and aerobic exercises. After finding out I had diabetes and taking my health seriously, I started exercising and tried running and walking but found that my excessive weight caused some real problems in my feet and joints. So I focused first on bicycling which proved to be a great way to lose weight and gain strength. The first couple of weeks I needed to get my body accustomed to it. My butt and thighs were aching even after only a couple of miles but I only allowed a maximum of forty-eight hours to pass before getting back on and working toward increasing my workout or my distance. It got easier each time I got on the bike and rode, and it's funny how I can now do forty or fifty miles without needing much time to recoup.

Bicycling is also fun because you can watch the scenery change and you can plan trips around your rides. I've ridden along Lake Michigan and in some beautiful Forest Preserves throughout Illinois. I've done the L.A.T.E. ride in downtown Chicago at one o'clock in the morning along with nine thousand other riders for a twenty-five mile loop. Once I got back to California, one of my favorite things was to take my bike on the train from my roommate's house up to Anaheim Stadium where I pick up the Santa Ana River trail. It is a paved trail that ends at the beach in Huntington Beach, and if the beach is your destination then you can do twenty-six miles round trip or go the entire length for fifty-six miles. I've done both and loved it.

I also have ridden my bike from San Juan Capistrano to Camp Pendleton, which is about a thirty to forty mile route with tons of hills depending upon how you map it out. The ride goes through San Onofre State Park which sports a beautiful view of the ocean from the bluffs as you ride. My next step is to complete my one-hundred-miler which is to ride through Camp Pendleton to San Diego.

I have also found that some rides are great to go on with clubs especially if you have health concerns or don't know the area. I have belonged to two riding clubs and through them was able to find ride locations that I would not have known existed. Being in the clubs also gave me backups in case I ran into trouble along the way, and being a diabetic this should be a major area of concern if you are just starting out.

I have hit major sugar lows on some of my early rides and once had to be escorted to safety by some fellow riders. The significant thing was they recognized it before I did and got something in me before I completely passed out. I was very lucky that day and it sunk in just how much I needed to pay attention to what my body was saying and what I needed to do to keep it from happening.

It's usually pretty easy to find a bicycle club if you're looking, and bike shops are often good resources. But if you don't ride with a club then it is advisable to ride on trails where there are other riders. The river trail I ride on is heavily traveled with avid riders so you can have backup that way, but it's not congested so you can travel at high speeds if you want as long as you're careful.

The simplest objective is to exercise and work your body at intensity levels it can accept at that moment, and remember that you're not going to undo the results from ten years of bad habits in one week of exercising no matter how badly you would like. Go easy and find any way to exercise and when you are starting to rack up the active minutes each week, then look at alternate routines but just make sure your body is as ready as your mind.

Eating and keeping your energy up is critical when you start to exercise; be sure to check your blood levels. Nothing is more disheartening than having a great exercise plan only to have it shut down because your body can't take it. I spent quite a while planning a bike trip on a beautiful trail in Illinois. My plan for the day was a thirty-mile round trip along the tree-lined and reasonably cool Fox River. I packed snacks which only consisted of two energy bars with plenty of water but I wasn't worrying about packing anything more because I felt great. I hadn't factored in the thirty-five minute drive to get there from where I was living and another ten to fifteen minutes for parking and prep once I got there.

I had eaten what I thought was a good breakfast and felt energized, so when I hit the trail I was really jazzed because I was pacing at between eighteen to twenty miles an hour and not even breathing hard. After about five miles I hit a low energy wall and almost passed out. I was very dizzy and had trouble walking. Once I was able to get to a bench I had trouble keeping my eyes open and was shaking. I was able to get some of my energy back by eating the snacks I had brought, but only enough to barely make it back my car and to a place where I could get some food. There were no stores along the trail.

I got to where I was on the trail in about twenty minutes, but it took me over an hour to get back at the same distance and I almost fell off my bike twice because I was so dizzy and weak. Too much time had passed since I had eaten. The two biggest problems for me that day were that I allowed too much time to pass between eating, and my meal and energy bar snacks weren't substantial or balanced. They were too high in carbs and not enough protein, so I was getting spikes from high to low. I should have had a PBJ and some cheese, and the water should have been much colder. It was a lesson learned but it wasn't a fun one. It was also a little scary because the trail wasn't heavily traveled so I didn't see anyone else the entire time I was there.

There was another factor about exercising that caught me off guard, the impact of heat. I noticed that on especially hot days I had trouble maintaining energy levels even when I was exercising inside, so I researched to see if there were any extra problems for diabetics trying to exercise when it was hot. I forgot that excess glucose in the blood can itself cause dehydration; the risk is greater if your levels are high on a very hot day. Dehydration is more likely if you are drinking caffeine or alcohol.

Diabetics and people with heart disease are more susceptible to overheating. Since I have both I can understand why I have at times felt the symptoms of heat exhaustion including dizziness or fainting, excessive sweating, muscle cramps, and clammy skin. Other symptoms include headaches, rapid heartbeat, and nausea.

The Joslin Diabetes Center recommends you move to a cooler environment and drink some water, juice or sports drinks and seek medical attention. They also recommend that you store your diabetic supplies in a cool, dry place and protect your insulin supply. For pump users there are additional precautions because of extra perspiration. You may need to pay attention to whether or not the adhesive is loosening and if the pump is exposed to too much heat. Of course, be sure to consult with your health care professional about the best courses of action for you, whether it is diet, exercise, or dealing with the heat.

Monitor Your Blood

Blood monitoring regularly is a really important part of helping you gain control of the disease. It's a method to tell you if what you're doing is working; if not, when you need to be getting in to the doctor's office. There don't appear to be consistent blood level table references, so it took me a while to understand what tables are the best ones to use and what levels should be concerning. I found differences of opinions even among my doctors. I also would check in with friends to see how their levels were and what their doctors were saying about it. I came to realize that a) I need to check my levels regularly, and b) start to worry when my levels are showing high readings. The NDIC shows this range as acceptable:

TABLE 11: Blood Monitoring	
Before meals	70 to 130 mg/dl
1 to 2 hours after the start of a meal	less than 180 mg/dl

Source: U.S. DEPARTMENT OF HEALTH AND HUMAN SERVICES, National Diabetes Information. Clearinghouse (NDIC) - *What I need to know about Eating and Diabetes (08-5043, 2007)*

I've seen tables indicate a tighter range of 70-110 mg/dl before meals and 120-140 mg/dl within two hours after eating. I have placed a ten-day log below to show how I tracked my progress. If you look, you'll see that with the exception of a few spikes my levels all fall into the ones in the chart. In general, I was happy with the progress, but it was the fasting levels that were particularly worrisome to me at that stage and I stayed focused on it. My average fasting levels over a thirty day period were at 135 mg/dl, so clearly I needed work but I was at least heading in the right direction. Believe me, if I had been seeing regular readings above 180 mg/dl I would have found some way to get myself to a doctor.

Over time, I have been able to maintain healthy eating in general but once I got the right parameters in place my biggest problem was being able to afford to eat right. Because of my unsteady earnings and lack of work, I wasn't always able to get fresh vegetables and good meats.

There were times when I could only eat what was left in the house until more money came in. At times I'd have to eat peanut butter and jelly or cheese sandwiches at least twice in a day. Other times were lunches and dinners of tortillas and refried beans for several days because that's all I could afford at the dollar store, or because it was left over by visitors who brought them. I would put on a little weight because of it, but would resume the right diet once I got paid.

That was a different lifestyle, but one I had no choice over because it was purely related to my circumstances. In the big picture, I was still eating healthier overall and my heart seemed to be in good shape. I could tell because my beats were steady and I had very few bouts of shortness of breath which used to be a big problem when I was heavier and under stress. Now the diet and routines were helping. High blood pressure was still a big problem though and I would feel it each time I ate the bean burritos or PBJs, but there wasn't much I could do.

Although I had to live that way for a while and endured the consequences of it, I was able to celebrate the fact that I had made some major strides in my eating behaviors as well as diet regimens. I was beginning to score more health victories instead of logging in failures. The tables below gives you a better look at how I was progressing based on a random ten day span which largely mirrored my everyday routines.

TABLE 12: 10-Day Table

Blood Sugar After Eating/Workout (unless noted)

DAY 1: Date: 8/27/2013

Fasting: 159 mg/dl
Breakfast: 139 mg/dl; low carb granola, 2% milk, 3 cups coffee
Lunch: 119 mg/dl; canned salmon, tomato, ½ cucumber, peeled, 1 large raw jalapeno, oil & vinegar
Snack: 172 mg/dl; unsweetened honey/chamomile/green iced tea, water, 1 slice Swiss cheese
Workout: 144 mg/dl 2.5 hours after eating; 25 pushups, 25 curls, 25 butterflies, 25 triceps, 26 mile bike ride (avg. 16 mph)
Dinner: 137 mg/dl; 121 mg/dl before eating, 2 baked chicken thighs, ½ cup brown rice with onion and garlic, iced tea

DAY 1: Date: 8/28/2013

Fasting: 139 mg/dl
Breakfast: 150 mg/dl; peanut butter and jelly sandwich on whole grain, 3 cups coffee
Lunch: 150 mg/dl; liver and onions, cooked carrots, unleavened bread, water
Snack: 113 mg/dl; unsweetened honey/chamomile/green iced tea
Workout: 109 mg/dl 2.5 hours after eating; 20 minute bike ride (avg. 16 mph)
Dinner: 137 mg/dl; Grilled Salmon, rice, roasted veggies, pita bread, lemon soup, iced tea (Daphne's)

DAY 3: Date: 8/29/2013

Fasting: 114 mg/dl
Breakfast: 106 mg/dl; 2 Turkey cheese burgers, plain no bun, pbj ends, 3 cups coffee
Lunch: 121 mg/dl; salad of 1 med-lg tomato, I jalapeno, cut up onions, 3 small thin-cut steaks, ½ cucumber
Snack: 114 mg/dl; ½ cucumber, unpeeled, unsweetened honey/chamomile/green iced tea
Workout: 115 mg/dl; 47 minutes on the exercise bike (avg. 16 mph) = 1 hour
Dinner: 130 mg/dl; 2 baked chicken thighs, water, iced tea

TABLE 12: 10-Day Table (continued)

Blood Sugar After Eating/Workout (unless noted)

DAY 4: Date: 8/30/2013

Fasting: 115 mg/dl
Breakfast: 84 mg/dl; 2 Turkey cheese burgers, plain no bun, 1 egg fried in olive oil, 2 cups coffee w/2% milk, 1 tbsp peanut butter
Lunch: *** mg/dl; tortellini with pesto, flat bread, cucumber/mint salad, water = did not take reading before or after lunch
Snack: 114 mg/dl; ½ cucumber, unsweetened honey/chamomile/green iced tea
Workout: 162 mg/dl 5 hours after eating; no workout
Dinner: 207 mg/dl; 2 steak kabobs, rice, roasted veggies, pita bread, lemon soup, iced tea

DAY 5: Date: 8/31/2013

Fasting: did not take reading, drank whiskey and three beers the night before
Breakfast: *** mg/dl; did not note breakfast, did not take reading
Lunch: *** mg/dl; did not note lunch, no reading before or after lunch
Snack: no snack
Workout: 128 mg/dl 2.5 hours after eating; 30 minute on exercise bike, cleaned house and yard for four hours
Dinner: 205 mg/dl; 2 slices pineapple / ham pizza, small sausage and cheese omelet, small ice cream sandwich, iced tea (note: I was starving at dinner time)

DAY 6: Date: 9/1/2013

Fasting: 109 mg/dl
Breakfast: *** mg/dl; sausage and egg burrito (homemade, whole wheat tortillas), 2 cups coffee, 2% milk
Lunch: 155 mg/dl; chopped chicken salad with cucumber, lite mayo
Snack: no snack
Workout: 125 mg/dl 2.5 hours after eating; 9 mile bike ride (avg. 17 mph) too hot to go further, energy was very low due to four hours of sleep the night before
Dinner: *** mg/dl; Peruvian Shrimp scampi, Italian bread, butter, Peruvian green hot sauce, water. Small frozen yogurt with toffee topping. No reading after dinner.

TABLE 12: 10-Day Table (continued)

Blood Sugar After Eating/Workout (unless noted)

DAY 7: Date: 9/2/2013

Fasting: 127 mg/dl
Breakfast: 181 mg/dl; chicken sandwich on whole grain with lite mayo, 2 slices of Swiss cheese, 3 cups coffee, 2% milk
Lunch: 132 mg/dl; PBJ on whole grain bread, 2 slices Swiss cheese, water
Snack: 139 mg/dl; 2 small carrot sticks, 1 tbsp potato salad, 1 tbsp guacamole, glass of iced green tea.
Workout: 161 mg/dl 2.5 hours after eating; 161 mg/dl 64 minutes on the exercise bike (avg. 16-17 mph)
Dinner: 151 mg/dl; roasted chicken –leg, thigh, wing with skin. 1 tbsp of potato salad, 1 tbsp guacamole. Cucumber/tomato/jalapeno salad, oil and vinegar. Water

DAY 8: Date: 9/3/2013

Fasting: 125 mg/dl
Breakfast: 93 mg/dl; 2.5 tbsps potato salad (Costco), 1 tbsp guacamole, 1 roasted chicken quarter and wing, 2 cups coffee, 2% milk
Lunch: 140 mg/dl; canned salmon, 15 bbq chips, chewy granola bar (peanut butter/chocolate chip)
Snack: 106 mg/dl; 106 mg/dl 5 hours after eating
Workout: 143 mg/dl 2.5 hours after eating; 1 mile slow walk, five hours of sleep the night before
Dinner: 140 mg/dl; baked Tilapia, 2.5 tbsp of potato salad, roasted vegetables. 2 glasses of red wine with diet 7-up, 140 mg/dl

TABLE 12: 10-Day Table (continued)

Blood Sugar After Eating/Workout (unless noted)

DAY 9: Date: 9/4/2013

Fasting: 121 mg/dl
Breakfast: 108 mg/dl; roasted chopped chicken, 2 tbsp of light mayo, 3 cups coffee, 2% milk
Lunch: *** mg/dl; ½ cup cold mac and cheese, water= no reading
Snack: *** mg/dl; none, no reading
Workout: *** mg/dl; Climbing the rocks with the nephews and neighbor kids for three hours. Significant climbs, worked up a good sweat, low intensity.
Dinner: 130 mg/dl; grilled salmon, steamed white rice, bok choi with onions and garlic. 1 Sam Adams beer. Strawberry cheesecake with whipped cream, later 2 glasses of red wine

DAY 10: Date: 9/5/2013

Fasting: 118 mg/dl
Breakfast: 135 mg/dl; roasted chopped chicken, 1.g tbsp of light mayo, 2 slices of swiss, 15 pringles chips 3 cups coffee, 2% milk
Lunch: 136 mg/dl; 2 small thin cut steaks with brown rice, garlic and jalapeno cooked in oil, water
Snack: *** mg/dl; none, no reading
Workout: 160 mg/dl; 25 pushups, 25 50-pound curls, 25 shrugs, 25 butterflies, and 25 triceps,
Dinner: 194 mg/dl; skinless chicken sandwich, light mayo, whole grain bread, 1 small tomato, one slice swiss, 5 bbq chips, water

As you might have noticed, I still ate desserts as a form of comfort food once in a while but I limited it. I lived mainly on fish, chicken, and raw or roasted vegetables with very little beef. I focus on healthy filling meals to at least help me maintain my weight as I push on to use diet and exercise routines to help me achieve the rest of my health and weight loss goals. Considering how far I've come, I am pleased with the progress.

It is also important to point out that when this sampling was logged, I had been without heart and diabetic medications for about one year simply because I couldn't afford it. I knew I was taking a risk, and as long as could keep my stress levels down and my exercise and diet routines in check I knew I had a reasonable chance of success.

But like with most life journeys, there were indeed more struggles to come and far bigger ones than I had already endured. There was no way I could have prepared myself for what was coming next, but I took steps anyway.

I armed myself with knowledge and practical use of what I learned but when it was all said and done; I didn't know how I survived not just the disease but the circumstances themselves. It took more than a year before things unraveled to the point where I was once again told that I almost didn't make it, and I missed disaster by only a few months.

NINE

What is Diabetes?

The short answer to the title question is diabetes is a group of metabolic diseases that result in one's body having excess blood sugar. This happens when either a body produces no insulin or its cells are insulin resistant. In both cases the blood sugar, or glucose, remains unprocessed which will lead to disastrous consequences including death. If you or someone you know has it or exhibits some of the symptoms get to a doctor and learn as much as you can about the disease.

Once I learned I had diabetes, I found there were ample resources available to help me understand this disease and I took comfort in that. After all, in order to know how to manage or defeat something that threatens your life and well-being the way this disease can, it is much better to form a strategy by knowing as much as possible about the enemy you have to deal with.

A quick note on the topic of resources though before moving on. Throughout the course of my research, I ran into plenty of resources that were more interested in selling me something based upon my fears rather than giving me what I really wanted which was a better understanding of diabetes.

Diabetes, as I've learned over time, is far too important to play games with. I found common threads among the reliable resources and noted consistent patterns in the discussions of the disease that were based upon the available studies. It's not like there isn't a large enough data pool to draw from. Twenty-nine million in the USA alone and counting should produce a pretty good crop of studies, which it has. So I confined my research for the book to what

I deemed reliable based upon the credentials of the resource and the fact that the data was confirmed and/or corroborated by other equally credentialed resources.

I provided a list of these resources at the end of the book so you can do your own research or spot check mine if you choose, and by the way, I strongly recommend that you do. Why? First is because what I got out of it were real eye openers. Before I started digging in I didn't really feel like anything was going on inside of my body.

The second is because this book is based on one man's interpretation of the research, and although I'm meticulous in presenting the facts as they are stated (at least I try to be), some things may be more important to me than they are to you. My objective here is to answer some of the basic questions and provide some details of the disease. My objective is also to provide some guides for you so when you ask the question: "but what about...?" You can have some resources to help you find the answer to that question or others.

A Short History Of Diabetes

From its history, diabetes has been known for thousands of years. Diabetes was named in 250 BC by Apollonius of Memphis, Egypt, a name which means "to go through". But it was also reported around the same time that a Greek surgeon named Aretaeus named Diabetes for the Greek word for "Siphon." It really doesn't matter who named it or when they named it but what does matter is that early physicians understood the disease caused people to get rid of more liquid than they could consume.

In 160 AD, a physician named Galen understood that diabetes was related to the kidneys; and hundreds of years later Galen's findings inspired an Arab physician, Avicenna, who added details, such as his observance of skin abscesses, to the growing knowledge of diabetes.

Various remedies were tried in the years that followed including vein cutting, slowing blood movement, exercise on horseback, and induced sweating among others. Exercise and diets, including starvation diets, were chief remedies. The starvation diets kept food intake down but provided almost no nourishment, often causing the patient to be under weight and even more sickly. It seemed that even back then doctors were catching on to the idea that diet had something to do with the disease, but what kind of diet really wasn't pinpointed until centuries later.

In the 1500s, diabetes was referred to as the "Pissing Evile" which denoted the large volumes of urine people with diabetes would secrete each day. In as late as the 1690s, doctors prescribed a jelly they called "viper's flesh" which consisted of broken red coral, sweet almonds, and fresh flowers of blind nettles, a plant from the mint family. As with nearly all of the prescribed remedies up until the late nineteenth century, it didn't work.

In 1796, a doctor named John Rollo used a urine glucose test, discovered twenty years earlier by an English doctor named Dobson, to develop what was considered the first effective treatment for diabetes: a diet high in animal fat and meat and low in grains and breads. This diet prolonged life for many diabetics who had type 2 diabetes, though the differences between types 1 and 2 were unknown at the time. What Rollo accidently discovered was the relationship between carbohydrates vs. proteins and how the body converts them.

Some doctors modified the diet in ways that we now understand doesn't make sense, such as that by Priory, a French physician, who prescribed eating large quantities of sugar. Overall, diet was the only treatment for diabetes until after the turn of the century. In 1869, medical student Paul Langerhans put forth his discovery of two systems of cells in the pancreas that later became known as 'The Islets of Langerhans' but sometimes called the 'Islands of Langerhans.' These islets are cell clusters within the pancreas that secrete insulin and other hormones into the blood system. This discovery paved the way to successful treatments for diabetes later on.

In 1897, the typical life expectancy of a child with diabetes aged twelve years or younger was only a little more than a year, and for diabetics who were older could only expect to live with the disease for somewhere between four and eight years depending on their ages at the time they contracted it.

In 1908, a German scientist named Zuelzer developed an extract called Acomatrol from the pancreas that, when injected, was able to suppress glucose levels in the urine. Acomatrol had extreme side effects; while it could keep a dying patient alive, they could only stay alive for as long Acomatrol was in the system. Once it was gone, the patient died.

In 1921 insulin was discovered by a young Canadian surgeon named Frederick Banting. After successful experiments on a dog,

Dr. Banting, along with Canadian doctors James Collip and John Macleod gave insulin to a young boy and saved his life.

In 1922, Dr. Elliot Joslin began overseeing the administration of insulin in a fourteen-year-old boy. Before the injections, the boy's treatments were starvation diets that kept his weight at just sixty-eight pounds. He was able to live a more normal life after receiving insulin, which kept him alive until he died of pneumonia at the age of twenty-seven.

Dr. Joslin went on to found the Joslin Diabetes Center which is still a major center for help and support for diabetics today. In the years following those first insulin injections much emphasis was placed on improving insulin which included attempts to come up with an oral version. Insulin breaks down once it's digested and, because of the side effects, the attempts toward an oral version were dropped.

In 1935, Roger Hinsworth concluded that there were two types of diabetes, type 1 which is insulin sensitive, and type 2 which is not. But that discovery was riddled with unanswered questions about which parts of the body, the stomach, liver, Langerhans' Isles, or the kidneys, were responsible for the disease. These questions were legitimate as all of those parts appeared to be connected to the disease in some fashion.

Since then, great strides have been made to where a diabetic can indeed live a normal life. Improvements continued for injectable insulin type 1 diabetics, and in 1955 oral medications for type 2 were discovered and although improved, some are still used today which strikes me as remarkable yet problematic.

For a disease that has been around for so long, how is it that we are still using remedies that are more than half a century old, can we not make strides that take us closer to a cure? For type 1 diabetics there is now an insulin pump which can be programmed to inject measured doses, but the user still has to monitor blood sugar levels.

Who Has Diabetes?

- » Among U.S. residents
- » Ages 65 years and older, 10.9 million, or 26.9 percent, had diabetes in 2010.
- » About 215,000 people younger than 20 years had type 1 or type 2 diabetes in 2010.
- » About 1.9 million people ages 20 years or older were newly diagnosed with diabetes in 2010.

» Between 2005-2008, based on fasting glucose or hemoglobin A1C levels, 35 percent of adults ages 20 years or older and diabetes 50 percent of adults ages 65 years or older had pre-diabetes.[18] Applying this percentage to the entire U.S. population in 2010 yields an estimated 79 million American adults aged 20 years or older with pre-diabetes.

What Are The Impacts Of Diabetes?

» Diabetes is the leading cause of kidney failure, non-traumatic lower-limb amputations, and new cases of blindness among adults.
» Diabetes is a major cause of heart disease and stroke.
» Diabetes is the seventh leading cause of death in the U.S.
» 231,000 died in 2007 because of diabetes.

The more disturbing aspect of these statistics is how the number of afflicted people went from 5.6 million in 1980 to over 17 million by 2007 and more than 25 million by 2010. This suggests that our unhealthy, stress-filled lifestyles and eating habits are taking their tolls and manifesting themselves in the form of diabetes, and it is showing up in the pre-diabetes statistics.

Too often though, once you've reached those levels you are very likely to get it unless you take action right away and change your lifestyle. These statistics are for the US population alone, and I don't know if any studies have been done to ascertain why the incidences of diabetes among Americans have risen so dramatically. I am only surmising the causes based upon my own onset as well as those I know among my peer group with type 2.

How Do You Know If You Have Diabetes?

There are a number of ways for you to know that something is wrong, although I have to say that I was completely unaware when it came to my own problems. Mine was caught while having tests done to determine the cause of numbness in my arm. The doctors

---

[18] Pre-diabetes is when your blood sugar is high, but not high enough to be considered diabetes. According to the Joslin Center, the new national guidelines for pre-diabetes are when people have a fasting blood glucose in the 100-125 mg/dl range, and if your doctor gives you an oral glucose tolerance test, and blood glucose is 140-199 mg/dl, two hours later, then you are considered pre-diabetic.

wanted to eliminate stroke as a reason for the numbness so they took all sorts of tests. It was later determined that the numbness was due to a crimped nerve but the blood tests showed that I was a diabetic and had been for at least a year. I was so used to feeling bad, looking bad, and consumed by my search for a job, I was too busy to notice that I was heading down the road to disaster.

What Are The Symptoms Of Diabetes?

People who think they might have diabetes need to see a doctor for diagnosis. You might have some or even none of the following symptoms and could have the disease without knowing it:

- Frequent urination
- Excessive thirst
- Unexplained weight loss
- Extreme hunger
- Sudden vision changes
- Tingling or numbness in hands or feet
- Feeling very tired much of the time
- Very dry skin
- Sores that are slow to heal
- More infections than usual

Nausea, vomiting, or stomach pains may accompany some of these symptoms in the abrupt onset of insulin-dependent, or type 1 diabetes. *(Centers for Disease Control, 2015)*

Type 1 Diabetes

Type 1 is an autoimmune disease affecting the insulin production in the pancreas. Autoimmunity is when agents in the blood attack invading cells. Some researchers believe that a virus may trigger the immune system to attack the cells involved in the insulin production and permanently destroy them, though it still remains a mystery. As a result, the pancreas can no longer make the insulin necessary for the cells to absorb the sugar in the blood and convert it so it can be used for energy. The end result is that sugar builds up in the blood over time and causes damage to the internal organs and blood vessels. When a diabetic has too much glucose in his or her blood they have hyperglycemia.

A person with type 1 diabetes either makes too little insulin or can't make any insulin at all. This form of diabetes generally occurs in the late 20s or early 30s, but it can happen at any age. It may be caused by a genetic disorder, but the origins of type 1 are not fully understood. One thing is known about the disease: type 1 sufferers require frequent insulin injections in order to survive. If everything is working right, the pancreas releases the right amount of insulin to move the glucose to our cells while lowering the blood sugar level.

What does this mean to a person who just found out they have type 1? It means he or she will have to take insulin to survive, every day for the rest of his or her life or until a cure is found. What the pancreas does automatically, such as monitoring blood glucose levels and introducing insulin to balance it, the person will now have to do manually. Although the thought of it is scary, having diabetes today is not the death sentence that it once was.

There is still a lot to learn about type 1diabetes, and not much is known about its risk factors. Some of the known factors to date include a family history of type 1 as well as genetics. There also appears to be evidence that geography may have an impact, currently people living in Finland and Sardinia have about two to three times greater rates of type 1 than do Americans, and much higher in other areas. There aren't many known risk factors for type 1 diabetes, though researchers continue to find new possibilities.

Other possible risk factors could be exposure to certain viruses, and certain diets, but nothing appears to be conclusive at this time.

Type 2 Diabetes

Someone with type 2 diabetes produces enough insulin, but their cells resist it and therefore they can't convert the glucose into usable energy. In contrast to type 1 which is an autoimmunity disorder, type 2 is a metabolic disorder which affects how food is converted to energy in the body. It usually occurs in people over age thirty-five, but it is an equal opportunity disease and can affect anyone, including children.

The National Institutes of Health (NIH) reports that ninety-five percent of all diabetes cases are type 2. Unfortunately, as was the case for me, it is a lifestyle disease often brought on by obesity compounded by a lack of exercise and increased age. There may also be a genetic component, but be sure to keep a diary of your habits and look in the mirror before making the argument that genetics might be the problem. Lifestyle is generally the culprit. Although type 2 diabetes is not caused by obesity, being overweight is a significant risk factor for developing the disease.

You have a higher risk for type 2 diabetes if you have any of the following risk factors:

- » Age greater than 45 years
- » Diabetes during a previous pregnancy
- » Excess body weight (especially around the waist)
- » Family history of diabetes
- » Persons from certain ethnic groups, including African Americans, Hispanic Americans, Asian Americans, and Native Americans, have higher risks for diabetes.
- » Given birth to a baby weighing more than 9 pounds
- » HDL cholesterol under 35 mg/dl
- » High blood levels of triglycerides, a type of fat molecule (250 mg/dl or more)
- » High blood pressure (greater than or equal to 140/90 mmHg)
- » Impaired glucose tolerance
- » Low activity level (exercising less than 3 times a week)
- » Metabolic syndrome
- » Polycystic ovarian syndrome
- » A condition called 'acanthosis nigricans', which causes dark, thickened skin around the neck or armpits

Of those thirteen contributing factors, eight applied to me by the time it was confirmed that I was a diabetic. Looking back at it now, I can see how easily I was dismissing the warning signs. When I gained weight I bought new clothes instead of getting motivated to get off my fat ass and start living a healthier lifestyle.

According to the NIH, everyone over age forty-five should have a blood sugar (glucose) test at least every three years. Regular testing of blood sugar levels should begin at a younger age and be performed more often if you are at higher risk for diabetes especially if you have any of the risk factors detailed above.

Diabetes as a metabolic disorder is also called diabetes mellitus according to some experts, and for anyone who doesn't know, the metabolism is the network and its process through which our bodies convert food into fuel. Our metabolisms are measured in part by how efficiently our bodies burn that fuel.

In short, our metabolism is responsible for how fast we burn calories and use up energy, and we know not everyone burns calories at the same rate. Certain factors affect metabolism like age, gender, and how much muscle you have. The more muscle you have, the more calories you burn. That's why many athletes have zero fat, because their muscles burn calories even at rest. Genetics can also play a role, and there can also be medical factors too.

There's also an interesting aspect of weight and metabolism. People who are overweight or obese have metabolisms that run pretty high; and because of it they tend to lose weight at the start of a diet but once they lose a good amount of fat and muscle, the rate of weight loss slows down because their bodies don't need as many calories to sustain themselves.

It has often been a common misconception that slow metabolism leads to weight gain, and it has been one that I've labored under as well. The facts show the opposite but special attention needs to be paid to this because of what happens once you lose the weight. In simple terms, the best way to lose weight is to burn fat and replace it with muscle. Too often though, people simply diet without exercising and that can lead to muscle loss which is often where your basic metabolic rate (BMR) will slow down.

This section is very important for you professional dieters, so take notes! If you have two people weighing in at two hundred and twenty-five pounds, but one got there by dieting down from three hundred pounds while the other one was always at two hundred and twenty-five, the dieter is going to have the slower metabolism.

Since a higher BMR is the key to efficiently converting food to fuel and ultimately to glucose, a slower BMR means you have to watch what and how much you eat because that glucose will not get used up as quickly as it should. And excess glucose in the system of course increases the danger of developing diabetes.

Gestational Diabetes (GD)

The risks associated with GD are similar to those associated with type 2, like obesity, high blood pressure, family history, age and ethnicity, but there are others that are specific to pregnancy like giving birth to a baby larger than nine pounds, a stillbirth, or a baby with birth defects, and whether or not you had GD in an earlier pregnancy. Yet about half of the women who get it don't have any of those risk factors.

GD is a form of glucose resistance that occurs in about four percent of all pregnant women, usually around the second trimester but generally disappears once the baby is born. It seems to happen more frequently among African Americans, Hispanic/Latino Americans, and American Indians. GD requires maintenance to stabilize blood sugar levels to avoid having complications with the baby. Right after the pregnancy, about five to ten percent of women with GD are found to have diabetes, usually type 2. And those who have had GD have about a fifty percent chance of developing diabetes in the next five to ten years.

If GD goes untreated, it can pose serious problems for you and your baby. Some of these problems include the baby growing too large for a normal delivery, the baby having too low a blood sugar, or the baby can develop jaundice and breathing problems.

GD is the result of changes that occur in women's bodies when they become pregnant. Higher levels of hormones such as cortisol, estrogen, and lactogen can interfere with the woman's body's ability to naturally manage blood sugar levels. GD is also like type 2 in that the cells are insulin resistant.

Women with GD may not have any symptoms at all which is why pregnant women, whether at risk or not, should be tested.

So I had many of the symptoms but ignored them because I was distracted and depressed. I had chalked these up to simple maladies caused by lack of exercise and stress. In actuality I wasn't that far off but I was making a potentially deadly mistake by not getting a doctor's advice. Once I understood the disease I realized how lucky I was, especially knowing that death wasn't the only consequence. If I had a stroke or became blind as a result of having diabetes our lives would have been so much worse, especially for my family. Knowing this shook me up like getting hit on the side of the head with a two-by-four.

So we know that diabetes results in high blood sugar levels, but exactly why is that a problem?

Complications Of Diabetes And What It Does To Your Body

The strange thing about diabetes is that you don't necessarily feel like anything is out of the ordinary, at least at first. It's not like you're in a lot of pain all the time. In fact, one of the ironic yet very disturbing aspects of it is neuropathy, which actually desensitizes your feet, hands, and legs so you don't feel pain as you should. That opens the door for infections that can lead to amputations because you can't feel what's happening, and diabetics often take longer to heal. Of all the non-trauma related amputations, sixty percent are due to diabetes.

I've had diabetes now for almost ten years, yet despite all the research I've done on the subject I'm still constantly having to remind myself that I'm playing with fire. It's precisely because you don't feel the disease happening that makes it hard for some people like me to take it seriously.

To illustrate this point I often experience severe chest pains, heavy enough to where I should go to urgent care to have them checked out. But most often I can't tell if what I am experiencing is a heart attack, complications from diabetes, gas pains or if I am overly stressed because I have no job and no money, or it could be something as simple as having slept in an awkward position the night before. Whatever it is when they have occurred, I didn't have them checked out because I didn't have health insurance nor did I have the money to pay for the visit.

When I didn't get checked out, I was taking a calculated risk because that wasn't the first time I had experienced such severe pains. The first few times I had them I did go to my doctor and got a better understanding of what might be causing the pains. That said, in reality every time I don't react to those pains I'm engaging in a crapshoot because of my diabetes and my other health problems.

Problems from diabetes start small while laying foundations for the more serious stuff. It can happen quickly or slowly over time.

First, diabetes is a problem because the excess glucose gets attached to proteins in the blood vessels so the vessels themselves are affected and change for the worse. One change is that they become thicker and less elastic, making it hard for blood to squeeze through. This in turn affects the organs which need the blood flow for oxygen and nourishment.

The first question I had was how does diabetes cause damage? Why this is worth noting is because it boils down to how we make certain decisions in our daily lives, like should I eat a sandwich or a salad, a muffin or an egg? Two of the decisions can lead to higher levels of blood sugar while the other two do not.

Ketone Levels

Diabetic Ketoacidosis (DKA) is a complication that occurs when the body doesn't have enough insulin and cannot process glucose to be used for energy. When the body isn't getting the fuel it needs it starts to burn fat. When this happens, chemicals called ketones are released into the blood. Some ketones, as well as some glucose, pass out of the body through the urine but not all. DKA occurs more often in people with type 1 diabetes, but can sometimes also happen to people with type 2 diabetes.

High levels of ketones in the blood can be a problem because they cause the blood to become acidic. Too much acid in the blood throws off the body's chemical balance and causes the following symptoms:

- » Thirst or a very dry mouth
- » Frequent urination
- » High blood glucose (blood sugar) levels
- » High levels of ketones in the urine
- » Constantly feeling tired
- » Dry or flushed skin
- » Nausea, vomiting, or abdominal pain (Vomiting can be caused by many illnesses, not just ketoacidosis. If vomiting continues for more than 2 hours, contact your health care provider.)
- » Difficulty breathing
- » Fruity odor on breath
- » A hard time paying attention, or confusion

DKA is a very serious condition that can lead to coma or death if it's not treated. The good news, though, is that it's preventable and can be treated so very few people actually die from it.

Hyperosmolar Hyperglycemic Nonketotic Syndrome (HHNS) HHNS is an opposite condition than DKA in which one's blood sugar levels become very high and ketones are not present in the blood or urine. It can happen to either type 1 or type 2 diabetics but more often in type 2 and is most common in older people. It happens when the diabetes isn't being controlled properly and is usually brought on by an infection or illness. It causes the body to get rid of liquid and will lead to dehydration. If the dehydration is not dealt with effectively it will lead to coma and then death.

While both DKA and HHNS can lead to comas if not treated properly, the causes of the comas are opposite. In cases of DKA a coma can occur when too many ketones are present in the blood due to burning fat for energy and not having enough insulin. Although the symptoms may appear to be similar, HHNS can occur mostly in older type 2 diabetics when no ketones are present in the blood and the body is severely stressed or dehydrated. So if you know someone in a diabetic coma, you have no way of knowing what caused it so you have to seek professional help immediately. You can't make any assumptions about what kind it is because the fix for a DKA coma can kill a person who is in an HHNS coma, and vice versa.

Eye Problems

Diabetic eye disease can often develop without symptoms, so regular eye exams are important for finding problems early. Many major health plans now include free eye exams for early detection of a number of diseases, including diabetes even if a vision plan isn't part of the health package. Some people may notice signs of vision changes, I have noticed it in myself and it makes me nervous.

I'm still ok, but at times I have trouble reading things that are close and sometimes my vision is blurred. Of course, that could be a result of sipping a little more Jack Daniels than I should. All kidding aside, something else to be concerned with is if you're seeing rings around lights, dark spots, or flashing lights. They could be indicators of serious eye problems.

Diabetic retinopathy is the most common diabetic eye disease and a leading cause of blindness in American adults. It is caused by changes in the blood vessels of the retina. In some people with diabetic retinopathy, blood vessels may swell and leak fluid. In other people, abnormal new blood vessels grow on the surface of the retina, the light-sensitive tissue at the back of the eye. A healthy retina is necessary for good vision. In cases of untreated type 2 diabetes, non-proliferating and proliferating retinopathy develops which might result in blindness. These are part of the stages of retinopathy from the mildest form (non- proliferative) to the most advanced form.

Eye damage caused by diabetes (proliferative retinopathy) happens when the blood vessels in the back of the eye form pouches. It normally doesn't affect vision at that stage, instead it happens when the damaged vessels close off and are replaced by newer, weaker ones. The new ones can leak blood which blocks vision, and they can also cause scar tissue to grow and distort the retina.

The retina can be irreversibly damaged before you even notice it's happening, but caught in time it can be treated by laser to minimize vision loss so the ADA recommends yearly screening to help catch it.

And there's more you can do to prevent eye problems. A recent study shows that keeping your blood glucose level closer to normal can prevent or delay the onset of diabetic eye disease, and keeping your blood pressure under control is also important. It is best to have an eye doctor give you a dilated eye exam at least once a year. He or she will use eye drops to enlarge (dilate) your pupils to examine the backs of your eyes. Your eyes will be checked for signs of cataracts or glaucoma, problems that people with diabetes are more likely to get.

If you have diabetic retinopathy, at first you may not notice changes to your vision. Over time, diabetic retinopathy can get worse and cause vision loss. Diabetic retinopathy usually affects both eyes. All I noticed was that I had trouble reading things close to me, and the words were really blurry.

So I kept going to Walmart and Walgreen's to buy various strengths of cheap reading glasses. I attributed the onset of poor eyesight to age, but in reality it was due to the diabetes. It didn't take long for it to get progressively worse, but once I got my diabetes under control, my eyesight stopped getting worse. Unfortunately however, it didn't get any better.

The Glaucoma Research Foundation states some interesting aspects regarding the relationship of glaucoma to diabetic eye disease. On their website they note that someone with diabetes is twice as likely as a non-diabetic to develop glaucoma, though they qualify it by suggesting that new research may suggest a different percentage. They also note that someone who has developed open-angle glaucoma, the most common form of glaucoma, is more likely to develop diabetes than someone who doesn't have it.

Kidney Problems

Diabetic nephropathy is another major complication of diabetes. The exact cause of it is unknown but it is thought that uncontrolled high blood sugar leads to it especially when high blood pressure is also present. In some cases, your genes or family history may also play a role, but fortunately not all persons with diabetes develop this condition.

Each kidney is made of hundreds of thousands of filtering units called nephrons and each nephron has a cluster of tiny blood vessels called a glomerulus. Together these structures help remove waste from the body. Too much blood sugar can damage these structures, causing them to thicken and become scarred. Slowly, over time, more and more blood vessels are destroyed. The kidney structures begin to leak and a protein, albumin, begins to pass into the urine.

This type of kidney disease starts when the kidneys become leaky and allow albumin to go out with the urine, which is how doctors detect it. Over time some vessels will collapse and put more pressure on the remaining ones until the kidneys eventually fail. In diabetic kidney disease cells and blood vessels in the kidneys are damaged, affecting the organs' ability to filter out waste.

The condition slowly continues to get worse once large amounts of protein begin to appear in the urine or levels of creatinine in the blood begin to rise. Creatinine is a byproduct after muscles use Creatine for energy. As the waste is produced, it gets filtered through the kidneys and passed through the urine. Blood creatinine levels are measured to test how the kidneys are functioning. Higher blood creatinine levels indicate renal dysfunction. Waste builds up in your blood instead of being excreted, and in some cases this can lead to kidney failure. When the kidneys fail, a person has to have his or her blood filtered through dialysis several times a week or has to get a kidney transplant.

There are things you can do to prevent kidney problems and controlling your blood sugar levels can help, and not surprisingly keeping your blood pressure under control is also important.

Don't ignore bladder or kidney infections. Symptoms include cloudy or bloody urine, pain or burning when you urinate, an urgent need to urinate often, back pain, chills, or fever.

Persons with diabetes who have the following risk factors are more likely to develop kidney problems:[19]

» African American, Hispanic, or American Indian origin
» Family history of kidney disease or high blood pressure
» Poor control of blood pressure
» Poor control of blood sugars
» Type 1 diabetes before age 20
» Smoking

---

[19] Courtesy: National Institutes of Health: National Institute of Diabetes and Digestive and Kidney Diseases (NIH/DIDDK).

Diabetic nephropathy generally goes along with other diabetes complications including high blood pressure, retinopathy, and blood vessel changes.

According to the NIH, diabetic nephropathy is a major cause of sickness and death in persons with diabetes, and it is the leading cause of long-term kidney failure and end-stage kidney disease in the United States.

Complications due to chronic kidney failure are more likely to occur earlier, and get worse more rapidly, when it is caused by diabetes than other causes. Even after dialysis or transplantation, persons with diabetes tend to do worse than those without diabetes.

Possible complications include:

» Anemia
» Chronic kidney failure (rapidly gets worse)
» Dialysis complications
» End-stage renal failure (kidney disease)
» Hyperkalemia (which occurs when the level of potassium in the bloodstream is higher than normal, and can lead to cardiac arrest).
» Severe hypertension
» Hypoglycemia
» Infections
» Kidney transplant complications
» Peritonitis (if peritoneal dialysis used. This is an inflammation of the peritoneum, the tissue that lines the wall of the abdomen and covers the abdominal organs. It can lead to other complications, including death).

Untreated diabetes gives way to kidney failure as detailed above; the lack of treatment also gives way to cardiovascular disorders leading to heart failure and chronic dental diseases.

Heart

Heart problems can be caused in a different way because high sugar levels can lead to blockages which can cause heart attacks. Diabetics are at two to four times the risk of developing heart disease than the general population. Blocked vessels in the legs can be painful and can impair circulation which can ultimately lead to amputations.

One particular area of concern for me is the cardiovascular impacts because it is the leading cause of early death among people with diabetes. In addition to the increased risk of heart attacks, adult diabetics are two to four times more likely to experience a stroke. Also, about seventy percent of people with diabetes have high blood pressure, a risk factor for cardiovascular disease.

People with type 2 diabetes often have high rates of cholesterol and triglyceride abnormalities, obesity, and high blood pressure, all of which are major contributors to higher rates of cardiovascular disease. I'm sorry to report that I still have most of these conditions at the same time though I'm doing my best with what I have to change that.

This combination is often called metabolic syndrome and is defined as the presence of any three of the following conditions:

1) excess weight around the waist
2) high levels of triglycerides
3) low levels of HDL, or "good," cholesterol
4) high blood pressure
5) high fasting blood glucose levels

If you have one or more of these conditions, you are at an increased risk for having one or more of the others. The more conditions you have, the greater the risk to your health.

Fixing this all centers around eating right, getting physical activity, avoiding smoking, and maintaining healthy blood glucose, blood pressure, and cholesterol levels. Choose a healthy diet, low in salt. If you can, get a hemoglobin A1C test at least twice a year to determine what your average blood glucose level was for the past two to three months. Get your blood pressure checked at every doctor's visit, and get your cholesterol checked at least once a year. Easier said than done for some of us, but well worth it either way.

Nerve Damage

Nerve damage, circulation problems, and infections can cause serious foot problems for people with diabetes.

Sometimes nerve damage can deform or misshape your feet, causing pressure points that can turn into blisters, sores, or ulcers. Something as simple as a hangnail or ingrown toenail can be catastrophic because of poor circulation and the infections they can cause. Having high blood glucose for many years can damage the blood vessels that bring oxygen to some nerves, as well as the nerve coverings. The damaged nerves can stop sending messages or send messages too slowly or at the wrong times. Numbness, pain, and weakness in the hands, arms, feet, and legs may develop.

And if that weren't enough, problems can occur elsewhere including the digestive tract, heart, and sex organs. Diabetic neuropathy (not to be confused with diabetic nephropathy which affects the kidneys) is the medical term for damage to the nervous system from diabetes. The most common type is peripheral neuropathy, which affects the arms and legs.

An estimated fifty percent of those of us with diabetes have some form of neuropathy, but not all with neuropathy have symptoms and that's a scary statistic because you don't know that you have it and might not know it until some damage has been done. People with diabetes can develop nerve problems at any time, and the longer a person has diabetes, the greater the risk. The highest rates of neuropathy are among people who have had the disease for at least twenty-five years.

Diabetic neuropathy also appears to be more common in people who have had problems controlling their blood glucose levels, in those with high levels of blood fat and blood pressure, in overweight people, and in people over the age of forty. Again and not surprisingly, keeping your blood glucose as close to normal as possible, getting regular physical activity, not smoking, taking good care of your feet each day can help you avoid it. Keeping your feet healthy is important because they can be the easiest things to be affected.

Here are some steps you can take for your feet (no pun intended): Look for cuts, cracks, sores, red spots, swelling, infected toenails, splinters, blisters, and calluses on the feet each day. It is recommended that you call your doctor if these wounds don't heal after a day or so. If you have corns and calluses, ask your doctor or podiatrist about the best way to care for them. Wash your feet in warm, not hot, water and dry them well. Cut your toenails once a week or when needed, and it's best to cut them when they're soft from washing. Rub lotion on the tops and bottoms of feet to prevent cracking and drying, and wear shoes that fit well. Break in new shoes slowly, wearing them one to two hours each day for the first one to two weeks to avoid blisters and sores.

Avoid going barefoot when it's easy to step on something that might hurt your feet, and protect your feet from extreme heat and cold. Keep the blood flowing to your lower limbs by propping your feet up and moving your toes and ankles for a few minutes at a time when sitting. Avoid smoking, which reduces blood flow to the feet. Most of all do everything you can to keep your blood sugar, blood pressure, and cholesterol under control by eating healthy foods, and staying active.

When diabetes remains untreated, it can cause severe damage to nerve cells that results in sexual dysfunction and can impact all involuntary functions. Foot problems and limb amputations are still other outcomes. Another significant complication is the impact diabetes has on blood circulation, something I was also faced with because of my heart problems. To sum it all up, not treating diabetes is similar to inviting death. Little did I know that my death wish had been very close to being granted.

Low Energy Disease

Diabetes is also a low energy disease; Low testosterone is common in diabetes but is often overlooked because it is very similar to other conditions, like arrhythmia. In reality though, you are twice as likely to have low testosterone if you have type 2 diabetes compared with someone who does not. Some symptoms of low testosterone can be diminished interest in sex, erectile dysfunction (ED), reduced muscle mass, depressed moods, and lack of energy. Checking testosterone levels is done with a simple blood test and it is easily treated. My doctor gave me a gel that I rubbed on my arms once a day after my shower. There are also other options like patches or injections. Once I started using it, I felt a difference in my energy levels almost immediately. But testosterone can also be produced naturally through muscle development and that is far less risky than the medications.

There is much more that is associated with diabetes and how it affects normal functions. In her book Healthy to 100 (Alexa Fleckenstein, 2006) Dr. Alexa Fleckenstein gives a detailed description of some of the physiological aspects of the disease. Seeing it helped me answer a lot of questions I had about some of the emotions I was feeling and why I was making some of the decisions I had made.

That isn't to say that I'm blaming the disease on any of my choices, but Dr. Fleckenstein's description gave me a much better perspective about how my thought processes, and more important, how my energy levels were being affected. I used to think it was all me and I no longer had the ability to exercise mind over matter. Once I knew the sources of my weaknesses, I was able to offset those weaknesses and begin a plan to overcome them.

One of the more striking perspectives offered by Dr. Fleckenstein relating to energy output among diabetics is this: "It is as if diabetics stack wood around the mitochondrial stove until that stove – buried under fuel that can't be used – is unable to function any longer."

So in her hypothesis, Dr. Fleckenstein uses a wood stove to illustrate the source of energy in one's body and notes that the unused sugar in the blood as it builds up can lead to catastrophic events like a stroke, heart attack or an infection. This can be brought on by something as relatively simple as eating large meals over a period of time.

More telling for me was Dr. Fleckenstein's commentary on how the onset of low energy caused by diabetes affects a diabetic's mental and physical faculties. "Exhausted as they are, diabetics scramble to make it through their daily activities – they just can't face going to the gym as well. Of course, exercise would use up some of the stacked fuel and reduce the fire hazard – but they can't bring themselves to move. Period."

Other Problems

Gastroparesis, otherwise known as delayed gastric emptying, is a disorder where, due to nerve damage, the stomach takes too long to empty itself. It frequently occurs in people with either type 1 or type 2 diabetes.

Symptoms of gastroparesis include heartburn, nausea, vomiting of undigested food, an early feeling of fullness when eating, weight loss, abdominal bloating, erratic blood glucose levels, lack of appetite, gastroesophageal reflux, and spasms of the stomach wall.

These are all extremely uncomfortable, and the reflux problem can scar your esophagus making it extremely hard to swallow. I have had to have my esophagus stretched five times over the course of about five years in order to be able to swallow food without choking.

My problems were not related to diabetes at the time, but they were related to extremely high levels of stress and very poor eating habits. And as we know, both are related to diabetes in one form or another.

Oral Health. Diabetes also affects oral health and diabetics are more likely to have problems with their teeth and gums because of high blood sugar. Like with all infections, dental infections can make your blood glucose go up and make it worse by letting bacteria into your blood stream. Sore, swollen, and red gums that bleed when you brush your teeth are signs of gingivitis. Periodontitis is another problem that happens when your gums shrink or pull away from your teeth.

People with diabetes can have tooth and gum problems more often if their blood glucose stays high. Smoking makes it more likely for you to get a bad case of gum disease, especially if you have diabetes and are age forty-five or older. Diabetics are also prone to other mouth problems, like fungal infections, poor post-surgery healing, and dry mouth.

Sexual Intimacy. Diabetes really affects sexual intimacy due in part to the nerve damage caused by the disease but also due in part to testosterone levels being low, excess glucose, poor circulation and obesity. It affects both men and women. Men can have trouble maintaining an erection and ejaculating, and women can have trouble with sexual response and vaginal lubrication. For men, there are prescriptions for Viagra, Cialis, and Levitra, but there can be side effects and there are risks with them. You need to talk with your doctor about these remedies before ever taking them if you have diabetes, especially if you have the other complications as well. In addition, both men and women with diabetes can get urinary tract infections and bladder problems more often than average.

Depression. Several studies suggest that diabetes also doubles the risk of depression, although it's still unclear why. The psychological stress of having diabetes may contribute to depression, but diabetes' metabolic effect on brain function may also play a role. At the same time, people with depression may be more likely to develop diabetes. The risk of depression increases as more diabetes complications develop. When you are depressed, you do not function as well, physically or mentally; this makes you less likely to eat properly, exercise, and take your medication regularly.

Psychotherapy, medication, or a combination of both can treat depression effectively. In addition, studies show that successful treatment for depression also helps improve blood glucose control. This affects a person's mood, their outlook, and their responses to sexual stimuli among other things.

Impacts of Common Ailments. Even things like a cold or flu take on new meanings once you become diabetic. Being sick can raise your blood glucose, and when you're sick you often don't eat right which further affects blood glucose. According to the American Diabetes Association, being sick can make your blood sugar levels go up high enough to put you in a coma. When you're sick your body releases hormones that help fight off the sickness, but they raise blood glucose levels while interfering with the sugar-lowering effects of insulin. This can then lead to an acid buildup (ketoacidosis) in the blood when your body is using fat for energy instead of glucose, and is especially concerning for people with type 1 diabetes.

For people with type 2, especially older people, there is Hyperosmolar Hyperglycemic Nonketotic Syndrome or HHNS which I covered earlier. This happens when your body tries to get rid of excess sugar by passing it into your urine. It causes you to go to the bathroom more often. Your urine can become very dark and you can get dehydrated. If HHNS continues, it is the severe dehydration that will lead to seizures, coma and eventually death. More important is that HHNS may take days or even weeks to develop. Both conditions are dangerous and can be life-threatening.

In the bigger picture, diabetes can make the immune system more vulnerable to severe cases of the flu and it may even be necessary to go to a hospital. It is recommended that diabetics get a yearly flu shot. The best time to get one is between October and mid-November, before the flu season begins.

Things to watch for and possible reasons to have someone call your health care provider or go to an emergency room if any of the following happen to you:

» You're too sick to eat or you're unable to keep down food for more than 6 hours
» You're having severe diarrhea
» You lose five pounds or more
» Your temperature stays over 101 degrees F
» Your blood glucose is lower than 60 mg/dl or remains over 300 mg/dl
» You're having trouble breathing
» You feel sleepy or can't think clearly

Major Organ Failure. Like type 2 diabetes, type 1 can affect major organs in your body, including heart, blood vessels, nerves, eyes and kidneys and probably more so because with type 1 your body has stopped making insulin. Keeping your blood sugar level close to normal most of the time can dramatically reduce the risk of many complications.

Long-term complications of type 1 diabetes develop gradually over years. Eventually, diabetes and complications from the disease can cause you to become disabled or cause death.

Osteoporosis. A few more items include osteoporosis for one. Diabetes may lead to lower than normal bone mineral density, increasing your risk of osteoporosis.

Pregnancy Complications. Another is complications during pregnancy. High blood sugar levels can be dangerous for both the mother and the baby. The risk of miscarriage, stillbirth and birth defects are increased when diabetes isn't well controlled. For the mother, diabetes increases the risk of diabetic ketoacidosis (DKA as referenced earlier in the chapter), diabetic eye problems (retinopathy), pregnancy-induced high blood pressure and preeclampsia.

Preeclampsia. Preeclampsia is a condition that typically starts after the 20th week of pregnancy and is related to increased blood pressure and protein in the mother's urine as a result of kidney problems. It affects the placenta, and it can affect the mother's kidney, liver, and brain. When preeclampsia causes seizures, the condition is known as eclampsia – the second leading cause of maternal death in the U.S. Preeclampsia is also a leading cause of fetal complications, which include low birth weight, premature birth, and stillbirth.

Hearing Impairment. And if that wasn't enough, diabetics are prone to having hearing problems. Hearing impairments occur more often in people with diabetes though why or in what percentages are largely unknown. I could probably blame diabetes for my hearing problems, but everybody who knows me knows the real problem is loud rock and roll and country music. There are some things in life that I just can't get enough of.

The bottom line, and frankly what this chapter should have told you is that diabetes touches on every area of a diabetic's life and body. Despite my overall feelings of normalcy, each time I research an area of the disease I come to realize that I'm sick and I need to remember that I am. The fact that I can't get help or medicine only underscores my need to remember what I'm up against. The stress and the skipped workouts aren't helpful and I need to develop a regimen now more than ever if I'm ever going to see a way out of it.

Below are some areas for you to explore if you want to learn more:

CDC publication, 'Take Charge of Your Diabetes' *(Centers for Disease Control, 2007)*:
- » Heart and Blood Vessel Problems
- » Learn About Heart Disease
- » Eye Problems
- » Kidney Problems
- » Nerve Damage
- » Foot Problems
- » Dental Disease
- » Feeling About Having Diabetes
- » Vaccinations
- » Lower Extremity Amputation in People with Diabetes. Epidemiology and Prevention, a professional journal article

CDC National Diabetes Statistics Report *(formerly known as the National Diabetes Fact Sheet)(Centers for Disease Control, 2015)*:
- » Prevention of Diabetes Complications
- » U.S. Department of Health and Human Services and the CDC (National Diabetes Education Program, 2015)
- » The Link between Diabetes and Cardiovascular Disease
- » Be Smart About Your Heart. Control the ABCs of Diabetes
- » Take Care of Your Feet for a Lifetime
- » Feet Can Last a Lifetime: A Healthcare Provider's Guide to Preventing Diabetes Foot Problems

From the National Diabetes Information Clearinghouse (NDIC) *(National Diabetes Information Clearinghouse, 2015)*:
- » Prevent Diabetes Problems: Keep Your Heart and Blood Vessels Healthy Kidney Disease of Diabetes, a fact sheet
- » Prevent Diabetes Problems: Keep Your Kidneys Healthy, a fact sheet
- » Prevent Diabetes Problems: Keep Your Nervous System Healthy, a fact sheet
- » Diabetic Neuropathies: The Nerve Damage of Diabetes, a fact sheet
- » Prevent Diabetes Problems: Keep Your Feet and Skin Healthy, a fact sheet
- » Prevent Diabetes Problems: Keep Your Nervous System Healthy, a fact sheet

From the American Diabetes Association *(American Diabetes Association, 2015)*:
- » Diabetic Retinopathy, a professional journal article
- » Nephropathy of Diabetes, a professional journal article
- » Preventive Foot Care in People with Diabetes, a professional journal article

From the National Kidney and Urologic Diseases Information Clearinghouse *(National Institute of Diabetes and Digestive and Kidney Diseases (NIDDK), National Institutes of Health , 2015)*:
- » Kidney Disease of Diabetes, a fact sheet
- » Prevent Diabetes Problems: Keep Your Feet and Skin Healthy, a fact sheet
- » Sexual and Urologic Problems of Diabetes, a fact sheet
- » Gastroparesis and Diabetes, a fact sheet

From the National Kidney Foundation: *(National Kidney Foundation, 2015)*:
- » Diabetes and Kidney Disease, a fact sheet
- » From the National Institute of Dental and Craniofacial Research: (National Institute of Dental and Craniofacial Research, 2015)
- » Diabetes and Oral Health

Healthline.com *(Healthline.com, 2015)*:
- » Microalbuminuria Test

TEN

Stress and Depression

Vacation's where I wanna be
Buddy on the beach where the fun is free
We don't need a holiday to start to celebrate
(I need a break; I need a vacation)

- Vacation-Pokémon (Colleen Fitzpatrick, 1999)

This is probably the most important chapter in this book because it relates to the silent but deadly killers we face every day of our lives. Stress has a direct impact on diabetes, and it impacts our bodies in virtually every major health and life area like heart, organs, blood, and emotional instability. Not to mention that living under constant stress makes for a very miserable life.

I had often thought that stress was the primary cause of my burnout and poor health. In fact, when I looked at the maladies caused by prolonged stress while doing the research, I saw that every one of mine, including flaky skin and hair loss, two of the relatively minor impacts, had and has direct links. It's funny though, while we were married and then later while we were trying to reconcile before the divorce, I showed Abby how stress affected me and others in general. But without realizing it, I gave Abby the key to knowing how she could do me in; it seemed like she and her thugs at Child Services used every bit of that knowledge to their advantage. Putting me back under stress became her favorite sport which I had to endure all over again for about five years before I could finally move away from it for good.

Stress comes at us in all forms. Some of the stuff that I blow right past now, public speaking, tough bosses, financial messes, is the kind of stuff that impacts people in the same way that my marriage and divorce impacted me. No matter what causes our stress, too much of it will lead to physical and mental health disasters. Stress and the depression that often follows are as silent as they are deadly, which is why we all have to be on the lookout. Otherwise one day you can wake up like me or worse.

Stress played a major role in most of my health problems and the research shows I was right about that all along. As I looked into it, I learned some important things. While I had correctly attributed my obesity, high blood pressure, and heart problems to stress, I learned stress can actually lead to the development of diabetes.

I also learned something that I hadn't realized about myself. As I looked back in time at my childhood and later years to compare with how things are today, I saw that I was raised in highly stressful environments from the time I was two-years-old until my mid-teens, and then again in my late twenties to the present. The stress back then contributed largely to my bed-wetting until the time I was about seven-years-old and to my depression as a teenager. But it never manifested itself through physiological health problems until after being married to Abby and having a family. My stress of course wasn't necessarily because of them (except in Abby's case), it was more the way I handled certain pressures when it related to them.

I wasn't an overweight kid and didn't have any kind of skin problems because back then I only had myself to worry about, and I could withstand a lot as long as I had some escapes. I had quite a few different escapes that I would run to, mainly because for a while I had nowhere else to turn. Those escapes weren't always the best for me, but over time I traded the drinking, drugs and smoking for rest, intense exercise, socializing and sex. I actually became a very relaxed, stress-free individual from about the time I was nineteen until my first marriage when I was twenty-eight.

Even in my first marriage, I didn't have the health or weight problems that I had in my second marriage and it wasn't until I was married to Abby that I started noticing problems with my skin and heart. My blood pressure problems and heavy weight didn't happen until after about ten years into my second marriage. I was always under stress because my only focus was that my family was well-provided for.

After Abby and I divorced, I was back under extreme stress over money and health, and it had really become hard to cope. Ironically though, I paid far closer attention than I used to knowing how great my risk was to having a stroke, my risk was about eight times greater than a normal person to be specific. So I forced myself to take calming breaks, deep breathing and doing anything I could to relax. I began looking at what my stressors were and it gave me a chance to see how I let those impact me to the point where I lost my health and my desire to live. In doing so, I was able to compare the stress I was under and how I reacted to it which allowed me to assess whether or not I had learned something from the experience; I was pleased to see that I was reacting to it so much better than I ever had in the past.

In the past when I was stressed out, I simply shut down or went to comfort food, then forced myself to complete whatever tasks were at hand. I drank a lot too and just kept taking it out on myself. In comparison, I now stop when I'm stressed, and I avoid doing bad stuff to myself like heavy eating or drinking, and instead I put on quiet music and take a break from whatever is stressing me. This also helps me to clear my head so when I do come back to the stressor I can see solutions instead of problems.

This was important because citing the studies from my research, it confirmed what I had always suspected: Stress kills, or in my friend Vince's case, stress maims.

I also learned to monitor the effects of the stress I was under, which in my case were visible and very apparent once I lost my jobs and Abby started trying to keep me away from my kids. The ringing in my ears was often very loud and at times I had chest pains at regular intervals. The skin on my arms, face and scalp also would become very flaky and inflamed, and I had sores that weren't healing. Worse, my blood sugar levels would spike and would keep getting worse. My blood sugar spikes were another source of stress since I didn't have medication to be able to control them. Strangely enough, the health problems the stress was causing caused me even greater stress.

Because of the health problems I was experiencing, the right thing would have been to see a doctor. But I barely had enough resources to be able to survive day-to-day, and I didn't want to spend what little money I did have on a doctor. My real estate deals kept falling out even after months of working them, and my unemployment insurance ran out so I couldn't justify a doctor visit because I often didn't even have enough money for food.

I kept applying for work, including temporary and contract work and circulated over forty-five hundred resumes since I started looking for a permanent job more than three years before when my contract with the FDIC ran out. I have the experience and background to run a half-billion dollar company but I couldn't even land a ten dollar an hour temp job in that economy. I wasn't alone though, many of my friends and former colleagues from the FDIC were in similar boats after their contracts ended.

The fact that I was under such intense stress really stayed in the forefront of my mind because I didn't want to end up like my buddy or anyone else who suffered a stroke for that matter.

As I mentioned before, one of the important lessons I learned was not to just keep barreling ahead while I was under that much stress, especially if it was only to make sure that I finish whatever task was in front of me. Now I give myself some breathing room and take some time out to remind myself that the world isn't going to end if I don't finish the task on time or even finish it at all.

One morning was especially tough because of the real estate transactions I was trying to close. That's a whole different kind of stress altogether because a lot of it can involve trying to keep opposing parties engaged and calm until the deal is finally done. The good news is I built a very successful career doing those types of deals, and based on some feedback from current clients it appears that I haven't lost my touch in terms of negotiating tough deals.

On that morning I noticed that my heart was beating pretty fast. The ringing in my ears was loud and I was very short of breath. I felt my limbs getting tingly and my skin was peeling much more than usual. I realized I was feeling this way because it seemed like what should have been a great transaction and an easy one to close might not happen for reasons beyond my control. It also made me realize that I may not get a paycheck for all the efforts I was putting in.

I recognized the signs of heavy stress and decided to let myself relax and drift into a short but deep nap. The brief respite gave me the break I needed. I didn't sleep long enough to be fully refreshed, but I was able to move ahead and get the problems with the transaction resolved.

Stress Impacts On Physical Health

There are a number of studies that point directly to the increase in blood sugar caused by stress, and there are those that also include how stress can affect or cause the ancillary complications like obesity, cardiovascular problems, and hypertension. These are all related and are dramatically impacted by stress, and the fact that anyone under a lot of stress is at a higher risk of stroke by having heart problems or diabetes. Those of us who are under severe stress need to recognize the relationship between stress and poor health. We also need to know what can be done to minimize the risks.

Stress is both mental and physical, and can cause your blood sugar to spike and stay spiked. If you have diabetes you have to do whatever you can to keep your stress at a minimum.

It's important to pay attention to what is stressing you out. It can be one thing or a combination of things, like work, family, finances, a rocky marriage, or, in my case, all of the above. When you are stressed your body secretes stress hormones like cortisol and adrenaline (also known as epinephrine). These stress hormones are designed to raise your blood sugar so you get the energy boost you need to either fight or flee whatever it is that is causing you stress.

Chronic vs. Acute Stress is also defined as acute, or short term stress, and chronic, or long term stress. Acute stress is brought on as a reaction to an immediate threat, whether real or perceived, and this is the fight-or-flight aspect of stress. Common short term stressors are loud noises, noisy crowds, being hungry, remembering or imagining a scary event or even playing a video game or watching an intense movie. In these cases you usually get the shot of adrenaline, or the 'rush' as we call it, but then you get back to normal once the stress has passed.

Chronic stress, on the other hand, doesn't let up and becomes a more dangerous form of stress, dangerous to your health. When you have chronic stress it means that you are in a perpetual fight-or-flight mode so your body is consistently pumping adrenaline and cortisol in your system without letting up. That means a lot of extra sugar in your blood.

The most common chronic stressors are mental stressors like pressure at work, relationship problems like with a significant other or kids, loneliness, or money problems. There are physical stresses like having the flu or various infections. One thing that often happens during periods of stress is stress-eating while simultaneously skipping the daily workout. For many it can be one or the other, but for me it's both and it is very hard for me to combat it.

It is a good idea to break down warning signs of stress based on the categories they impact. These signs aren't always going to appear together, but they are worth paying attention to so you can work at finding ways to relieve the tension.

One category that is often affected is cognitive or one's ability to reason and function intellectually. Signs of stress can show up in memory problems, an inability to concentrate, poor judgment, and negative or anxious thoughts.

Another serious area is one's emotional well-being, something I struggled with for quite a while. It can show up as moodiness, irritability or short temper, loneliness, feeling overwhelmed, and depression. Irritability and short-temperedness are also symptomatic of diabetes.

While behavioral areas might be lumped in with emotions, they are really a separate category since one's emotional state is all about how one feels whereas behavioral areas are relegated to how one is acting based upon those feelings. Excessive stress can lead to eating problems, sleep problems, procrastination or avoidance, escapes like smoking, drugs or alcohol, isolation and nervous habits like nail biting.

Then there are actual physical symptoms to look for like aches and pains, problems with bowel movements, nausea and dizziness, chest pains and rapid heartbeats, and loss of sex drive.

I can attest to most of those symptoms which I chose to ignore for so many years without realizing just how much damage I was causing myself.

Keep in mind that the signs and symptoms of stress can also be caused by other psychological and medical problems. If you're experiencing any of the warning signs of stress, it's important to see a doctor for a full evaluation. Your doctor can help you determine whether or not your symptoms are stress-related.

There is an interesting side note here about adrenaline. Earlier I talked about the positive effects of exercise because it gets your adrenaline up and helps you achieve a better outlook. Getting that adrenaline does a lot for lifting people out of their depression but if your adrenaline is always being pumped into your system because of chronic stress, then it will harm your body because of the added sugar in your system and other harmful effects.

I rely on certain habits and routines to help at least offset the harmful effects of stress-eating or skipping workouts, like sticking to a healthy menu but throwing in some chips, an ice cream bar or a frozen yogurt. At times I'll overeat some of the healthy stuff and then have a small amount of the bad stuff which was completely opposite from before.

In the past, I'd eat a big steak with a baked potato and rolls, appetizers, salad with extra dressing, two or three regular beers, and finish it off with some carrot cake or cheesecake and regular coffee. My heart would beat like crazy and I'd be so stuffed I'd have trouble breathing sometimes.

In contrast, now on the really stressed days I might have two tuna-sized cans of salmon prepared with low-fat mayo, chopped onions, avocado, tomato, and chopped jalapenos with a big handful of Pringles and a one-hundred-calorie ice cream-sandwich. The latter still isn't the best for me but it is a lot better than what I used to do and it gives me that stress-eating outlet. To compare calories, what I used to eat would be anywhere from twenty-five hundred to three thousand calories in a high-fat meal vs. less than one thousand calories low-fat meal that I gravitate to now. My ultimate goal is to purge stress-eating from my life cycle, but for now I'm happy to keep the stress eating on the healthier side.

Prolonged Illness Or Distress

Something else that diabetics need to watch for is prolonged illnesses or long periods of distress or deep depression. This will keep blood sugar levels up for a long time. As crazy as it might sound, I don't always recognize that I'm under stress until I start noticing certain physiological changes like my heart beating faster or erratically accompanied by shortness of breath, my blood pressure is higher, or my skin starts to flake and peel.

It might be hard to imagine, but there are a lot of things in our world that can be sources of long-term threats. One source can be surgeries that have normally short recoveries but instead take a long time to recover from become or are stressors to your body, and the stress hormones that are normally designed to defend against short-term danger become activated for long periods and can elevate your blood sugar levels.

Other long-term stressors can be mental and you end up with

the enemy in your own mind. I do this all the time. How many times have you stayed angry over something that happened on a phone call, at work, or while stuck in a traffic jam? If you carry grudges or keep reliving the event in your mind then you are creating a long-term stress problem and your body will keep pumping sugar in your blood. My mental stress is the worst and it definitely impacts my physical health. If I can't go to a better place mentally then I can't sleep, I eat poorly, and I won't exercise.

There is research on this topic that points to those effects of stress. In diabetics, stress alters blood sugar in two ways, and one of them is exactly the same as when you are depressed:

1)People under heavy stress usually don't take good care of themselves, they tend to drink alcohol more and exercise less, and they don't check their glucose enough or at all.
2)Cortisol and adrenaline are known to increase blood sugar levels.

Managing Stress

Stress can actually be a good thing under certain circumstances. There's nothing like a shot of adrenaline to boost you over the finish line when you're in a friendly competition. The same can be said when you need it to help you get out of harm's way. Those kinds of things are what our stress hormones were designed for. Think of your body as a finely tuned car engine.

You start it up in the morning and give it the gas to get where you need to go, and you give it extra gas when you need to get somewhere fast or out of the way fast. Once you get where you're going, you turn the engine off and give it a rest. And that's the way our bodies were designed. We have to fuel them by eating the right foods, we have internal mechanisms to give us the boosts of energy that we need, and we have to get plenty of rest so that we can recharge.

Let's look at an alternative, and for argument's sake let's assume that our gas engine has an unlimited fuel supply which, in our case, it does through eating and burning fat and muscle for fuel. What do you think would happen to that finely tuned engine if we started it in the morning and kept our foot on the gas even when we got to where we were going?

Vital parts of the engine are going to wear out until the engine eventually breaks down. That is exactly what happens to our bodies when we are under chronic stress. We are constantly in a revved state so things will eventually breakdown. Anyone dealing with stress has to start analyzing what kind of stress they're dealing with and what the stressors are. Then you can start to take a look at what you can do to deal with the stress the right way as opposed to drinking or eating it away. You might even look at whether or not you can eliminate it.

Sometimes people are under stress because they don't like their jobs. It doesn't mean you can't take steps to move ahead in the job you're in. There is an abundance of online classes, so work on getting a degree. If money is a problem, look at ways to supplement your income. Despite all of my stress and worry about money that you've read me gripe about, I'm networking with friends and getting real estate leads as a result so that I can generate income. Soon I'll be doing that for insurance leads as well. Some stress can be relieved simply by changing the scenery or breaking old, bad habits. Exercising for fun is a great way to relieve stress and so is joining new social groups and making new friends.

As I mentioned in Chapter 7 I was very fortunate to be referred to Dr. Deidre Alexander who counseled me for nearly a year, and the results were great. She answered my first question by telling me that, in her opinion, I wasn't crazy. I took that to mean we were off to a good start. Dr. Alexander helped me sort through the olio of emotions that was brewing inside me and was causing me to act in ways that were very unlike me. More importantly she helped me find ways to get control of my emotions.

As a testimonial to this is my current situation, my current financial mess is largely due to not finding work and due to the havoc that Abby has continued to cause to suit her vile disposition. Despite having to live with it, I'm not consumed by it like I used to be and I'm actually able to look beyond those events and see ways to overcome them.

I can't stand the sight of Abby now that I've seen the kind of person she really is, but seeing or hearing her doesn't ruin my day like it once did and I don't have the same physiological responses that I use to have. I treat her cordially for Austin's sake, but beyond that I don't think about Abby much at all except when I'm forced to.

Coping With Stress

How we cope with stress can be a big deal and the means I use to cope with it now are dictated by my circumstances. A while ago I was faced with having to pay for a major repair on my Suburban, but if I were to get it fixed I would still be driving a vehicle that only gets eleven miles to the gallon. My other option was to buy another vehicle. There was no way that I could afford even a used car, so I took the money that it would have cost to make the repairs and bought myself a motorcycle. It's an old Honda which gets more than fifty miles to the gallon, and not only is the insurance cheap but it lowered the insurance on my Suburban since I'm driving it fewer miles. I was able to really lower the stress that I had from seeming to never have enough money to buy gas.

I also like riding the Honda and it became a kind of fun therapy. One day I just took off and rode it along the beach and then on a mountain road nearby, the same mountain road I thought of when I was deciding how I wanted to kill myself. This time, I was enjoying the scenery and loving the way the motorcycle was handling on the curves. Better yet, I hit the beaches, the mountains, and visited with friends over many miles, and it only cost me less than twelve dollars in gas.

That is one of the ways I learned to relax, but other people have different yet equally effective ways. It really depends upon who you are, what your environment dictates, and how much control you are able to gain when dealing with your stressors. Some people treat stress as a problem that can be solved, so they first look at their options then try to change what needs to be changed. That's what I did when I saw Dr. Alexander and when I bought my motorcycle.

Others decide to accept the problem for what it is and then live with it. This too can have a calming effect. But if acceptance is how you choose to deal with a problem, then I will offer this bit of caution: Make sure you really understand what the problem is and what the consequences are for accepting it.

Let's say you are stressing over your adult son or daughter's decision to buy a car that was different than the one you hoped he or she'd buy. Is that such a bad problem? Probably not, and it certainly isn't going to cause you any impact unless you're seven feet tall and can't fit in it or you are the one making the payments. In other words, analyze the problem to see if it is a problem at all or is it just something in your head? If it is just in your head, the best fix is to simply accept it and move on.

But how about if you were like me and resolved yourself to being obese instead of taking steps to fix it by losing weight? When I bought new clothes instead of losing weight, I was only considering how bad I looked when I was that heavy. I didn't notice any health changes so I never considered that I was going to have heart trouble, high blood pressure and diabetes by accepting my excessive weight.

Solving the problem or accepting the problem can be great ways to reduce stress and lower your blood sugar, but just be sure it's a problem you can accept without long-term consequences. These two methods of coping are usually helpful. People who use them tend to have less blood glucose elevation in response to mental stress.

There's also a deeper issue for diabetics under stress, especially type 2 diabetics. Stress causes blood sugar levels to rise, but it also can block the body from releasing insulin. This isn't a problem for type 1 diabetics since they already have problems with insulin production, but you can see how it can be an added problem for people with type 2. If someone with type 2 stops releasing insulin, there are a host of problems that could occur but not least of which is becoming insulin dependent or a type 1 diabetic. Studies show that relaxation can help offset the blockage.

Breathing exercises is one way. Sit or lie down in a comfortable, relaxed position and make sure your limbs are uncrossed. Breathe deeply and slowly, in and out for as long as you want or need. Relaxation therapy is yet another, based on tensing then relaxing your muscles. Lately I have been focusing my thoughts on, "everything is going to be ok." It's short and sweet, and is the line that I used over many years to get me through very dark times.

How Do You Deal With Stress When It Is Related To Diabetes?

In life, there will always be some sort of stress no matter where you are or what you do. Even in the most peaceful of existences, stress will find its place in our lives and that is something we all have to accept. For us diabetics, diabetes is one of those stress sources that won't go away, but it doesn't mean that the stress of it can't be reduced.

Talking with others who have it can be a way to find relief, especially if you trade tips on how to deal with it effectively. You might want to consider joining a support group. My niece's son Timothy is a type 1 diabetic and one of the many ways she supports him is by being an active organizer for the Junior Diabetes Research Foundation (JDRF).

It's a way to help raise money for research while getting exercise and making new friends. Some people get stressed by having to deal with diabetes care issues, and I've known type 1 diabetics who have had these issues at times. And who wouldn't? We are all human and while some really grab on to the regimen of blood glucose monitoring and insulin injections, many often become resentful and stressed. The idea of having to monitor my blood doesn't stress me out, but when under a lot of stress I have a tendency to abandon all of my regimens including that one so I really have to work on dealing with it better.

This is where others may be able to help. Friends, family, fellow diabetics or counselors can all help to calm the storm, lend a shoulder or bring you back to reality so you don't go too far off the edge. I have been very lucky with my friends and family, and while I'm very cognizant of my potential to become burdensome, I do reach out when I feel my levels of stress are at a point where I'm physically sick and just need to take a break.

Chronic stress often presents physical symptoms. Sometimes they're mild like headaches or being extra vulnerable to colds or flu. I think back over many years where I would get these bad flus, usually around the holidays. I would sometimes sleep for thirty hours straight then start to recover; that should have been a warning sign.

But like in the gas engine analogy I used earlier in the chapter, persistent, chronic stress will often lead to more serious symptoms and health problems. These problems can include:

1. *Depression*
2. *Diabetes*
3. *Hair loss*
4. *Heart disease*
5. *Hyperthyroidism*
6. *Obesity*
7. *Obsessive-compulsive or anxiety disorder (OCD)*
8. *Sexual dysfunction*
9. *Tooth and gum disease*
10. *Ulcers*

Put me down for numbers 1, 2, 3, 4, 6, 7, and 8.[20] Number 9 is a possibility but it also runs in our family. The added weight also led to my getting a hernia in my stomach which was unsightly. Earlier I talked about the importance of adrenaline and cortisol, but too much cortisol in your system can impact some very important body functions including glucose absorption, blood pressure maintenance, insulin production, immune system functions, and how your body reacts to inflammation.

Cortisol usually appears in higher levels in the morning, and is normally lowest at night. Stress isn't the only reason your body secretes cortisol, but it's referred to as a stress hormone because it is activated in higher levels in response to stress and can actually be beneficial.

Cortisol secretions can result in quick bursts of energy or help the immune system react. It can also help lower your sensitivity to pain. To make it work best for you, it's critical that you learn to relax and relax often or you can end up learning the hard way like me.

I listed some of the consequences of excessive cortisol secretions, but there are more which are caused by prolonged stress, ones that I didn't pay attention to but should have. Too much stress can cause you to have impaired performance, can decrease bone density and muscle tissue.

It can slow wound healing and more importantly can cause you to have increased belly fat which is the worst kind of fat to develop. Increased belly fat can lead to heart attacks, stroke, increase levels of LDL (bad cholesterol) and reduced levels of HDL (good cholesterol) and we don't need to be geniuses to know that cholesterol leads to a whole other set of health problems.

Relaxation is really the key, and like I discussed before you need to identify what you can do about your stressors to keep them from happening or to keep them from impacting you, but don't wait until you remove, change, or accept them before learning to relax. Relaxation is a whole separate but necessary function to utilize while you are choosing the best way to deal with your stressors. I recommend it as good therapy.

There are also studies that show how people who are chronically stressed tend to eat more, and the food is often high in carbohydrates. We've all seen it right? I did it myself; I had a tendency to run to

---

[20] This cluster of health disorders is known as the X syndrome or Metabolic syndrome which is a direct result of cortisol secretion caused by chronic stress.

comfort food when I used to have those hard days. I know someone who would drink a minimum of two bottles of wine a night on those hard days. So how bad is that for a combination of assaults on your body due to chronic stress? Let's see, chronic stress puts more sugar in your blood while reducing the amount of insulin needed to process it. You put more sugar in your blood on top of it through eating and drinking, then not exercising due to stress and low energy. Whoops, I said you, I should have said me. I was and am extremely sensitive to stress and now that I know about it, I know exactly how I became so sick and out of shape.

My goal along with hoping to reverse my diabetes is to get to where I can live a very low-stress life. Not so coincidently, each of the goals has a tremendous impact on the other. It is estimated that ninety percent of doctor's visits are for problems in which stress has had some kind of impact.

In an excellent article titled *The Effects of Stress Overload and What You Can Do About It (Melinda Smith, 2015)* stress is broken down into very simple terms and the consequences of long term chronic stress is laid out and as I know firsthand, the results are not pretty. In it, Psychologist Connie Lillas uses an analogy similar to the one I used before to describe the three most common ways people respond when they're overwhelmed by stress foot on the gas, foot on the brake, or foot on both.

In fact, many of the immediate health problems that are a direct result of stress themselves lead to other health problems such as what I have, heart disease and diabetes. Helpguide.org has put together much more than just a good article, its website features a whole life plan and road map to understanding stress and its causes, complications, and more importantly proven remedies while bringing the subtleties of it to the forefront.

Stress however, doesn't always look stressful. If you frequently find yourself feeling scattered or overwhelmed, then you need to take the time to get back into balance. You can teach yourself to recognize stress symptoms so you can take action to reduce the harmful effects.

Physical and psychological threats are recognized separately when your body starts to react. If you happen to be agonizing over bills, job problems or an ugly confrontation, your body can't tell the difference from those events versus one where somebody is threatening your life. And if your mind is filled with lots of stress inducing thoughts, then your response system is going to be on most if not all of the time. Worse, once that stress mode is triggered, it becomes very hard to turn off. It can also make you much more susceptible to depressions and panic attacks.

How Much Stress Is Too Much?

This is a question that can only be best answered by the individual, but with that said it is a very important question to ask because of how much damage stress can cause. What causes you stress may have no impact on me and vice versa. As an example, I'm comfortable standing in front of a room with a hundred people in it and giving an impromptu speech, yet public speaking is the number one greatest fear in this country.

Additionally how you cope with stress is also a major factor in surviving it and often boils down to things we might not think of like genetics, how well you control your emotions or the strength of your key relationships. Some people get freaked out in a five mile –an-hour fender bender while others barely escape death without giving the event a second thought.

These things can and do influence how well we tolerate stress, and while some of them seem basic it is a pretty good bet that most people don't realize how much they are really being impacted by some of these influences.

Strong relationships with family and friends can be a great source of support, whereas lack of relationships can actually be a source of stress. And so can meddling from some of those who are usually well-intended.

Self-confidence and self-esteem can help you withstand significant challenges, but lack of them can lead to added stress.

Optimism and positive feelings are powerful antidotes to heavy stress, and so is your ability to control your reactions to everyday events. Right along-side of optimism is how well you can prepare yourself for what comes next, knowledge is power but wishful thinking is a recipe for disaster. The more you can learn about what is causing you stress, the better equipped you will be to deal with it and even possibly eliminate it.

One of the areas that took me quite a while to deal with was whether or not I could control my stress. The truth of the matter was

I couldn't which is why I went to counseling. There are questions we all need to ask ourselves in order to determine the right courses of action, like do I know how to relax, or can I release my anger? There are more questions like who can I turn to, and how am I feeling when I get home at night? Am I depressed or am I in a good mood?

The bottom line is you need to take an emotional health inventory on a pretty regular basis so you can spot the signs, especially if you find yourself in one or more of the common stress inducing events.

The Holmes-Rahe Life Stress Inventory (The Holmes and Rahe Stress Scale) lists the following as the **Top Ten Stressful Life Events:**

1. *Spouse's death*
2. *Divorce*
3. *Marriage separation*
4. *Jail term*
5. *Death of a close relative*
6. *Injury or illness*
7. *Marriage*
8. *Fired from job*
9. *Marriage reconciliation*
10. *Retirement*

Stress can come from just about anything, in fact something as simple as change, or your perception of change, can be a major source of stress. Looking at the top ten list; it's interesting to see that five of the ten involve marital relationships, four of which are dealing with marital strife. I have a friend, Jim, whose wife of eight years refused to be happy, but not surprisingly she wasn't happy before they were married nor was she happy after they were married or divorced. She wasn't happy with the affair that led to her divorce either. After the dust settled from the divorce Jim found Tamara who seemed to be the perfect match, so much so that they have had serious talks about getting married.

Something happened to cause him to rethink whether or not marrying Tamara would be a good idea. Jim had been putting more time and money into his house to make her happy and not only incorporating Tamara's ideas but pretty much using her ideas instead of his. It was his way of helping her to feel as though the house is more hers than his ex-wife's. Not only did Tamara not live there, she had openly said that she doesn't like the house and when they get married she wants them to buy something bigger and use his as a rental.

Jim had been very accommodating until one day he wanted to finish a room that had been under reconstruction for months because of a leak. When it came time to pick the paint, Jim talked with Tamara about the color and asked her to come with him to pick it out. Tamara refused because she said she had things she needed to do.

At the hardware store Jim sent Tamara pictures of the various colors he was considering, and four of the five she hated but said she could live with the fifth. Jim bought that paint and spent many hours prepping the room for painting. When Tamara saw the small section he painted the next day she blew up at him saying the paint was unacceptable and accused him of not giving her any opportunities to choose the paint with him. HUH?

The reaction surprised all of us who are close to them, but it went far beyond heated arguments. Tamara was relentless and would try and rally support for her side from anyone who would listen. Jim stopped working on the room for a week while they argued and finally he gave in to the paint that she wanted which cost more than double. Tamara was also fine with the idea that Jim couldn't get his money back for the paint he'd purchased previously.

Here is the kicker: Once he finally gave in after a week of ugly fighting and a week of lost time during which he could have finished the room, she told him he could use the original paint that he picked. She told him that it really had nothing to do with picking the paint; it was only about whether or not she could get him to change his mind.

This whole scenario resonates so deeply with me because he looks like I used to, slim, fit, and most of the time calm. But I can already see the physiological changes because of the toll these sorts of things are taking like his hands shaking and the involuntary twitches. He is a guy who is willing to share a life he worked hard to build with someone he thought was ready to accept it as the gift it is. Instead he is learning that it is only about whether or not he can be controlled by Tamara, and that is putting him under a lot of stress.

I know others who are dealing with similar mates and they have developed heart problems despite leading a very healthy lifestyle but with daily doses of massive stress. What causes us stress depends a lot on how we perceive it, but stress also has direct sources. I don't know of anyone who is not stressed by an overbearing mate who is all about themselves no matter who gets hurt.

We looked at the Holmes-Rahe survey for the top ten sources of stress, but there are many others whether external or internal. Kids and family can be major sources of stress whether internal or external. When Austin told me he was put in a headlock by Ralph1, that caused me a tremendous amount of stress because I was thousands of miles away and who knows what else this guy was going to try and do to my kid when I wasn't around. I was also stressed because that could have been true of Abby's other boyfriends for that matter.

I was eventually able to deal with it through my court action, but it was a significant source of stress until I got it resolved. When family is sick or when you are arguing, these events can also be highly stressful.

Other things are very impactful, like dealing with uncertainty, being pessimistic and pummeling yourself with negative talk, setting goals too high or trying to be perfect when perfection is beyond your control, or letting others control you. I am often guilty of generating my own stress through any number of the above.

Some people thrive on having a deadline to meet while others panic at the thought of it. Some people have no problem dealing with a conflict like deflecting a false accusation or bringing a problem to someone's attention, while others cringe at the thought of any confrontation.

Some people thrive by leading a team and having to deliver actionable items on short notice; others are consumed by it and can't move ahead. When I was with the FDIC one of the first things they told us in orientation was how much they needed us to be flexible. I had been called to action on several occasions where we had to be ready to go in and take over a bank at a moment's notice. In order for us to make that happen, those of us selected to manage the field teams had to conduct an in-depth analysis of the bank structure and then devise a strategic plan as to how we would conduct the closing. And there was no room for error.

Once a bank employee was angry with his bank's management so he posted some derogatory comments about the bank and said it would be closing. In doing so he almost caused a run on the bank and so we had to assemble a team ready to go in and close the bank as soon as the regulator directed us to do it. Within just a few hours of being notified that it might happen, we were ready. Some of the people who were asked to do it couldn't handle the stress of it, others, including me, were raring to go.

The reason a bank run is so critical is because it can be a potentially dangerous environment because of, are you ready? The stress the depositors are under; and it can take on mob-like scenarios. The FDIC is one of the best quasi-government organizations that I'm aware of and they are well equipped to handle those problems and do so with care specifically to alleviate the stress caused by a run or bank closing. It all ended well, we sat in the shadow ready to assist but the bank management team kept cool heads and took care of its customers and everyone stayed calm. And the idiot who nearly caused the run? He faced federal charges because what he did violated federal laws.

There are many references and studies regarding depression and the link to diabetes. The conclusions are pretty basic, at least on the surface:

1) People who are in deep depression[21] often develop a lifestyle that leads to diabetes. Through their feelings of hopelessness, they often abandon healthy living.
2) People who have diabetes often become depressed because of the maintenance that is required for survival.

I fall into the first category, though during the early months after my diabetes diagnosis I found myself becoming angry instead of depressed. I was angry because it finally sunk in that I wasn't the superman I thought I was, and I couldn't keep hammering at my body the way I had been without suffering the consequences. I didn't like having to restrict myself now that I had the disease. You would think I would have drawn that conclusion when I found I had heart problems, but I ran into so many people who had the same heart problems that I didn't take my own very seriously.

My lifestyle and habits deteriorated over many years of daily stress. Before I got married I was an avid bicyclist and jogger. My regimen was about two to five miles a day on runs and between fifteen to thirty miles on bicycle almost every other day. As a result

---

[21] Deep depression is when one can no longer see any positives around them, regardless of how many upsides there might be within their grasp. Deep depression is a feeling of total hopelessness that can lead to dire consequences like self-destruction and suicide.

I was in good shape and could eat almost anything I wanted. I also got a lot of sleep, generally in bed between 8:30 and 9 p.m., then up at 5 a.m. for my early morning run.

The rest of my life back then consisted of going to school, to which I rode my bike, and working in undercover security at a department store. I had a tight regimen that was easy to maintain, and if for some reason I missed a bike ride or a morning run, it was easy to make up for it by doing a workout at a different time of day.

That all changed not long after I was married and our oldest son was born; and boy did my life change. Since I had a whole new responsibility of having a family to feed, I found myself working two jobs and carrying a full course-load in college. It took a lot out of me physically, but after Alex was born I found new purpose and direction, so I poured everything I had into building a life for us.

We lived in a tiny one bedroom apartment then later upgraded to a two-bedroom while struggling financially the entire time. I tried to incorporate my exercise regimen into my daily life but between two jobs and carrying fifteen to eighteen college units at any given time it was next to impossible. I hated the life we were living and the fact that we were so poor. I had a financial vision of where I wanted us to be but that vision would get cut short every time the phone or electricity would get cut off because we were past due.

While I was in school and later when I got out, I kept focused on finding a career that would help me take us out of poverty and I found the mortgage banking industry. For the first part of it, I worked on straight commission with a small draw against commissions to help keep our income and bill payments steady. In the early years I sometimes would have a paycheck of as little as twenty-five dollars for the month. Although rare, it usually happened because some of my loans that I needed to close so I could get paid got cancelled or postponed. The job demanded many late nights and weekends, and because I made no money unless a transaction closed I was constantly on the search for new ones. So I found it very hard to relax especially on the weekends if no one was calling me to meet with clients.

The stress load was heavy and by the time we had two boys who were seventeen months apart, I never reestablished a workout regimen. I was too tired all the time, both mentally and physically, and I wasn't the easiest person to get along with. This was mainly because of my job, my schooling, and all of the other stuff my wife kept dumping on me. That other stuff consisted of her never wanting to help shoulder the burden and instead would just come to me with all of her problems and expect me to make her happy. The stupid part was that I did. I took on every single responsibility for our well-being, and that included housework, baby duty and yard chores on top of going to school and earning a living.

After about five years of roller coaster riding with finances and career, I got a big break. I was recruited by a competitor because Myrna, one of their top agents wanted me out of her territory. After I was there for a short while I got promoted and our financial stress eased a lot, but I traded that for a different kind of stress. Not only was I being held accountable for some lofty production goals, I also had to manage a hostile and mercurial group of producers and turn a perpetually money losing region into a profit center.

I was able to do that by forcing my team to break their bad habits and teaching them to work smarter. But while I was doing that, I was actually developing some new and very bad habits of my own and growing heavier as a result. But I wasn't paying attention because I was looking externally at our living situations instead of internally at my own health.

While this was happening there was another problem brewing that I also chose to ignore. It was intimacy with Abby, or should I say lack of it. In all my stupidity and arrogance, I could not or would not see what I looked like through her eyes. Because of that blindness, I became angry that I no longer excited her and sometimes was angry with her for not being excited. Instead of fixing it, I resigned myself to feeling entitled to sex because I was such a great provider. That just sent me into deeper depression and added stress. I found out during the divorce however that she never did have an interest in me from day one; I was mainly the way for her to get out of living at home. Even if I had been paying attention it probably wouldn't have made a difference anyway.

Though a good financial provider with a promising future, I should have also been focused on balancing my life for my sake as well as my sons'. One of my problems was I looked at the past so I could compare where we were in that moment to the poverty we had come from, so of course we looked great. We had a nice house with a pool, new cars, and money in the bank. I looked at my physical appearance differently. Knowing what I used to look like and how many miles I used to run every day, I lulled myself into believing that it wouldn't take much to be physically fit again. I was always too busy and ignored thinking about all the effort it took to build solid workout routines which included endurance exercises, good diet and lots of sleep; none of which was a part of my current lifestyle. Had I given it more thought, I would have started the process by making small changes toward a bigger goal of trimming down.

Despite our overall lack of intimacy we did manage to connect at some point and so came our third child Austin, one who took nearly three years before he would sleep through the night. I'm both blessed and cursed with an ability to sleep for twenty to thirty minutes then waking up refreshed for several hours. This served me well when I needed sleep while driving long distances or even when taking power naps during the day before important presentations and meetings.

Yet it proved to be a nightmare at home because Austin would wake me up at two in the morning and I would be awake for the rest of the day. I could get through one or two days of it just fine, but I would be exhausted beginning about the third consecutive day. Everything for me was impacted during that time; I had no energy and was irritable most of the time. By about the fifth day though, I would usually collapse in to a deep sleep and wake up refreshed only to begin the vicious cycle all over again.

Soon after I was promoted to VP, we were taken over and by the time our company was sold I weighed over three hundred pounds because of all of the stress and bad habits I accumulated while earning the promotion. I was out of a job because the new company didn't have a position I could transition to; and it wasn't long before I was fending off even deeper depressions.[22]

The first few months after I lost my job though, we were pretty secure financially because as an officer I got a golden parachute that was pretty substantial. Instead of working on me, I painted our house, played with Austin who was then eighteen months old, and I did try some running and biking but none of it stuck as a regimen.

---

[22] One interesting side note was that the bank who bought my bank was one that we closed down while I was at the FDIC, and many who had careers there were decimated financially because of the closure. So even if I had gotten a job there, it would have only delayed the inevitability of my job loss. I joined the FDIC a little under a year later and became part of the team that administered portions of the shutdown.

Ironically about two years after I lost my jobs with other banks, WAMU, the bank that took my previous company over offered me a job in their Newport Beach Office but rescinded it when they shuttered their entire mortgage operations throughout the country. It was incredibly hard to see any positives in my life by that point because my whole career was based on products and operations that were perceived to be responsible for all the shut downs that were taking place all over the country. It wasn't because I had done anything wrong, but the market had turned and killed off all of the opportunity we had been looking forward to.

I now understand for myself the correlation between depression and diabetes, at least in the link that shows how depression can lead to a lifestyle that causes diabetes. Through my feelings of self-loathing and worthlessness, I abandoned what little self-control I had and was secretly trying to kill myself through poor health. Despite having plenty of time on my hands, my state of mind was so congested with all that self-hatred that I couldn't find a routine to help myself, nor did I want one.

I learned this time that eating right, exercising and sleep were important keys to warding off depression, and I figured high doses of prayer couldn't hurt either. There is also a lot to be said for just exchanging negative self-talk with positive self-talk. I really didn't attach these things to my problems before, but now I was able to see their impacts more clearly. Oddly enough, those key items were the keys to many other cures for things like obesity, skin problems, high blood pressure, and virility.

I had problems early on though as I was trying to find the right balance. By eating smaller portions more frequently I found that I ran out of energy quickly. That kind of took the wind out of my sails since I had recently built up enough stamina to do twenty and thirty mile bike rides, but after working on my new diet plan of smaller meals, I petered out at twelve miles on my first try. That was depressing, but I eventually overcame it.

Another aspect of a diabetes and depression was one that I hoped I wouldn't experience. It is depression caused by being held prisoner to the disease itself and envying fat people who could eat candy all day and not have the disease. I'm exaggerating of course, but the point is that once you have to force yourself into a box in order to survive; it can have a debilitating effect on your outlook if you don't find a way to stay upbeat. And it's even worse for people who have type 1.

Experts have a lot to say about depression and diabetes. One is how research shows that blood sugar changes and mood swings impact and worsen the other and can become a fatal combination. A more recent study by the University of Connecticut shows how diabetics who are depressed don't benefit as well by drugs or insulin. But when treated for both diabetes and depression at the same time, diabetics benefit more from the medications and their symptoms seem to lessen.

One other disturbing piece to this connection is that type 1 diabetic children are more likely to experience depression as adults. It's hard enough being a kid as it is, but so much tougher when you have type 1. My little nephew Timothy is type 1 and because of his mother's strength and attention to detail, he is great at living with the disease. But you can also see it have an effect sometimes.

What a vicious cycle depression sets off. When you are depressed, your body releases cortisol which we know causes problems. Another hormone depression messes with is serotonin which influences our moods, sexual desire, appetite, sleep, memory, and even social behavior. These hormone interruptions can result in many bad mood swings and weaken your immune system.

Here is one ugly rub; a lot of us eat comfort foods when we're stressed, depressed, or just in a bad mood. Those eating habits can actually lead one to getting diabetes, hence the vicious cycle. That was indeed a big part of my problem which was eating comfort food or simply going somewhere to eat just to get a break from all of the turmoil that was going on at work and often at home.

Here's a sobering statistic: a University of Washington study (MedResources Inc., 1996-2015) concluded diabetics with minor depression have a sixty-seven percent greater chance of dying, and diabetics in major depression have a one hundred and thirty percent greater chance of death than they would if they weren't depressed or diabetic. The diabetics who were depressed had more diabetic symptoms than those who weren't depressed. When you look at those statistics you can really see yourself as a walking time bomb, but the statistics themselves are so much more depressing.

The study didn't say why those with both diabetes and depression died; researchers believe it could have been a number of factors. Whatever their conclusions, the fact that they died makes a lot of sense to me. I often battled very severe bouts of depression which sapped my energy so much that I nearly was consumed by it.

What happened to me with tremendous frequency is that just when I started to get a little peace and some optimism about the future, I would get hit from all sides relating to my financial outlook, my ugly divorce and my health setbacks.

The paths that I was taking to try and live a normal life while battling a vile ex-wife and several deadly health conditions were often hard to navigate and I'd often wonder how I was going to survive any of it. I wanted desperately to show my sons that I could beat this but at the time all of the doors kept slamming shut. I needed to know that I could accomplish something especially in the face of what appeared at the time to be near insurmountable odds, and I needed a reason to hang on and keep working to fix myself.

There are symptoms of depression, and I've learned to notice most of them even though I often feel powerless to do anything about it. One that I never experienced though was loss of appetite; that would have actually been a plus for me. Other symptoms occurred; especially within the past few years starting with mood swings, and sadness or anxiety along with feelings of hopelessness and pessimism. Feelings of worthlessness and helplessness are common with depression and have intermittently been my life for the past ten years or so. Other symptoms are lack of concentration, insomnia, irritability and thoughts of suicide. These are all common symptoms of depression and those were what I experienced on most days. There are others like weight changes or no interest in sex, but those don't apply to me like the others do.

Depression researchers suggest that if five or more of these symptoms are in your daily living for at least two weeks then you should get professional help. Let's see, I counted nine for at least two months so based on the recommendation I should have been seeing a professional, but there was one more item to depress me. I didn't have any money to pay for a visit.

I guess one possible bright spot is that I don't have to feel so alone. I'm being facetious of course; this is a bad place to be. It is estimated that sixteen million diabetics are dealing with depression, and there are depressed people who are now at greater risk of developing diabetes because of it.

Research also shows how depressed people function poorly in their mental and physical capacities and are less likely to follow a mandatory diet, medication, or workout plan. I can attest to that because it's something that I had to grapple with daily and often lost the fight.

Why this happens is not entirely known, and it is thought that depression might be caused by stress, but it might also be caused by the metabolic issues associated with diabetes and the impacts on the brain. Even with so much known about depression, once it has set in, it still goes on undiagnosed and untreated.

Sometimes it's because people around you aren't always interested in your inner thoughts, and sometimes it's because when we're depressed we often do a good job of hiding it so we don't bring others down. If you asked me how I was doing on any given day, I guarantee you wouldn't know anything was wrong unless I made it a point to tell you there was something bothering me.

Treatments For Depression

If you don't happen to be in the desperate financial situation I was in, it's a good idea to get a professional's help. Sometimes depression can be treated by talking it through with a counselor. I did when I was a teenager and I saw a counselor a couple of years ago when I was going through some of the ugliest parts of my divorce. Those sessions help tremendously, and if I could afford it, I'd be going to a counselor right now to help me deal with an additional onslaught of problems.

Other times depression is treated with drugs. I mentioned earlier that I never did take my prescriptions, but that doesn't mean that this type of treatment isn't effective. For some people it is hugely effective, so this is an important discussion to have with your doctor or mental health professional. Scientists have reported that some of the medications have positive effects on mood swings as well as glycemic control. Indeed, it is worth looking into.

An important note especially if you are taking any kind of medication, be sure to talk with your doctor before taking any herbal or over-the-counter remedies because some of these, while appearing harmless enough, can have nasty interactions with medications so knowing what you are taking is vital if you are a diabetic.

If you are depressed, get help. I know it's something that many of us joke about at times but in reality depression drains you of the energy and strength you need to survive. I have built a network of close, trusted friends and family who have vested interests in my well-being. I can talk openly with them and they know me well enough to flag any issues that I may not have noticed. The fact that I can talk and vent, the fact that I have set some goals for myself that I can actually achieve, and the fact that I have my kids close are all factors that give me reasons to live and resources to help me get through the painful stuff.

If you don't have hope, do everything you can to find it and then pursue it. We're human so we will succumb to fear and helplessness at times, no matter how strong we used to be or could be. Don't let those feelings dictate who you are or cause you to think that there is no way out. There is always a way out, but for some of us it can be harder so we just have to brace ourselves and head straight into the storm.

One day I found myself complaining about my circumstances to my good friend Vince, who is permanently disabled because of strokes caused by stress. I closed my rant with my usual tag line, "Well, I shouldn't complain because I know it can always be worse."

Vince looked at me with a smile of compassion and said with labored speech, "I know. You could be like me." Whew! His comment brought me right back down to earth to where I finally got my head out of my ass. I often think of that response and while I don't dwell on it, it helps to snap me back into reality so that I don't get consumed and overwhelmed by what is getting me down. No matter what, things can always be worse.

I can tell you that no matter what, life is indeed worth living so don't waste time worrying about things you can't control. I'm living proof that you can focus on those things around you that are good and use them to pull you up so you can see what a great life this really is. Regardless of anything you can't change, the thing you can always change is your attitude. Chin up, because life is what you make it!

ELEVEN

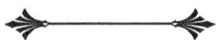

Myths, Misinformation, Medications and Lawsuits: All About Diabetes

Diabetes is the seventh leading cause of death in the U.S. That statistic alone should tell you what a serious disease this really is, but as I discussed in previous chapters, there are those who often don't take it seriously enough.

In this chapter, I've compiled a list of some of the most common myths associated with diabetes along with common medications. I separated the misinformation from the myths so I could make some clear distinctions. Bear in mind that a good number of myths reflected conventional wisdom at the time they began to circulate and some still do. I break apart myths from misinformation because a myth is mainly a belief but generally not something one uses to act upon. Misinformation however is something that someone can run across when trying to gain insights and that information could be harmful.

Here are two examples of myths: Sharks don't get cancer, a statement which was often heard at various health food and vitamin stores. The Discovery Channel says they do and proved it by showing a Great White with a tumor, but whether they do or don't is of no consequence to the average information consumer either way. Another myth was the cabbage soup diet which went as far back as the 1950s. Whoever followed the diet probably lost a little weight but not for long, not to mention the loss of essential nutrients needed for survival. Other than going hungry for a week this too had little consequence for the dieter.

On a more sinister scale however, are these two examples of misinformation: In as recently as the early 1980s it was common knowledge that giving a child aspirin when they had a fever or flu was helpful. Instead it was found to cause Reyes Syndrome which can be a child killer. Sadly it happened to some friends of my first wife whose twelve year old daughter died after being given aspirin for her flu. Another stark example of misinformation (in criminal form) was the Tapeworm Diet. The diet was marketed in the 1940s as a miracle diet pill which was actually a tapeworm egg. People lost a lot more than weight with that diet because they were ingesting a parasite that kept growing inside while slowly killing the host. Incredibly it surfaced again in the 1980s, this time as a tapeworm diet and people still used it as a means of dieting, and did so as recently as just a few years ago.

Some misinformation can result from the best information on hand at the time. It wasn't all that long ago that someone diagnosed with diabetes or heart condition was often relegated to only eating special diabetic foods as detailed in previous chapters, mainly sugar-free fare, but it wasn't until the early mid to late 20th century that diets and nutrition planning began to offer more freedoms and choices. Prior to that, as a general rule and depending upon the type of diabetes you had, you ate what the doctor and the nutritionist told you to eat and that was much harder to do because the food wasn't all that great. Science is forever evolving and that often results in a better picture overall.

I remember when my father had one of his several heart attacks in the late 1970s. The doctors ordered him to stay sedentary and not do anything strenuous. Now we know that regular exercise is far better than none in those cases provided you're under doctor supervision. It's possible that we'll see some of what we currently accept as best practices today may later themselves become myths, but that's something we really have no control over at this point. We simply have to work with the best information we have at hand and do our best to ensure that it will help and not hurt us.

That said, myths and conventional wisdoms should be scrutinized using viable, reputable, and credible information resources to confirm or contradict them.[23]

---

[23] There are some of what I feel are excellent resources noted in the bibliography, and if you don't find what you're looking for in them those resources can point you to other areas that may help.

With the many myths currently circulating about diabetes, people may believe some of them as truths, like whether or not it's a serious and deadly disease. It is serious, since diabetes causes more deaths than AIDS and breast cancer combined; two-thirds of them from heart problems or stroke. Here are some of the more common myths about diabetes and diets:

Myth: Don't eat sugar.
Fact: Sweets and sugars are ok if they are part of a balanced meal plan and combined with exercise.
Myth: The best diet is a high protein diet.
Fact: Some studies indicate that too much animal protein can cause insulin resistance. Once again, a balanced diet should include protein, carbohydrates, and fats.
Myth: Avoid Carbs (different from a high protein diet).
Fact: Carbohydrates are essential, but there are good and bad carbs. Simple sugars that are found in deserts and sugary drinks break down easily and should be avoided. But whole grains and legumes are complex carbs and break down slowly which helps your body to use the fuel it provides more efficiently.
Myth: Diabetics can't eat like normal people.
Fact: Moderate and monitor what you eat, talk with your doctor or nutritionist periodically but no reason you can't enjoy yourself.

I talk about how the way to eliminate the impact of type 2 diabetes is to lose weight and watch what you eat if you are overweight or obese. That is widely discussed in a number of resources but obesity lends itself to another myth: being overweight or obese will make you eventually develop type 2 diabetes. Weight is certainly a risk factor and losing it plays a definite role in reversing or managing it, but there are other risk factors that contribute to getting the disease.

Other factors, like family history, age, lifestyle, and ethnicity, can cause it to develop regardless of weight. Simply being overweight isn't a guarantee that you'll become diabetic, but it's a good idea to lose the weight anyway. If you are overweight and don't have diabetes, pretend that you will develop it so you have a greater incentive to get to a healthy weight and lifestyle.

In my family we had and have two type 1 diabetics and three type 2s so far in our history as well as heart disease, cancer and leukemia, and deaths from all of them except type 2.

Anybody remember a commercial in the early 1980s for the "Thirsty-Two Ouncer?" It featured a singer belting out her song about how she wants her 32-ounce Coke in the morning in a convenience store ad. To me nothing could be grosser, but people were actually drinking 32 ounces of regular Coke in the morning instead of a cup of coffee or two. Talk about sugar overload.

I've known people who told me they thought drinking coffee in the morning was really bad and wouldn't dream of it, while cracking open their can of Dr. Pepper at 6:00 a.m.. This all came to mind because I was recently watching a message from Coke at the movie theater about how they were taking a stance against obesity. Hmm, too little too late? One of the guys in my office at my last gig drank several of those thirty-two ounce Cokes a day from a cup about the size of a Jacuzzi. He was a good guy and I liked him, so I wanted to tell him that he wasn't doing himself any favors but never found the right opportunity. He ended up finding out on his own and learning the hard way. He developed type 2 about a year after I got to know him, and one of the big reasons was his soda habit.

Not surprisingly, the American Diabetes Association (ADA) cautions people, diabetic or not, to watch their intake of sugary drinks like sodas and fruit juices. Read the label and ask yourself if it's worth the 200 calories or more per 12 oz. drink in some cases. Anything sweetened with any form of sugar is going to be high in calories and carbs; whether it's soda, sport drinks, fruit juice, or sweet tea; it pays to take a look at what you're drinking. It also pays to limit your intake because your body can only take so much abuse before it starts to get overloaded.

Another myth is limiting the starches that you eat, like pasta, bread or potatoes. I have a tendency to do that because at one time I was on a low-carb diet and lost a lot of weight that went right back on from stress. One thing I've learned since being diagnosed with the disease is that our bodies like what they were intended to get naturally. We're omnivores so vegetables and grains are a part of the plan. Whole grain breads and pastas are usually best, and potatoes are good sources of nutrients, but for diabetics it depends upon what kind you're eating and how they're cooked because of the high starch content. The main point is portion control and balance.

If you're sitting down to eat a mashed potato sandwich on white bread with a side of corn and yams, you're going over the top. But a little potato with a piece of fish or chicken and a side of peas can be part of a healthy meal plan.[24] Sometimes I am offered sweets or chocolate and I'll say "thanks, but I really can't because I'm diabetic." That's a myth of course. The reality is that we diabetics can eat chocolate, sweets, and desserts, whether we have type 1 or type 2, but like everything else we need to watch the portions, make sure we get exercise, and type 1 diabetics need to plan ahead so their insulin shots are sufficient.

Here's another myth: Diabetes is contagious. No one really knows what causes it and yes there are genetic links, but it is a metabolic or autoimmune disease which is confined to the individual so you won't pass it to your neighbor by sneezing or any other way. It's not contagious.

Another myth is diabetics are more susceptible to other illnesses. In reality if a diabetic catches something like a cold or flu we can then develop more serious complications as a result of what we've caught, but we're not going to necessarily get sick just because we're diabetics. So for that reason, it is usually recommended that people with diabetes get flu shots and take extra precautions during the sick seasons.

Here's one, "I have a touch of diabetes". Huh? Diabetes is a metabolic disorder, resulting in either your body's inability to process the glucose in your blood because your cells are resistant, or because your body no longer produces the insulin necessary to process the glucose.

I don't know if this has ever happened to you, but I've been at parties and outings where people have learned that I am diabetic. It's not anything that I wear on my sleeve but every once in a while the host or someone else will make a reference to my having diabetes that others overhear. I've had people come over to me on the sly, usually women, who say something like, "I don't eat carbs because my glucose goes too high." So I'll take the bait and ask if they're diabetic and the answer is usually no, but it's almost like they wish they were so they can get extra attention. The fact of the matter is that carbs will elevate glucose levels in diabetics and non-diabetics alike, it's what our bodies use as fuel. The differences between the two are how that fuel is processed.

For some reason, some people think that only adults get type 2 diabetes. If only that were true, but unfortunately more and more children are contracting it and the culprit seems to point to poor diet and childhood obesity.

---

[24] Refer to the guide on portions in Chapter 8.

There is some question about whether or not diabetes is reversible. It used to be thought that once you had diabetes you were stuck with it forever. Results following gastric bypass surgery pointed to reversal of type 2 due to extreme weight loss. So to be sure, it's not the bypass surgery that led to the reversal but it was the extreme weight loss as evidenced by much more than just gastric bypass. It's not really being cured or reversed; the reversal is really the diabetes going dormant once you get it under control. The fact is, once you have it, you have it. The severity of diabetes will differ but that mostly applies only to type 2.

There is a member of my family who believes that diabetes drugs like insulin are the same or better at controlling diabetics as diet, so she opts for the drugs rather than change her lifestyle. Granted she's in her 70s and lived a long hard life, so I don't necessarily fault her for not wanting to take on new challenges. If that's the case, at least admit why you don't want to change. There's no question that meds can be lifesaving, but they're not going to do what's really needed in the case of type 2s. Bottom line is you have to lose the weight and change what you do to ensure you keep it off. Drugs help with the maintenance and in type 1 diabetes, insulin is an absolute must; but taking off the weight and eating right are the keys to better health.

And on the subject of drugs, a lot of people don't seem to be concerned about their side effects, and in some cases diabetes meds are thought to be free of side effects. All one really needs to do is look these drugs up on the FDA or WebMD websites. There is quite a bit of information on certain drugs that have had warnings issued and are subjects of pending lawsuits which I've listed later in the chapter. Don't fall in the trap of believing this myth. That's not to say you should stop taking your prescriptions, absolutely not, if your doctor is telling you to take them then by all means you have to take them. Don't let that stop you from eating right and developing your workout regimens, because evidence points to diet and exercise as being the surest paths to fixing the problems.

Going back to the 1980s and long before people often believed that diabetics couldn't lead active lifestyles, and surprisingly I've met a few people who still harbor those same beliefs. In fact the opposite is true, subject to the precautions like talking with your doctor as I've mentioned about in previous chapters. We now know that exercise and activity leading to weight loss are essential as long as you are paying attention to your body and talking with your doctor about the kinds of exercises you're doing.

Walking, stretching, yoga, and Tai Chi are all great ways to ease into exercise routines, and they can be moderate or intense depending on your desire and energy levels. I'm working my way up to 100-mile bike rides, but it's funny yet self-satisfying to hear my varsity-track-star-letterman son tell me he won't ride with me on the long rides because he lacks the stamina to go the distance. I'm pretty sure Austin was just trying to make me feel good.

One myth that should cause people some concern is that you will develop telltale symptoms of the disease once you have it, except there often are none at first. One of the scariest things about this disease is its stealth. When it was confirmed that I had it, my doctor told me that based on my test results I had had it for at least a year. Obviously I didn't realize it, but by having it for that long it was already doing its damage. Worse, had I not gone in to the hospital for a pinched nerve I likely would have gone much longer before being checked and who knows by then what damage I would have incurred. The diabetic symptoms I was feeling were also associated with my heart problems which I already knew about. Those were symptoms like fatigue and low energy, shortness of breath so I never bothered to get myself checked for anything else.

I have a friend named Tom who found out about his diabetes only when it had reached very dangerous levels which is anything over 400 mg/dl. Tom was at a family gathering and his sister noticed that he was slurring his words and appeared as though he was losing consciousness. When they got him to the hospital Tom's blood glucose tested at 650 mg/dl. Tom was probably heading into a diabetic coma without realizing it. In his case, I guess there were telltale signs of the disease, but seriously, do you really want to wait till you nearly go into a coma?

What scared me about the disease as I started looking into it was there really are no telltale signs, and my friend Tom is a good case in point. Tom must have had it for quite some time before his glucose levels got that high, and who knows what damage had been done by then. Unfortunately no one can really tell. Alternately he was lucky that he didn't have a heart attack or stroke because of the damage already done. Regular checkups are pretty good ways to avoid these kinds of unpleasant surprises.

Another myth out there is the one about how most diabetics will eventually end up having to get kidney dialysis or incur some other debilitating complications. The risk of these things certainly exists once you have the disease but it's not a guarantee. A lot can depend on how seriously you take it and what you do to manage it. Get regular checkups, monitor your blood sugar, and begin a healthy lifestyle. These are the best ways to prevent things from getting worse. Diabetes is just too important to dismiss, and even though I'm feeling pretty good these days and certainly feeling so much better than when I first found out I had the disease, my blood sugar levels tell me I still have it so I have longer to go before I can sit back and think I'm doing ok. The fact is I'll never be able to sit back and know that I'm ok, even if I'm able to reverse it because it could come back if I were to fall back in to my old ways.

The myths I addressed here are samples of what is circulating about the disease, and there are more if you want to look. Do your homework, and consider the source of the information. Above all, don't take just anyone's word for it, and don't even take my word for it, find out for yourself especially if you have it or if you think someone you know may be headed in that direction.

I have the dubious benefit of my day-to-day experiences after having diabetes for nearly ten years and observing diabetic family members over the past forty years yet there was so much I had to learn once I found out I had it.

Remedies And Medications

The best thing for you to do is to get engaged and develop your own trusted resources for information. There is plenty of it out there to say the least; my job here is to show you what can happen once you have this disease, how you can set targets to help yourself to overcome it and where you can go to get help on your own. I'm also showing you there are a lot of snake-oil salesmen out there, so don't fall for just anything because you fear diabetes. The best defense is to be on the offense. If you run across somebody telling you something that sounds too good to be true, then it probably is so do your homework and keep following your doctor's advice. Above all, stay focused on getting and staying healthy by doing the things you can control.

The simple answer is that it might help to ask your doctor or health care provider some important questions about the drugs you are taking or might be taking. It wasn't that long ago that of the eight prescriptions I had, two of the manufacturers of the drugs prescribed were subjects of class action lawsuits because of deaths involving those drugs. This underscores why you should want to ask informed questions to get the answers you need. Don't forget that doctors and health care providers are themselves human, and no matter how good they are at what they do, they can't be expected to know all of the information each time you ask a question. Sometimes your questions will help jog a health-care provider's memory regarding a recent change about an item that they only briefly scanned when they got the information, if they got it at all.

When I was taking Metformin which is one of the more common medications for type 2 diabetics, I let my doctors know that I would often join my colleagues for drinks and asked if there were any problems with doing that. Each of my doctors on the west coast and in the mid-west said there were no issues, but when I mentioned it to my pharmacist, she pretty much convinced me that I was going to die if I drank often; that was the first time I had heard of lactic acidosis. After looking it up, I realized that although it was rare, alcohol and Metformin could become a deadly combination under certain circumstances like simply having one drink too many, so to be safe I had to modify my lifestyle. Here's an odd twist; I have seen a number of references from various sources that say diabetics could benefit from one but no more than two glasses of red wine on an occasional night, but I never saw one that issued the caution about the possibility of it triggering lactic acidosis. My pharmacist was the only one who brought it up. One would think that this should be a standard caution or a least a caution instead of none at all.

WebMD has an excellent library identifying the basic information about various medicines, highlighting warnings, known interactions, uses, and side effects. That is where I found the possibility of side effects and lactic acidosis with Metformin. Like the ADA they are careful to note that they do not make any recommendations about any of the drugs, deferring instead to conversations that should take place between you and your health care provider. As you probably figured out by now, I can't stress that enough. Use this chapter for what it is and the resources for what they are, sources of valuable information but for everybody's sake don't try and become your own doctor once you access it.

I had a friend who was constantly going to places online like the Merck Manual and finding diseases that listed symptoms indicated by any number of pains she was having at the time. Armed with that information Francine would go into depressions because she was sure she was going to die based on the information she found. Francine would get all of us friends involved by talking with us and appointing which of us to take over as mother, housekeeper, etc. if she died, but then would ignore our advice about going to see a doctor. Fortunately for her husband, kids, and everybody around her who loved her, Francine never got any diagnoses right and we all figured later that she was an attention hog. But she was lucky because she never got sick.

There's also a bigger reason to not self-diagnose. I used to have an esophageal problem and at times when it acted up the symptoms were exactly the same as that of someone who was having a heart attack. So one day I called my cardiologist thinking I was having a heart attack. After she checked me out she sent me to a gastroenterologist who fixed me up, and that's when I found out that the problem I had experienced was often confused with heart attacks. The GI doctor said that some patients came to him thinking they were having GI issues but he'd have to send them to the hospital because they were having heart attacks. Then he told me some patients tried self-diagnosing their symptoms as GI problems but ended up dying of heart attacks.

I'm telling you this to drive home the point while reminding myself that simply because we have access to this valuable information, we're not trained professionals who should be making our own judgments about how to use what we learn. And while I'm on the subject, don't do what some of my other friends have done which is to take other people's prescription medicines.

One of the dumbest things anyone can do is to take someone else's prescription. You don't know how those prescriptions will interact with any medications, including those prescribed for diabetes like insulin or Metformin. If you look at the information about some of the drugs more closely you'll also find that some of them react negatively with certain over-the-counter meds as well as vitamins and supplements.

According to the ADA, all diabetes pills sold today in the United States are members of six classes of drugs that work in different ways to lower blood glucose levels:

» Sulfonylureas
» Meglitinides
» Biguanides
» Thiazolidinediones
» Alpha-glucosidase inhibitors
» DPP-4 inhibitors

The ADA is careful to point out that by highlighting the types of medications, it does not endorse their use but advises that all matters relating to medications and the treatment of the disease be taken up with your doctor or health professional. The ADA is but one of a number of excellent resources available to anyone who wants to learn more about the causes, treatments, effects, and prevention of diabetes.

If taking combinations of medications is something that you and your doctor feel is right for you, the ADA has a free medication monitoring service called My Medicine Tracker. It helps you to:

» Track and print a list of all your medications, both prescription and over-the-counter
» View safety information regarding side effects and when combining medications may not be advisable
» Receive email alerts and updates on important safety information about medications
» Interact with others to share experiences with medications

If you learned anything in this book so far, it should be that preventing or managing type 2 diabetes is all about healthy lifestyle choices which include diet, exercise and weight control. But if you have to take medications or in the case of type 1 where you always have to take medications, it's best to know what you are taking and why so you can understand the importance of taking it and the associated risks. The table below compares, at a glance, the most common diabetes medications and how they work.

Some meds work by stimulating the pancreas to produce more insulin; some inhibit the release of glucose from the liver. Others block the action of stomach enzymes that break down carbs, and some like Metformin improve the sensitivity of cells to insulin. Some of those are taken orally, and some are injected.

The tables below are a compilation of the most common treatments for type 2 diabetes *(MayoClinic Staff, 2014)*.

TABLE 13: Oral Medications

Medication	Action	Advantages	Possible Side Effects
Meglitinides			
Repaglinide (Prandin) Nateglinide (Starlix)	Stimulate the release of insulin	Work quickly	Severely low blood sugar (hypoglycemia); weight gain; nausea; back pain; headache
Sulfonylureas			
Glipizide (Glucotrol) Glimepiride (Amaryl) Glyburide (DiaBeta, Glynase)	Stimulate the release of insulin	Work quickly	Hypoglycemia; weight gain; nausea; skin rash
Dipeptidyl peptidase-4 (DPP-4) inhibitors			
Saxagliptin (Onglyza) Sitagliptin (Januvia) Linagliptin (Tradjenta)	Stimulate the release of insulin; inhibit the release of glucose from the liver	Don't cause weight gain	Upper respiratory tract infection; sore throat; headache; inflammation of the pancreas (sitagliptin)

TABLE 13: Oral Medications (continued)

Medication	Action	Advantages	Possible Side Effects
Biguanides			
Metformin (Fortamet, Glucophage, others)	Inhibit the release of glucose from the liver; improve sensitivity to insulin	May promote modest weight loss and modest decline in low-density lipoprotein (LDL), or "bad," cholesterol	Nausea; diarrhea; rarely, the harmful buildup of lactic acid (lactic acidosis)
Thiazolidinediones			
Rosiglitazone (Avandia) Pioglitazone (Actos)	Improve sensitivity to insulin; inhibit the release of glucose from the liver	May slightly increase high-density lipoprotein (HDL), or "good," cholesterol	Heart failure; heart attack; stroke; liver disease
Alpha-glucosidase inhibitors			
Acarbose (Precose) Miglitol (Glyset)	Slow the breakdown of starches and some sugars	Don't cause weight gain	Stomach pain; gas; diarrhea

TABLE 14: Injectable Medications

Medication	Action	Advantages	Possible Side Effects
Amylin mimetics			
Pramlintide (Symlin)	Stimulate the release of insulin; used with insulin injections	May suppress hunger; may promote modest weight loss	Hypoglycemia; nausea or vomiting; headache; redness and irritation at injection site
Incretin mimetics			
Exenatide (Byetta) Liraglutide (Victoza)	Stimulate the release of insulin; used with metformin and sulfonylurea	May suppress hunger; may promote modest weight loss	Nausea or vomiting; headache; dizziness; kidney damage or failure

When you talk with your doctor about developing the best treatment strategy, it is best to be completely honest about your lifestyle, especially about other drugs or vitamin supplements that you're taking or are planning to take.

Vitamins: The Good And The Bad

You will find all sorts of new vitamin ads that will tell you how their products can be used to cure diabetes, but don't rush out to buy them without checking first.

Let's take a look at potassium to illustrate how not only a good thing but a necessary thing for your body can be deadly if not handled properly. According to the University of Maryland Medical Center, potassium is an essential mineral needed for the proper function of all cells, tissues, and organs in the human body. It is also an electrolyte, which is a substance that conducts electricity in the body, along with sodium, chloride, calcium, and magnesium.

Potassium is crucial to heart function and plays a key role in skeletal and smooth muscle contraction, making it important for normal digestive and muscular function. The good news is that many foods contain potassium, including all meats, some types of fish (such as salmon, cod, and flounder), and many fruits, vegetables, and legumes. Dairy products are also good sources of potassium.

According to Medicine Net there are a variety of ways that low potassium can occur, from vomiting, diarrhea, through the kidneys, and from side effects of taking certain medications, including diabetes meds. When that happens, you can develop something called hypokalemia. The symptoms can include abnormal heart rhythms (especially in people with heart disease), constipation, fatigue, muscle damage, muscle weakness or spasms, or paralysis.

Too much potassium in the blood can lead to an opposite condition known as hyperkalemia and it can lead to deadly consequences fairly quickly or over time. Some of the problems caused by hyperkalemia are weakness, slow heart rate, or abnormal heart rhythm. It is difficult to diagnose which makes it more troubling since it mimics other ailments.

I'm picking on potassium because I was one of those self-diagnosing fools who did exactly what I've been warning against. Fortunately I covered it with my doctor shortly after I started taking potassium supplements and he stepped in and told me what I was doing wrong. This was a case of me trying to find alternatives because I was tired all the time and I wanted to have energy to work out and lose weight. In my research I saw that low potassium could be a cause so I started taking it without exploring the possible side effects or how it could impact my heart, high blood pressure, and diabetes. Indeed I've been very lucky so far.

I have already highlighted the fact that care should be given when looking at supplements and alternatives because finding reliable information about the benefits and safety of these products is not so easy. There must be hundreds of diet and vitamin supplements; with the manufacturer of each claiming special health benefits. Unfortunately for us there is no system for testing these supplements to not only see if they work, but to see if they can cause any harm. In a general sense, most of these supplements are harmless by themselves. Again, they can do just the opposite for diabetics as well as people with heart and kidney problems which can result from complications of having diabetes. They appear to be sold everywhere, like pharmacies, grocery stores, vitamin and health food stores, websites, mail-order catalogs, and at retailers such as Target and Walmart. The main types include fatty acids, vitamins, minerals and botanicals which are derived from plants and possibly including herbs.

The biggest cause for concern is that diet supplements seem safe because they're natural or naturally derived. Many people think that something natural couldn't hurt them. Here are a few examples of some potential side effects:

» Things like aloe vera, fenugreek, and vanadium may cause excessive bleeding during surgery or interact with anesthetics.
» Some vitamins can interfere with prescription medications. Ginseng can be used to treat diabetes, but can lessen warfarin's ability to prevent blood clotting. This is especially dangerous for people with arrhythmia. Warfarin is a primary ingredient in rat poison but also a very effective blood thinner and the main ingredient in Coumadin. Heart patients are often on Coumadin to help prevent strokes.
» St. John's Wort is often taken for depression but it can actually interact with antidepressants as well as with other prescription medications.

This only underscores my previous cautions to be open and detailed when talking with your doctor about treatment for diabetes.

Lawsuits Involving Diabetes Medications

There are a number of active websites detailing current lawsuits, and these can be accessed through a variety of keyword searches. Or just watch any afternoon news channel and you'll see some of those ads about them. It was actually the ads that got me thinking about this.

One in particular was an ad from an attorney's group citing studies showing that a popular cholesterol medication may cause diabetes. Among the drugs and groups that appear to have lawsuits forming against the manufacturers are:

» Thiazolidinediones – Actos and Avandia
» Exenatide (Byetta, Bydureon)
» Sitaglptin (Januvia, Janumet, Janumet XR, Juvisync)

- » Liraglutide (Victoza) Saxagliptin (Onglyza, Kombiglyze XR)
- » Alogliptin (Nesina, Kazano, Oseni)
- » Linagliptin (Tradjenta, Jentadueto)

The FDA issued an early communication entitled: Incretin Mimetic Drugs for type 2 diabetes: Early Communication - Reports of Possible Increased Risk of Pancreatitis and Pre-cancerous Findings of the Pancreas. The communication was issued on March 14, 2013 and was based upon unpublished reports of side effects of some drugs used to treat type 2 diabetes. The report names specific drugs and drug groups and states the communication is mainly to serve as a notice to the public but it has not as of that time formed any opinions regarding the safety of the drugs. This communication sparked a number of websites prepping for lawsuits, even though in its statement no conclusions were drawn. Here is the official statement from the communication:

> RECOMMENDATIONS: FDA has not reached any new conclusions about safety risks with incretin mimetic drugs. This early communication is intended only to inform the public and health care professionals that the Agency intends to obtain and evaluate this new information. FDA will participate in the National Institute of Diabetes and Digestive and Kidney Diseases (NIDDK) and National Cancer Institute's (NCI) Workshop on Pancreatitis-Diabetes-Pancreatic Cancer in June 2013 to gather and share additional information. FDA will communicate its final conclusions and recommendations when its review is complete or when the Agency has additional information to report.
>
> The Warnings and Precautions section of drug labels and patient Medication Guides for incretin mimetics contain warnings about the risk of acute pancreatitis. FDA has not previously communicated about the potential risk of pre-cancerous findings of the pancreas with incretin mimetics. FDA has not concluded these drugs may cause or contribute to the development of pancreatic cancer.
>
> **At this time, patients should continue to take their medicine as directed until they talk to their health**

care professional, and health care professionals should continue to follow the prescribing recommendations in the drug labels.

It is not by accident that I haven't provided details of the lawsuits in terms of the claims, merits, validity, or probability of success. That was never my intention when raising the issue, nor was it my intention to evaluate the drugs or comment on them because of the respective lawsuits. I think the FDA comment in bold sums it up well when it advises to keep taking the medications as prescribed, but talk to your doctor or health care professional about it. Seeking out problems with certain medications is somewhat of a double-edged sword, kind of like Francine who used to search the medical catalog until she found a disease that fit. The people bringing on the lawsuits are not necessarily doing it out of the goodness of their hearts, they're very likely looking to make a profit and often go after large, well-financed targets. Now that is not to say that a lot of good hasn't come out of these lawsuits either, much has and frankly sometimes the only way to punish a company for doing bad and get its attention is through major lawsuits and big damage awards.

But on the subject of lawsuits a funny thing happened to me on one of my doctor's visits. Because of my A-fib condition, my doctor recently prescribed a blood thinning medication which was different than more common drug Coumadin to mitigate the risk of stroke. A nurse pulled me aside and told me to look at the drug very seriously knowing my interest in outdoor activities since, as she pointed out, the drug could turn me into a bleeder if I fell.

I discussed it with my doctor (without throwing the nurse under the bus) and he suggested I give up the activities so I could take the drug. I wasn't convinced and was adamant that I wouldn't give up the activities but I would be careful once I started taking it. Fate however decided for me by way of copayment for the prescription: $310 at Walmart.

I called him and let him know that I wouldn't be taking it because I couldn't afford it, and then requested an alternative which was aspirin. Less than a week later I heard on the news that the makers of the drug were facing hundreds of complaints with the FDA and class action suits. The reason? Unlike other drug thinners, according to the lawsuit summary there are no antidotes to reverse the thinning of the blood caused by this drug, so the claim is that people can bleed to death over minor cuts. This will make the third drug that I've been prescribed over the past ten years that became subjects of class action lawsuits due to defects.

No doubt there are lessons to be learned here. The best prescription in my view, whenever possible, is to live healthy and as stress free as you possibly can so your body can heal naturally. But it would still be a while before I was in a position to do that, and it would be at least once more that I would hear about how close I came to dying even though I had achieved so many health victories.

TWELVE

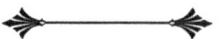

Diabetes and the ACA: The Politics of Healthcare

Ordinarily politics wouldn't belong in this particular discourse because they would detract from the main objectives which are to inform, educate and possibly entertain. In addition; and especially due to a deeply divided nation as it currently stands, politics can also be the source for bitter emotions. Yet the reality is the politics of our healthcare system has affected us all in a big way so it would be foolish on my part to try and ignore it. The impact, whether through higher taxes and costs, cut in pay or an inability to find work, has left us with serious implications. In my case the impact has affected me both in good and bad ways.

But before we talk about me, let's talk about healthcare by asking what is so bad about what we call Obamacare? For starters it changed the national economics in such a way that it has kept millions from finding permanent work, including me. The often ignored employment number in news reports is the "not in labor force" number. At first glance it looks like unemployment keeps going down, but in reality there are more than 92.8 million people out of work today (Bureau of Labor Statistics, 2015) up from 78.5 million when Obama took office, and up from 77 million when the Democrats first took over Congress in 2006.

Today's unemployment numbers of 5.5 percent don't factor in how many people ran out of benefits or stopped looking for work, and so to the average person they look pretty good. In stark reality there are 15 million more people out of work since the stimulus took effect that aren't showing up in the statistics. I have gone to work on contract eight times for five different companies in a little more than two years. But I keep getting let go (along with as many as 100 or more of my colleagues at a time) because the tax penalties of Obamacare keep many companies from hiring permanent full time employees.

Is there anything good about Obamacare? I'd be lying to you if I didn't admit that having access to health insurance because of it saved my life. Here's how it happened. I went without access to healthcare and medications for diabetes, high blood pressure and atrial fibrillation for nearly two and a half years since my contract job with the FDIC ended. For nearly two years of that time; I was able to effectively control my health through diet and exercise.

But the high stress of not finding work, real estate deals not closing and loss of unemployment benefits continued to intensify and eventually took its toll. The clincher was when Child Services tried to take away my insurance and real estate licenses because of Abby's deception. Child Services already took the money I set aside for healthcare and starting a business, but then they had my licenses suspended over $800. It didn't matter that, in addition to her substantial inheritance, Abby had just made $175,000 in a single month just two months before they tried suspending my licenses. The suspensions almost prevented me from working a contract that was going to give me enough money for a few months to keep me from having to live out in the street.

Psychologically and physically I went into a downward spiral that lasted for months. The events described above were only part of an onslaught of even more stressful events that kept happening without any relief in sight. Those events started one July and pounded me heavily before finally letting up in mid-January of the following year.

The consequences were nearly fatal. I could tell my body was going through major changes and the stress affected my breathing and sleep patterns for days and in some cases weeks without letting up. I knew that I was in serious trouble health-wise but there was nothing I could do about it, mainly because I had no money coming in and my unemployment payments had run out again.

Miraculously I was able get my licenses back and I landed a two week contract in mid-December and by mid-January I was able to begin playing catch up with my finances. And shortly after a small real estate transaction that I started more than a year and a half before finally closed which helped me to catch up a little more.

At the gentle prodding of my friend and colleague, Eric, I signed up for Obamacare or the Patient Protection Affordable Care Act (ACA) or Covered California for those of us in California. Eric did a great job with my enrollment and soon after I had health insurance. By early February I was able to pay my premiums and received my cards so I made an appointment with a doctor right away. A few days before going to my doctor's appointment I met with a friend who appeared to have symptoms of diabetes so I bought her a cheap monitor and showed her using my kit on me how to check her blood. My reading shocked me since it was at 364 mg/dl, a figure I hadn't reached since first being diagnosed with it in 2009, and up until the bad events started happening my sugar levels stayed fairly steady in the 105mg/dl to 145mg/dl ranges without meds.

I knew I was in trouble before I made the doctor's appointment but now I was even more thankful that I had health insurance. When I did see the doctor he did preliminary tests then sent me straight to the emergency room where I spent the entire day getting tested and medicated before they finally released me that evening. By the time I got in, my blood sugar was at 375 mg/dl and my blood pressure was erratic in a range from 120 /90 to 163 /120. The only thing that was ok was my heart rate which was ranging between 60 and 78 BPMs. They expected it to be much higher due to the atrial fibrillation.

My new doctor told me that, based upon what he had seen before getting me back on meds, I most likely would have had a stroke or died before summer. I was shattered because it was a total reversal of everything I had achieved over the previous years since I began working to get myself healthy. I hadn't put on any more weight, but I hadn't lost any more either once all of my routines got cast aside during my times of extreme stress. It was stress that got me sick in the first place, and it ended up putting me right back there all over again.

I was smart enough to know how bad things had been getting so I didn't wait too long to get help for myself once I was in a position to get help. But even though I had access to health care the day still cost me $298 out of pocket plus the $140 I had to pay for the premium. It was unrelenting stress, a big part of it coming from Abby and her minions at Child Services that got me sick all over again, and it was lack of work and lack of money that kept me from getting help.

So yes, in this case the ACA saved my life and I am indeed grateful for it. But in terms of Obama and the Democrats, can or should my experience be viewed as their mission accomplished? Well that would depend on one's point of view. Because of my business background and my knowledge of the insurance industry since I hold a health insurance license, I had a definite bias against it. I held that bias because the ACA was the result of a partisan effort to force people to become dependent while changing the entire workforce dynamic in a negative way.

Yes having access to healthcare saved my life, but because of the way it was forced upon businesses it was instrumental in keeping me from getting a job that would have given me access to healthcare before my health got out of control. Let me illustrate it this way. Let's say I was putting a pool cover on my pool to keep debris out from an upcoming storm, but I don't bother to notice that the neighbor's dog is in the pool. Since the cover sits on the water and leaves no airspace the dog starts to drown while frantically gasping for air. Once I hear the panicked scratching on the cover, I remove the cover and save the dog. I take the credit for saving it while ignoring the reality that the dog wouldn't have needed saving if I would have bothered to check the pool in the first place and made sure he wasn't in harm's way.

Furthermore, as in the case of the Democrats and Obama highlighting how many people have signed up for healthcare, they ignore how many of those signing up had to because the plans they already had were taken away due to Obamacare. Not to mention the end of nearly a half-million dental plans that were connected to the health plans that were also canceled because of it.

I don't mean to say that Obama and the Democrats are responsible for my health problems but had they not imposed the penalties that kept companies from hiring me full time I could have had access to health care much sooner and avoided the near death experience altogether. How do I know that I would have been hired? Because on the first contract job I took I was winning awards for performance within the second month I was there, and after being there for only three months they had me training workers who had been there for over a year. And they kept offering me contracts to come back but never on a full time basis. Still, I would be a total hypocrite if I didn't emphasize how much worse off I would have been had I not gotten healthcare through the ACA when I did.

All of that in mind, I went to work on trying to get some questions answered and found things that were good about the plan. Surprisingly many Democrats and Democrat politicians themselves didn't know. I say Democrats because it was their plan and they completely excluded the Republicans when they put it together then later passed it.

Conversely many in the Republican ranks have pointed out what things are wrong with the plan but never bothered to educate the voting public on what they were trying to do to fix it. But had the Republicans been given the opportunity to submit their ideas in a true bi-partisan way, a lot of the problems might have gotten resolved before the act was passed.

Here are some of the good aspects of the plans:

» If someone is in my situation (unemployed, broke, diseased, and without healthcare) it can actually be a godsend. Why? Because I have access to a Silver Plan and the subsidies would pay for most of my premiums. I pay $140 for a plan that I would have to pay $593 a month for without subsidies.
» The above is true of any family who is poor and need health care. The current poverty level for a family of four is $24,250 and 400 percent of that is $97,000 which means they will still qualify for a government subsidy if their incomes fall within that range. It doesn't mean their healthcare costs are lowered; it just means the government simply pays their way like it does with mine.
» Kids or adult kids can stay on their parents' plans longer, until age twenty-six.[25]
» Pre-existing conditions are eliminated through the ACA.
» In some states, the cost of health care is now very low and readily accessible to individuals who need them.
» Lifetime maximums have been eliminated.
» Wellness and preventative care at no charge by insurance plans have been mandated by the law.
» Someone having trouble making their health premiums can have up to ninety days before their coverage is cut off.

These are good things, right? Indeed most of them are so why the bias? It's because there is a bigger picture here that has been ignored so no one will be the wiser. The fact is that we already had a national health plan which wasn't only for seniors, but for the poor and disabled as well. Medicare and Medicaid were plans offered nationally and through individual states, and offered an alternative if someone couldn't get access.

The American Public Health Association (APHA) provided a good comparison of Medicaid before and after the ACA (Berwick, 2012). Before ACA, a person had to meet two requirements in order to qualify for Medicaid, 1) belonging to an eligible group, typically children, pregnant women, parents, blind or disabled persons, and elderly people, and 2) they had to meet the financial test set by the state.

It was already mandatory that children and pregnant women would receive coverage if they were at least 100 to 133 percent of the poverty level. But it was up to the states to decide the qualifying poverty levels so until the ACA was passed those levels could be lower for parents, plus states didn't have to cover adults without dependent children. To date, many states set those financial levels at pretty low thresholds, so for a family of four to qualify for Medicaid they had to be earning below $23,100 or essentially anyone making minimum wage.

Some of those things changed with the ACA, and they were good for people who really needed it like those of us who were sick and had no money. So I can say in all honesty that there are many elements of the plan that I like and I'm not one who supports a total repeal unless the alternative plan fixes those parts which need fixing but keeps many if not all of the good parts. You see, I agree that the Medicare expansion part of the ACA could be a good thing in these very bad economic times, but it could have been achieved through bi-partisan legislation instead of one party imposing a plan that caused more than nine million people to lose the plans they were happy with. And that number continues to climb.

---

[25] Much noise was made about this, but buried in the rhetoric was that the age was already set at twenty-five before the ACA was enacted, and in some states the dependent age was as high as age 31. Some might think this is a good thing, but in many cases it meant that adult kids began opting to stay on their parents plan rather than getting their own health insurance. By them doing that it means the young healthy adults aren't paying their share of the ACA pool which is needed to offset the costs of servicing older more sickly participants. Proponents of the ACA also fail to mention that health insurers are not required to provide coverage for dependents. While it is unlikely that any insurer would not offer dependent coverage this entire scenario speaks to the merits of free market conditions and State regulations being considerably more beneficial than Federal Mandates.

Did the ACA affect me as a diabetic? Yes it did because it gave me lifesaving access to healthcare. Beyond that however, there was nothing for diabetics in the ACA plan that wasn't available in the health plans offered by private employers and private insurance plans.

But for all of the touting that Obama and the Democrats try to claim about them passing the law for everybody's sakes; that is about as true as Obama's line about you being able to keep your plan.

How do I know? The same way that many people know, first and foremost was how they excluded the Republicans from the dialog. But even if you don't buy that, then take a look at a guy named Johnathan Gruber, former Democrat darling.

Johnathan Gruber was one of the Affordable Care Act architects and healthcare consultant to many states across the country (Dayen, 2014). He was paid millions in taxpayer dollars to help Congress and some states design and put the ACA plans in place. Johnathan Gruber, Ph.D and professor of economics at MIT, was caught on tape multiple times for almost two years after the law had passed telling panel audiences how the Democrats relied on, in his words, " the stupidity of the American voter" to ensure the law would pass. Gruber went on to say how he helped write the law in "tortured" language to ensure that the fact that it was a tax wouldn't get noticed. Hmm.

Mitt Romney also pointed out in one of the debates that there was no way "Obama Care" could deliver anything Obama was promising, like average yearly savings of $2,500. Romney went on to say that it would actually raise annual costs per family by about $4,600, and he would know given that he worked with a Democrat majority in Massachusetts to deliver Romney Care. Not only was Romney right, almost to the dollar, Gruber's comments showed that Obama himself knew it well in advance of the debates but had no qualms getting out there and lying about it.

Make no mistake; Gruber was not a whistle-blower, not even close. He was speaking as a panel expert at different colleges around the U.S. and kept patting himself on the back about how he and the Democrats pulled such a big wool over the country's eyes. An investment adviser named Rich Weinstein was the one who found Gruber on video while he was searching for answers about his own health insurance (Weigel, 2014).

Weinstein's insurance policy was canceled because of the ACA and his new insurance premiums were costing double the amount from before. After sitting through many tedious hours of video taken at conferences he found about five in which Gruber made his claims.

Gruber testified in front of Congress and spent much of his time apologizing for his comments but also found himself in very hot water for admitting to what amounted to was fraud, at least in terms of the way it was presented to the voters. As of this writing, the testimonies have just begun and subpoenas appear soon to follow. A recent poll after his taped comments show 58 percent now want the ACA repealed, surprising considering the Democrats' and Gruber's assumptions about voters being too stupid to be able to make their own choices.

How else do I know the Democrats weren't sincerely trying to give us a plan that would be for the greater good? Because in 2008 through 2010 when the Democrats had a filibuster-proof majority in both branches they could have fixed the Veterans' Administration (VA) health system and used it as a center-piece for the ACA but didn't. In addition to the two national healthcare systems we already had in place, there was actually one more. So we already had three national plans available, the VA for Veterans and Military, Medicaid at the state levels for the poor, and Medicare for the elderly or anyone who was permanently disabled.

The Democrats failed to fix the VA when they had a chance to do it entirely with or without a single Republican vote whether for or against. For those of you who may not remember, the VA was caught lying about the average wait times for veterans needing medical attention. Managers at the VA were forcing staff to lie about the wait times and were showing about a fifteen-day waiting period, on average, when in reality it was one-hundred and fifteen days. The managers collected efficiency bonuses while more than forty veterans died because they didn't get the attention they needed. The fraud didn't become public until a number of whistle-blowers comprised of VA doctors and nurses went public.

The lack of sincerity from the Obama administration toward fixing the VA and penalizing those managers for how they treated our veterans should be one of our greatest shames.

This also speaks directly to what everyone should have been looking at before the passage of the ACA. When the issue of fraudulent wait times within the VA was first exposed, Obama held a news conference in 2013 and said he knew nothing about the problems at the VA, but videos of his campaign speeches in 2008 proved otherwise. He not only talked about the problems there but he blamed George Bush for the problems at the VA.

As a Senator though, Obama served on the Veterans Affairs Committee (VAC) from 2005 to 2008 and saw the problems firsthand since the VAC oversees the VA. Although he did nothing to fix it while serving on the committee, he made it part of his 2007 campaign promises and said he would fix the VA if elected. Obama was elected in 2008 with a filibuster-proof majority in both houses, but as of 2013 he not only did not fix the problems he told the public he knew nothing about them.

Had he and his fellow Democrats cared an ounce for our vets or their constituents for that matter, they could have fixed the VA during the two years when they had a guarantee that they could do it regardless of how many Republicans might have opposed. Given the number of Republicans who are veterans themselves though, it's likely that many would have been on-board if what the Democrats had been proposing made sense.

Had the Democrats fixed the VA like Obama said they would in his campaign speeches, their actions could have served two very important purposes. One, they would have addressed an Obama campaign promise that had real meat to it so our vets would not have to suffer as they continue to do. Two, they could have used their remedies at the VA healthcare system to show the rest of the country that their ideas indeed work, and the VA resolutions could have been their showcase. Instead, they chose to do nothing and many vets died because of it.

With all that in mind, there are many questions one could and should ask about healthcare and the administration of it, but the first question really should be: "what do politics have to do with Healthcare"? The answer is supposed to be "nothing" but that isn't true anymore, especially in light of Johnathan Gruber's captured comments about how he and the Democrats were deceiving their voters. I'm even more convinced that government should stay the hell out of our private lives and instead incentivize the private sector to hire and insure employees.

This topic became relevant to me because of the mandatory ACA roll-out that had taken place and was already affecting every adult in the US whether employed or not. As I began to research the ACA, I found that as a California-licensed insurance agent I was eligible to become certified to enroll people in Covered California which is the ACA in California. I went through the training and obtained my certification while also becoming an enrolling agent for private sector plans. My duties as an enrolling agent were performed while under contract with a group that specializes in assisting private employers sign their employees up for benefits.

Having done so, I was allowed opportunities to explore both private and public sector treatments of healthcare benefits while getting a better understanding of how these things work.

I was able to directly compare the effects of a private healthcare enrollment and a public healthcare enrollment before and after the implementation of the ACA. The comparisons were dramatic in some cases (Ehley, 2014). In a year's time I saw deductibles go up significantly in private plans in order to be ACA compliant, from about $2,000 a year for families before ACA to $12,600 a year after.

Before the act took effect, private plans usually offered two or three options (depending on which state the employee lived in) with great coverages and gave employees choices within the plans. The very healthy employees could opt for higher deductibles and lower premiums while people who needed to use the services more, higher premiums with lower deductibles were available. In some cases, the employer funded individual health savings accounts (HSAs) which helped offset copays and deductibles. By law, employees could add pretax dollars to add funds to the accounts and years later could keep and reinvest what they didn't use.

In contrast, after the ACA was enacted the Covered CA and other health exchanges offered similar coverages but for significantly higher premiums and much higher deductibles. There were no options for HSAs, but for people below the updated poverty lines there were tax credits and subsidies.

In reality, the plans offered by the ACA help those like me who truly need it, but the real consequences, whether intended or not, were the complete disruptions of people's lives in order to achieve something that could have been reached in a much better way.

I frankly don't believe that when the Democrats passed the ACA they wanted to disrupt the nation and the economy the way they did, but I do think they wanted to control what we could and couldn't do with our healthcare and because they were driven by an agenda they didn't take the time to explore all that could happen. Instead of forcing companies to insure more employees by lowering the work week to thirty hours instead of forty like the act was intending to do, the ACA caused companies to shorten employee work hours and hire part-time or contract employees so they wouldn't have to pay the mandatory fines for having uninsured workers.

The ACA also changed the employment dynamic to where it is now far more cost effective for companies to hire non-permanent or part time employees instead of full time. Ten years ago just the opposite was true. In fact benefits used to be a recruiting and retention tool for many big companies but once the ACA was enacted employees got their hours cut or lost their jobs, and many retirees watched their plans get canceled so they had to get the government plans.

What is evident is that while at some point early on the development of the ACA may have been well-intended, its mandates and execution scream out an ugly power-grab by the Democrats aimed at creating an even more dependent class and holding the country hostage. At the current number of ninety-three million unemployed, there are as many people unemployed as there are employed in our country today, the first time in a very long time.

So with the Democrats controlling the number of people who have to depend on Welfare, Unemployment Insurance, Welfare to Illegal Aliens, and Food Stamps, Healthcare became the next key to total dependency. Some of these social welfare programs were instituted going as far back as the Great Depression to help destitute people get a hand until they could get back on their feet, but the Democrats have turned it into a resource pool to get votes for their party.

Furthering the example of a power grab is how the ACA appointed the IRS as the overseer of who gets healthcare. The IRS can barely manage itself much less oversee the health of our nation's citizens. If you look closely, ask yourself what will best control the masses? Healthcare or income by themselves are significant enough to hold every citizen hostage, but the two together?

When France declared a 75 percent tax bracket to pay for its social programs the declaration made big news because actor Gerard Depardieu declared that he became a Russian Citizen so he could avoid the heavy tax burden. Around the same time the country of Cypress, heavily burdened by Greece's high unemployment rate and excessive benefit payments, confiscated the wealth of its individuals by simply seizing funds right out of their bank accounts.

Many financial wizards at the time these events took place

expressed deep concerns that with the ACA and the Democrats in charge, it would only be a matter of time before it happens here in the US. For any of you thinking the ACA was borne out of the goodness of the Democrats' hearts, you might want to take a deeper look. The way it stands now, you might be denied health insurance if the IRS decides you didn't pay enough in taxes.

On its face, the ACA is designed to ensure that everyone has health insurance, either through the government exchanges or a private employer or the individual will pay a fine if they choose not to be insured. ACA incorporates Medicare, Medicaid, and private sector insurance plans into the mandated coverage and it offers subsidies in the form of tax credits for those who can't afford it. The coverage is not optional choices; it's based upon what you qualify for. The basis of the ACA as a new national health plan was to broaden the pool of insured, charging more for younger, healthier people to help pay for costs associated with insuring older, sicker people.

My information on health coverage comes from my personal circumstances as well as my experience as an enroller, but for the average consumer I think it's hard to find straight answers on how the ACA works. One site that was very helpful to me is ProCon.org, it helped me get a better understanding of the ACA and I was able to see the Act itself on their site.

The ACA and healthcare has become an emotional topic, so when people start talking about it they get side tracked and enveloped in the politics rather than what it should be doing for us. That's probably because the ACA mandated the type of coverage that could be offered, which is how so many millions of people lost their plans.

In general, setting standards is not always a bad thing whether done by the government or by industry consortiums or combinations of the two. But with something as critical as people's lives and health, studies should have been done to measure the impacts of the changes before any mandates were enacted. And transition plans should have been developed and implemented to offset any losses that could occur once the changes were put into place.

No matter that the plans were doing what the individuals who owned them wanted before the ACA came into effect, apparently that wasn't good enough for the Democrats. In my estimation, it's only a matter of time before the Democrats force us to eat the way they want us to, drive their mandated cars, and of course vote only for Democrats.

Contrary to popular opinion, before the ACA there were 133 alternative healthcare bills introduced by Congress, many of them by Republicans including the Coburn-Burr-Hatch Act which took the best parts of the ACA and eliminated employer penalties which could have stimulated hiring. Yet the argument from the Democrats was that Republicans weren't offering alternatives, and even though the updated Patient Care Act known as Upton-Burr-Hatch is a far better alternative in my view as well as an analysis in Forbes indicates (Roy, 2015), the Democrats have nothing good to say about it.

And when the Republicans did offer alternatives out of the House, Senator Harry Reid, a party-line Democrat wouldn't bring them up for a vote in the Democrat-controlled Senate. That also exposed a huge problem on the part of the Republicans by not communicating it effectively to the general public.

The really scary part is, for all of the ACA training I went through, I learned nothing about the plans or the act itself. There were about 43,000 of us in California who took the same ACA classes and what we learned boiled down to a few things like who qualifies, how to sign them up, and how to price the plans. We know they have to be U.S. citizens or have valid Visas, and they can't be in jail. One of the trainers, after highlighting the "can't be in jail" aspect for about the nineteenth time as was required throughout the presentation, said it was because prisoners get better coverage than we do through the plan. The regional director for the Covered CA said nothing in protest. Joke or not, that's pretty scary.

The list of things that were achieved through the ACA could have been fixed far less invasively through legislation if both parties would come together to fix it. Most, if not all, of the fixes brought about by the ACA could have been done through legislation to benefit individuals instead of forcing it down everyone's throat and causing millions of health insurance policies to be canceled at a time when people needed them most.

Further proof of a Democrat agenda was when the government shutdown happened on October 1, 2013, the Republicans were holding out for two simple things but Obama refused. First the Republicans asked Obama to delay the requirement that all individuals sign up for the ACA for one year as he had done for the nation's largest employers and unions. They stated very clearly that it wasn't fair to require citizens to sign up on a system that didn't work, and be faced with a fine if they didn't. Most people would never know that Obama said "absolutely no" to the Republicans, but he did.

Second, the Republicans proposed that if all citizens were required to abide by the mandate, then all government employees and politicians including all members of Congress, their staff, and the president and his family should be required to lose their insurance and sign up for the ACA. Because of that proposal, the Republicans really faced Obama's wrath and he tried to make sure that we all felt it by allowing the federal government shutdown then blaming the Republicans for it. Imagine those mean Republicans suggesting that Obama sign up for his own plan, the nerve of them!

The Aca Lowering Healthcare Costs – Fact Or Fiction?

Obama sold his voting public on the idea that healthcare costs would be lower because of his plan, but nothing could be more naïve. He was attempting to lower premium costs by forcing companies and employers to eat certain costs like annual physicals and coverage for preexisting conditions, thus causing the costs of deductibles and premiums to skyrocket. But that has nothing to do with lowering the costs of healthcare. There are three basic things that would have dramatic impacts on lowering overall healthcare and premium costs across the board:

1. *Tax incentives for employers and insurance companies,*
2. *Allowing insurers to pool across state lines, and*
3. *Tort reform.*

Any or all of these could go miles toward lowering actual costs and premium costs, while keeping the government from controlling everything we do. Legislation could have been passed to incorporate those individuals and families who currently don't have access to health care by working with the systems that were already in place.

Here are a few examples:

Tax incentives and subsidies could have been implemented to help insurance companies offset the costs of individual plans and pre-existing conditions. With those incentives in place, the free market system would have taken over to develop programs that made sense for most everyone involved.

Businesses could have also been incentivized with tax credits in exchange for hiring more people and offering them insurance plans and Health Savings Account subsidies. Health care in the past was often a major recruiting tool for companies but now, thanks to the ACA, it has become a major liability.

Tort reforms have always been on the table, but the Bar Association Lobby is powerful and helps to make sure tort reform gets blocked every time, and the ACA does nothing to resolve that. Why is that such a big deal? In Chapter 11 I touch briefly on the sharks already circling the drug makers as a result of the FDA announcement about possible problems and ready to file class action suits.

Here's an example of why tort reform is needed. I drove myself to an urgent care facility to be checked out. The doctors determined I needed to be admitted to the hospital across the parking lot for tests. Although I could have driven or walked, or have someone push me in a wheelchair, they insisted on an ambulance at a cost of $1100 for a one minute ride. Why?

Because of the ambulance chasers who would sue them for who knows what if something happened to me along the way. Remember John Edwards, the former Democrat presidential candidate? He made about $23 million from just four cases involving medical lawsuits which included hospitals and doctors. Even if the doctors or hospitals win their cases, they often spend hundreds of thousands of dollars defending these cases and we're the ones who pay for it in the form of increased costs. Because of the suits, costs of malpractice insurance goes up considerably and doctors often will order unnecessary tests as attempts to avoid lawsuits if something unforeseen were to occur. Or they order $1100 ambulance rides for a one minute trip when at the very least they could have ordered a $20 taxi.

Ever see the warning label on an iron telling you not to wear your clothes while ironing them? That didn't get there out of the goodness of the manufacturer's heart. It got there because some attorney sued them for a client who wasn't able to figure it out on his own.

The other item is opening up insurance across state lines to increase the pool size; not surprisingly which is exactly what the ACA attempted to do. Bigger pool sizes allow more people to pay in the system, especially healthy ones to offset the costs of taking care of the sicker ones in the pool. By going across state lines the pools would get much larger and very likely more efficient. In the case of the ACA however it failed because the majority of the people signing up were going after Medicaid because they were sick and they were poor while many of the younger healthy ones were staying on their parents' health plans because the ACA was charging them too much.

Politics don't belong in a discussion on healthcare much less diabetes and politicians have no business telling insurance industry experts how to run their businesses, yet we are stuck with exactly that. If the political agenda had been cast aside, then the two sides could have worked together to carve out a plan that can indeed help the greater good without upsetting the overall dynamic of the economy or penalizing those it was supposed to help. That was the case with Mitt Romney in Massachusetts with a Democrat Congress and a Republican governor who came together for the people of their state.

The Democrats including Obama didn't do that when they had the opportunity to reach across the aisle and enlist the aid of real experts instead of academicians like Johnathan Gruber. So instead, we have a single-sided plan that forces certain events to take place while attempting to close out free-market conditions. In doing so, it has changed the whole employment paradigm.

Instead of expanding as companies often do when tax credits and incentives are put in place, companies are contracting in order to conserve and reduce costs, and to try and avoid the penalties as a result of the ACA being enacted. More devastating though is all of the companies that are cutting work hours and letting people go in order to avoid the calculations for penalties per employee that the ACA imposes. Others are opting to simply pay the fine because it's cheaper than insuring the employees under the current conditions. Many businesses stopped their plans to expand because of the ACA and the increased costs.

The White House will tell you that these consequences are simply baseless stories concocted by people who want the ACA to fail, and that shows just how out of touch Obama and the Democrats are. One of the most disturbing aspects of the ACA is how it expressly penalizes small companies from paying employees more and expanding. As an example, a company employing twelve people at $25,000 per year each will qualify for the full subsidy. But if any employee gets more than a ten percent raise, they and the company will no longer qualify for the full subsidy and if they don't report it in time they risk having to pay back the entire subsidy for a year.

Huh, now there's some real incentive to promote your employees and look for ways to expand your business.

But I would be lying to you if I didn't admit that I'm alive today because of the ACA, and talk about an unintended consequence coming from Obama and the Democrats. As a lifelong conservative, I'm probably the last guy they'd hope to save.

THIRTEEN

Introspection and the Next Steps

I asked God for strength, that I might achieve.
I was made weak that I might learn humbly to obey...
I asked for health, that I might do greater things.
I was given infirmity that I might do better things...
I asked for riches, that I might be happy.
I was given poverty that I might be wise...
I asked for power, that I might have the praise of men.
I was given weakness that I might feel the need for God...
I asked for all things, that I might enjoy life.
I was given life that I might enjoy all things...
I got nothing that I asked for, but everything I had hoped for.
Almost despite myself, my unspoken prayers were answered.
I am among all men, most richly blessed!

-Anonymous

It has been six years almost to the day since I began this project, and this chapter marks the end of it. For me, it's much more than simply bringing closure to something that I started long ago, it is an important milestone that lets me know I can trust myself again to achieve what I set out to do. When I started this, I was at the lowest point in my life and completely unsure that I could achieve anything significant ever again. Yet here I am with a finished book, and feeling better now that I have that hardest part behind me. Looking back in reflection, strangely enough I ran across some other milestones I hadn't seen before which also happened at six year intervals.

In the six years following my marriage to Abby, I had more than quadrupled my income, was studying for my bachelor's degree and I was in a new career as a branch manager for a lending unit of a local bank. In the six years following that, I was hired by a Fortune 100 bank as Vice President with a starting salary of $109,000, and six years later I filed federal tax returns showing earnings for the year at $568,000. But that six year interval was also the beginning of my downward spiral.

Over the past six years I've been mired in a vicious cycle of no job and no money to live on, which caused me a tremendous amount of stress and a whole slew of other problems. That stress not only reversed all of my successes on the health front, it nearly killed me. And I've also been stuck in an ugly, vicious divorce after being separated for more than six years.

Incredibly though I've managed to see a bright spot through all of what has been thrown at me, at least in the way I am looking at it. Six years ago I started rebuilding my life from the ruins, and what made starting over again seem so much harder was my emotional state because I had lost everything after having accomplished so much. I was afraid of losing my kids because of the divorce and because of Abby's attempts to sway them to her side, but thanks to their efforts along with their generous and unsolicited displays of love I no longer have that fear.

I continue to get hit with all sorts of problems, some natural and some deliberate, but I have reached a point where I can see that what I'm getting hit with are simply obstacles like those anyone would face when pursuing serious goals. Twenty years ago when I was building a life for my family and me I had many obstacles to deal with and the prospects of an uncertain future, just like I do now.

So the problems haven't changed, but what has changed is how I deal with those problems internally, and that was the change I needed the most. I can't change the things or the people around me but I can change how I deal with them and that is exactly what I have been able to finally do. I know that dealing with stress is vital to my survival, so I now make sure to take myself to a calm place through exercise and relaxation. It has become a no brainer, especially since I am at eight times greater risk of stroke than the average person if I don't find ways to relieve stress.

When I started my research there were seventeen million diabetics estimated in the US and thirty nine million pre-diabetics, but in approximately six to eight years' time that number has grown to twenty-nine million diabetics and a whopping eighty-six million pre-diabetics. And with more than three hundred and eighty-seven million worldwide, there doesn't appear to be any sign of slowing down.

Why is this the case? I'm no doctor, but it seems basic to me especially as I continue to work to reverse my own disease. We live our lives under constant stress and processed food diets, along with sedentary and sometimes liquor filled lifestyles for which our bodies are not designed. For most of us, from the day we were born, our bodies started out as finely tuned vehicles to house and transport our minds and our spirits. And while these bodies are tough, resilient and quick to heal they have to be maintained properly otherwise they start breaking down. By not taking care of myself, my body started breaking down in a big way but once I started with the right maintenance I have seen important results that keep leading me in the right direction.

Six years ago when I started this I was over 300 pounds with a size forty-eight inch waist and I was in financial ruin. Worse, I couldn't see any hope that my life was ever going to get better. Those were the darkest moments I've ever experienced and wouldn't wish it on anyone, much less ever want to live through it again. I reached the bottom of a very deep and dark hole but once the descent stopped, I could feel the hard surface and knew it was indeed the bottom and not a plateau in an abyss. The bad news about hitting the bottom of a hole that deep though, is that it's never a soft landing. Despite the ample cushion provided by my very fat ass I hit that bottom hard and it took me a while to recover from it.

The upside though is that once you hit bottom and unless you want to stay there, the only place you can go is up. At that point it's simply a matter of starting your climb then moving ahead without stopping. Once I got to a point where I could see bits of light peeking through, I found lifelines being tossed my way by my sons, my family, and old and new friends. Some of those lifelines came as a place to rent with flexible terms, or short term loans. And some were as simple as a few words of encouragement with little reminders that at one time I made a difference in someone's life.

Evidence of things getting better came by way of an interesting twist during my recent meetings with the Child Services agents. One of the agents looked over my case completely and compared my circumstances with Abby's then walked me through the legal process so I could take the right action against Abby if that's what I chose to do. I'm not sure what she saw that made her decide to help me, but if I had to guess she probably saw an injustice taking place which is what I had been pointing out to the agency and the court all along. It wasn't lost on me to note that her choice to give out advice was not something she would have done for a deadbeat husband who posed any kind of threat, nor would she likely have advised anyone who wasn't being taken advantage of. That agent's comments and advice gave me new hope and it helped me to move ahead in matters relating to Austin.

So even with the many things to block my progress of getting healthy and rebuilding my life, I eventually broke through the darkness and kept breaking through while getting stronger as I went.

Indeed, the stress of everything that had been happening nearly killed me because I couldn't afford to access the medications I needed to offset the unhealthy conditions I was forced to live through. But what I learned about the disease is what saved me until I could get the right kind of help.

My waist is now thirty-eight, I'm more than fifty pounds lighter than I was and I'm now back to the routines and diets that should take me the rest of the way to better health. I learned the hard way that for me, stress has to be avoided at all costs regardless of what's causing it. So my best defense has become quiet times with consistent affirmations of me telling myself that everything will be all right. There was no way I could say that to myself six years ago; because after what I had just been through there was no way I could believe that anything would ever be all right. But now, it doesn't matter if I believe it or not because I no longer have a choice.

I have a lot of work left to do and many goals yet to accomplish, but unlike when I started this journey, I have the benefit of seeing myself achieve some of the new goals I had set for myself, and not just the small ones. This means that I've laid a foundation upon which I can rebuild new and better successes.

So for me, the next steps are to use what I've learned to become even stronger, still setting small milestones and using those achievements to catapult myself to bigger successes, not least of which is reversing diabetes.

But had I not gotten diabetes in the first place, I never would have had the motivation to take it this far.

the end

bibliography

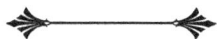

GENERAL INFORMATION

Alvarez, D. M. (2014, November 4). *How To Reduce Your Risk Of Diabetes.* Retrieved March 8, 2015, from Fox News Health: http://www.foxnews.com/health/2014/04/25/how-to-reduce-your-risk-diabetes/

Barnard, N. D. (2008). *Dr. Neal Barnard's Program for Reversing Diabetes: The Scientifically Proven System for Reversing Diabetes without Drugs.* Emmaus: Rodale Books

Diabetic Connect Online. (2015). *Diabetic Connect.* Retrieved March 8, 2015, from Online Community: http://www.diabeticconnect.com/

DLife.com. (2015). *For Your Diabetes Life.* Retrieved March 8, 2015, from: http://www.dlife.com/

Health Media Ventures, Inc. (2015). *16 Ways to Lose Weight Fast.* Retrieved March 8, 2015, from Diet & Fitness: http://www.health.com/health/gallery/0,,20501331_last,00.html

Health.com. (2008). *15 Websites That Can Help You Cope With Diabetes Every Day.* Retrieved March 8, 2015, from Living With Diabetes: http://www.health.com/health/condition-article/0,,20189189,00.html

International Diabetes Federation. (2015). *What We Do.* Retrieved March 8, 2015, from: http://www.idf.org/whatwedo

Whitaker, J. (2009). *Reversing Diabetes* (1 Rev Upd). New York: Grand Central Life & Style.

CHAPTER 8

National Institute of Diabetes and Digestive and Kidney Diseases (NIDDK), National Institutes of Health . (2015, March 4). *National Institute of Diabetes and Digestive and Kidney Diseases (NIDDK), National Institutes of Health.* Retrieved March 4, 2015, from National Institute of Diabetes and Digestive and Kidney Diseases (NIDDK), National Institutes of Health: http://kidney.niddk.nih.gov/

Alexa Fleckenstein, M. (2006). *Healthy to 100*. Deerfield Beach, FL: Health Communications, Inc.

American Diabetes Association (ADA). (1995-2015). *Eating Out*. Retrieved March 7, 2015, from American Diabetes Association (ADA) Food and Fitness: http://www.diabetes.org/food-and-fitness/food/what-can-i-eat/food-tips/eating-out/

American Diabetes Association (ADA). (2013, August 1). *Diabetes Meal Plans and a Healthy Diet*. Retrieved March 7, 2015, from Food and Fitness - Planning Meals: http://www.diabetes.org/food-and-fitness/food/planning-meals/diabetes-meal-plans-and-a-healthy-diet.html

American Diabetes Association (ADA). (2013). *Glycemic Index and Diabetes*. Retrieved March 7, 2015, from ADA - Food and Fitness - Understanding Carbohydrates: http://www.diabetes.org/food-and-fitness/food/what-can-i-eat/understanding-carbohydrates/glycemic-index-and-diabetes.html

American Diabetes Association (ADA). (2015). *Fats*. Retrieved March 7, 2015, from Food and Fitness > Food > What Can I Eat > Making Healthy Food Choices: http://www.diabetes.org/food-and-fitness/food/what-can-i-eat/making-healthy-food-choices/fats-and-diabetes.html

American Diabetes Association. (2015, March 4). *American Diabetes Association*. Retrieved March 4, 2015, from American Diabetes Association: http://www.diabetes.org/

Burke, D. (2015). Microalbuminuria Test. Retrieved March 7, 2015, from What Is a Microalbuminuria Test?: http://www.healthline.com/health/microalbuminuria-test#Overview1

Centers for Disease Control. (2007). Take Charge of Your Diabetes 4th Edition. Atlanta: U.S. Department of Health and Human Services.
Centers for Disease Control. (2015, Mar 4). *Diabetes Home*. Retrieved Mar 4, 2015, from Centers for Disease Control: http://www.cdc.gov/diabetes/home/index.html

Centers for Disease Control. (2015, March 4). *Factsheets*. Retrieved February 1, 2010, from Diabetes Home: http://www.cdc.gov/diabetes/library/factsheets.html

Elaine Magee, M. R. (2008). *Good Carbs, Bad Carbs: Why Carbohydrates Matter to You*. Retrieved March 7, 2015, from WebMd - Food & Recipes: http://www.webmd.com/food-recipes/carbohydrates

Fell, J. (n.d.). *Exercise and Eating Connection*. Retrieved March 7, 2015, from Ask Men: http://www.askmen.com/sports/foodcourt_600/684_exercise-and-eating-connection.html

Fiona S. Atkinson, K. F.-P.-M. (2008 - 2015, February 3). *Glycemic index and glycemic load for 100+ foods.* Retrieved March 7, 2015, from Harvard Health Publications - Harvard Medical School: http://www.health.harvard.edu/diseases-and-conditions/glycemic_index_and_glycemic_load_for_100_foods

Gardner, A. (2014, September 16). *Lactic Acidosis and Excercise: What You Need to Know.* Retrieved March 7, 2015, from WebMd - Fitness and Exercise: http://www.webmd.com/fitness-exercise/guide/exercise-and-lactic-acidosis

Garippo, G. (2013, July 22). *Foods That Cause Plaque Buildup in the Arteries.* Retrieved March 7, 2015, from HealthGrades: http://inhealth.healthgrades.com/taking-cholesterol-seriously/foods-that-cause-plaque-buildup-in-the-arteries?did=t9_outrss1&tp=2

Health.com. (2015). *15 Exercise Tips for People With Type 2 Diabetes.* Retrieved March 7, 2015, from Health A-Z Type 2 Diabetes Condition Center: http://www.health.com/health/gallery/0,,20425548,00.html

Healthline.com. (2015, March 4). *Healthline.com.* Retrieved March 4, 2015, from Healthline.com: http://www.healthline.com/health/microalbuminuria-test#Overview1

Jill Weisenberger, R. (2011). *12 Diabetes Food Tips to Avoid.* Retrieved March 7, 2015, from Diabetic Living - Nutrition: http://www.diabeticlivingonline.com/food-to-eat/nutrition/12-diabetes-food-tips-to-avoid

Joslin Diabetes Center. (2015). *Exercising with Diabetes Complications.* Retrieved March 7, 2015, from Diabetes Information & Resources » Diabetes & Exercise: http://www.joslin.org/info/exercising-with-diabetes-complications.html

Kress, D. (2009). *The Metabolism Miracle: 3 Easy Steps to Regain Control of Your Weight... Permanently.* Boston: Da Capo Lifelong Books.

Lyon, D. M. (2004). *How to Prevent and Treat Diabetes with Natural Medicine.* New York City: Riverhead Books.

Marilyn Kruse, R. (2013). *Top 25 Power Foods for Diabetes.* Retrieved March 7, 2015, from Diabetic Living - Nutrition: http://www.diabeticlivingonline.com/food-to-eat/nutrition/top-25-power-foods-diabetes

Maya W. Paul and Melinda Smith, M. (2015). *Diabetes Diet and Food Tips.* Retrieved March 7, 2015, from Diabetes Diet and Food Tips - Eating to Prevent, Control and Reverse Diabetes: http://www.helpguide.org/articles/diet-weight-loss/diabetes-diet-and-food-tips.htm

Mayo Clinic Staff. (2012, November 17). *Chart of high-fiber foods.* Retrieved March 7, 2015, from Healthy Lifestyle - Nutrition and Healthy Eating: http://www.mayoclinic.org/healthy-living/nutrition-and-healthy-eating/in-depth/high-fiber-foods/art-20050948

Mayo Clinic Staff. (2013, June 25). *Reading food labels: Tips if you have diabetes.* Retrieved March 7, 2015, from Mayo Clinic - Diabetes and Conditions: http://www.mayoclinic.org/diseases-conditions/diabetes/in-depth/food-labels/art-20047648

Mayo Clinic Staff. (2014, February 22). *Diabetes and Exercise: When to monitor your blood sugar.* Retrieved March 7, 2015, from Mayo Clinic - Diabetes and Conditions: http://www.mayoclinic.org/diseases-conditions/diabetes/in-depth/diabetes-and-exercise/art-20045697

Melone, L. (2014, November 6). *13 best and worst foods for people with diabetes.* Retrieved March 7, 2015, from Health: http://www.foxnews.com/health/2014/11/06/13-best-and-worst-foods-for-people-with-diabetes/

Nancy Klobassa Davidson, R. a. (2013, May 8). *Know your blood glucose target range.* Retrieved March 7, 2015, from Mayo Clinic - Living with Diabetes blog: http://www.mayoclinic.org/diseases-conditions/diabetes/expert-blog/blood-glucose-target-range/bgp-20056575#post

National Diabetes Education Program. (2015, March 4). *National Diabetes Education Program.* Retrieved March 4, 2015, from National Diabetes Education Program: http://www.ndep.nih.gov/

National Diabetes Information Clearinghouse. (2015, March 4). *NDIC.* Retrieved March 4, 2015, from NDIC: http://diabetes.niddk.nih.gov/

National Institutes of Health. (n.d.). Retrieved from National Institute of Diabetes and Digestive and Kidney Diseases (NIH/DIDDK).

National Kidney Foundation. (2015, March 4). *National Kidney Foundation.* Retrieved March 4, 2015, from National Kidney Foundation: https://www.kidney.org/

National Institute of Dental and Craniofacial Research. (2015, March 4). *National Institute of Dental and Craniofacial Research.* Retrieved March 4, 2015, from National Institute of Dental and Craniofacial Research: http://www.nidcr.nih.gov/

Natural On. (2104, March 9). *16 Cancer Causing Foods You Probably Eat Every Day.* Retrieved March 7, 2015, from Health News: http://naturalon.com/10-of-the-most-cancer-causing-foods/17/

Ph.D, H. J. (2007). *The Duke Diet: The World-Renowned Program for Healthy and Lasting Weight Loss.* New York: Ballantine Books.

Sanford-Burnham Medical Research Institute. (2011, August 5). *How fatty diets cause diabetes.* Retrieved March 5, 2015, from Science Daily: http://www.sciencedaily.com/releases/2011/08/110814141432.htm

Sharecare.com. (2010-2015). *8 Best Workouts for Diabetes.* Retrieved March 7, 2015, from Living Younder with Diabetes-Diabetes & Exercise: http://www.sharecare.com/health/type-2-diabetes/health-guide/living-younger-with-diabetes/best-exercise-for-diabetes

Team, H. E. (2012, Novemeber 8). *8 Restaurant Meals That Are Bad for Your Heart.* Retrieved March 7, 2015, from Health Central.com - Cholesterol: http://www.healthcentral.com/cholesterol/cf/slideshows/8-restaurant-meals-that-are-bad-for-your-heart?ap=825

Trimdown Club. (2014, March 26). *5 Foods to Never Eat.* Retrieved March 7, 2015, from Info Trimdown Club: http://www.info.trimdownclub.com/

Walk, V. (2014, October 17). *6 superfoods to cut your cravings.* Retrieved March 7, 2015, from Prevention: http://www.foxnews.com/health/2014/10/17/6-superfoods-to-cut-your-cravings/?intcmp=obnetwork

Watson, S. (2014, August 5). *How to Boost Your Metabolism With Exercise.* Retrieved March 7, 2015, from WebMd fitness and execise: http://www.webmd.com/fitness-exercise/how-to-boost-your-metabolism

WebMd. (2014, September 2). *Sleep Apnea.* Retrieved March 7, 2015, from WebMd - Sleep Apnea Health Center: http://www.webmd.com/sleep-disorders/sleep-apnea/sleep-apnea

WebMd. (2014). Type 2 Diabetes and Exercise. Retrieved March 7, 2015, from WebMd - Diabetes Health Center: http://www.webmd.com/diabetes/guide/exercise-guidelines

CHAPTER 9

About Health. (2015). *Type 2 Diabetes.* Retrieved March 7, 2015, from About Health: http://diabetes.about.com/

Alexa Fleckenstein, M. (2006). *Healthy to 100.* Deerfield Beach, FL: Health Communications, Inc.

American Diabetes Association (ADA). (2013). *DKA (Ketoacidosis) & Ketones.* Retrieved March 7, 2015, from Living With Diabetes - Complications: http://www.diabetes.org/living-with-diabetes/complications/ketoacidosis-dka.html

American Diabetes Association (ADA). (2013). *Hyperosmolar Hyperglycemic Nonketotic Syndrome (HHNS)*. Retrieved March 7, 2015, from Living with Diabetes - Complications: http://www.diabetes.org/living-with-diabetes/complications/hyperosmolar-hyperglycemic.html

American Diabetes Association (ADA). (2013). *Low Testosterone*. Retrieved March 7, 2015, from Living With Diabetes > Treatment and Care > Men: http://www.diabetes.org/living-with-diabetes/treatment-and-care/men/low-testosterone.html

Arthur Schoenstadt, M. (2013). *Type 2 Diabetes*. Retrieved March 7, 2015, from Type 2 Diabetes: http://diabetes.emedtv.com/type-2-diabetes/type-2-diabetes.html

CDC/National Center for Health Statistics. (2015, February 6). *FastStats*. Retrieved March 7, 2015, from Centers for Disease Control and Prevention (CDC) - Diabetes: http://www.cdc.gov/nchs/fastats/diabetes.htm

Centers for Disease Control. (2007). *Take Charge of Your Diabetes 4th Edition*. Atlanta: U.S. Department of Health and Human Services.

Centers for Disease Control. (2015, March 4). *Factsheets*. Retrieved February 1, 2010, from Diabetes Home: http://www.cdc.gov/diabetes/library/factsheets.html

Centers for Disease Control and Prevention (CDC). (2014). *Basics About Diabetes*. Retrieved March 7, 2015, from What is Diabetes?: http://www.cdc.gov/diabetes/basics/diabetes.html

Centers for Disease Control and Prevention (CDC). (2014). *Complications Due to Diabetes*. Retrieved March 7, 2015, from Living with DiabetesDiabetes - Complications: http://www.cdc.gov/diabetes/living/problems.html

Centers for Disease Control and Prevention (CDC). (2014). *Diabetes in Men*. Retrieved March 7, 2015, from Who's at Risk?: http://www.cdc.gov/diabetes/risk/gender/men.html

Clinical Key. (2012). *Diabetic Ketoacidosis*. Retrieved March 7, 2015, from Endocrinology: https://www.clinicalkey.com/topics/endocrinology/diabetic-ketoacidosis.html

Cogen, D. F. (2014, September 3). *Hemoglobin A1c Guidelines: Latest American Diabetes Association® Recommendations*. Retrieved March 7, 2015, from Injectables for Type 2 Diabetes: http://www.healthcentral.com/diabetes/c/651280/171472/guidelines-recommendations/?ap=835

Diabetes and the Environment. (2014 (e)). *Diabetes Incidence and Historical Trends*. Retrieved March 7, 2015, from Diabetes and the Environment: http://www.diabetesandenvironment.org/home/incidence

Diabetes.co.uk. (2015). *Diabetes and Hot Weather - Staying Safe in the Heat.* Retrieved March 7, 2015, from Diabetes and Hot Weather: http://www.diabetes.co.uk/diabetes-and-hot-weather.html

Diane Kress, R. C. (2013 (e)). *The Quiet Symptoms of High Blood Sugar.* Retrieved March 7, 2015, from diabetes symptoms: http://diabetes.answers.com/symptoms/a-new-look-at-symptoms-of-high-blood-sugar-its-not-just-excess-thirst-and-urination-anymore

Health Central. (2011). *Autoimmune disorders.* Retrieved March 7, 2015, from Health Encyclopedia: http://www.healthcentral.com/ency/408/000816.html?ic=506048

Houghton Mifflin. (2011). *Diabetes Mellitus.* Retrieved March 8, 2015, from The Free Dictionary: http://www.thefreedictionary.com/diabetes+mellitus

Jorge Alvarado, M. (2011). *Diabetes and Your Eyesight.* Retrieved March 7, 2015, from Glaucoma Research Foundation: http://www.glaucoma.org/glaucoma/diabetes-and-your-eyesight.php

Joslin Diabetes Center. (2015). *Diabetes-Friendly Tips for Handling the Summer Heat.* Retrieved March 7, 2015, from Diabetes Information & Resources - Managing Diabetes: http://www.joslin.org/info/Diabetes_Friendly_Tips_for_Handling_the_Summer_Heat.html

Joslin Diabetes Center. (2015). *Milestones in Joslin Care and Education.* Retrieved March 7, 2015, from Joslin History: http://www.joslin.org/about/care_and_education_milestones.html

Kulas, M. (2013). *Shakes & Sweating With a Drop in Blood Sugar.* Retrieved March 7, 2015, from Diseases and Conditions - Blood Conditions - Blood Health: http://www.livestrong.com/article/446196-shakes-sweating-with-a-drop-in-blood-sugar/

Madeline Vann, M. (2012). *Summer Heat and Type 2 Diabetes.* Retrieved March 7, 2015, from Everyday Health: http://m.everydayhealth.com/type-2-diabetes/summer-heat-and-type-2-diabetes

Mayo Clinic Staff. (2013, January 30). *AC1 Test.* Retrieved March 8, 2015, from Tests and Procedures: http://www.mayoclinic.org/tests-procedures/a1c-test/basics/definition/prc-20012585

Mayo Clinic Staff. (2014, July 31). *Definition.* Retrieved March 7, 2015, from Diseases and Conditions - Diabetes: http://www.mayoclinic.org/diseases-conditions/diabetes/basics/definition/con-20033091

Medicalook.com. (2007-2015). *Hormones Anatomy.* Retrieved March 7, 2015, from Hormones: http://www.medicalook.com/human_anatomy/organs/Hormones.html

Nancy Klobassa Davidson, R. a. (2012, June 7). *Heat and Diabetes.* Retrieved March 7, 2015, from Living with diabetes blog: http://www.mayoclinic.org/diseases-conditions/diabetes/expert-blog/heat-and-diabetes/bgp-20056563

National Center for Chronic Disease Prevention and Health Promotion, Division of Diabetes Translation. (2014). *Prepare for diabetes care in heat and emergencies.* Retrieved March 7, 2015, from CDC Features: http://www.cdc.gov/features/DiabetesHeatTravel/

NIH Publication No. 12-6129. (2012, July). *Type 2 Diabetes.* Retrieved March 2015, 2015, from Diabetes A-Z List of Topics and Titles: Type 2 Diabetes: What You Need to Know: http://diabetes.niddk.nih.gov/dm/pubs/type2_ES/

Silvestre, J. (2007). *Metformin-induced lactic acidosis: a case series.* Retrieved March 7, 2015, from Journal of Medical Case Reports: http://www.jmedicalcasereports.com/content/1/1/126

Siteman Cancer Center. (2013). *Your Disease Risk.* Retrieved March 7, 2015, from Diabetes - Risk Factors: http://yourdiseaserisk.wustl.edu/YDRDefault.aspx?ScreenControl=YDRGeneral&ScreenName=YDRDiabetesRisk_List

Stanford Health Care. (2015). *What Is Atrial Fibrillation?* Retrieved March 7, 2015, from Atrial Fibrillation: https://stanfordhealthcare.org/medical-conditions/blood-heart-circulation/atrial-fibrillation/treatments.html

Stone, B. (2011). *Blood Sugar Count Over 1000: Risks and Treatments.* Retrieved March 7, 2015, from Diabetes Complications: http://www.healthguideinfo.com/diabetes-complications/p108854/

Swidorski, D. (2014, January 22). *Diabetes ABC.* Retrieved March 7, 2015, from Defeat Diabetes Foundation: http://www.defeatdiabetes.org/diabetes-history/

Wanjek, C. (2015, January 23). *How genes and environment conspire to trigger diabetes.* Retrieved March 7, 2015, from Fox News - Health: http://www.foxnews.com/health/2015/01/23/how-genes-and-environment-conspire-to-trigger-diabetes/

WebMd. (2012). *Creatinine and Creatinine Clearance Blood Tests.* Retrieved March 7, 2015, from A-Z Guides - Information Resources: http://www.webmd.com/a-to-z-guides/creatinine-and-creatinine-clearance-blood-tests

WebMd. (2014). *Blood Sugar, Diabetes, and Your Body.* Retrieved March 7, 2015, from Diabetes Health Center: http://www.webmd.com/diabetes/how-sugar-affects-diabetes

WebMd. (2014). *Diabetes Insipidus.* Retrieved March 7, 2015, from Diabetes Health Center: http://www.webmd.com/diabetes/guide/what-is-diabetes-insipidus

WebMd. (2014). *Diabetic Coma and Type 2 Diabetes.* Retrieved March 7, 2015, from Diabetes Health Center: http://www.webmd.com/diabetes/guide/hyperglycemic-hyperosmolar-nonketonic-syndrome

WebMd Medical Reference. (2015). *Gestational Diabetes -- the Basics.* Retrieved March 7, 2015, from Health & Pregnancy Guide: http://www.webmd.com/baby/guide/understanding-gestational-diabetes-basics

CHAPTER 10

American Psychological Association, American Institute of Stress, NY. (2014, July 8). *Stress Statistics.* Retrieved March 8, 2015, from Statistic Brain: http://www.statisticbrain.com/stress-statistics/

Healio Psychiatric Annals. (2014, September 2). *Signs of Depression.* Retrieved March 8, 2015, from Psychiatry-Depression: http://www.healio.com/psychiatry/depression/news/online/%7Bdc27c480-9470-43d0-b247-45ec84a724f4%7D/signs-of-depression?gclid=CKXU55Cz5MECFQcKaQodum4A9Q

Joseph Napora, P. L.-C. (2013). *Managing Stress and Diabetes.* Retrieved March 8, 2015, from Living With Diabetes - For Parents & Kids - Everyday Life: http://www.diabetes.org/living-with-diabetes/parents-and-kids/everyday-life/managing-stress-and-diabetes.html

Julie A. Wagner, H. T. (2010, June). *Lifetime Depression and Diabetes Self-management in Women with Type 2 Diabetes: A Case Control Study.* Retrieved March 8, 2015, from US National Library of Medicine - National Institutes of Health: http://www.ncbi.nlm.nih.gov/pmc/articles/PMC3086788/

Lifespan. (2014). *5 Habits That Lead To Depression.* Retrieved March 8, 2015, from Lifespan: http://www.lifespan.com/5-habits-lead-depression/

Lloyd CE, R. N. (1991, Feb-Mar). *The relationship between stress and the development of diabetic complications.* Retrieved March 8, 2015, from US National Library of Medicine - National Institutes of Health: http://www.ncbi.nlm.nih.gov/pubmed/1827400

McCarthy, M. (2013, May 23). *Depression raises diabetics' risk of severe low blood sugar episodes.* Retrieved March 8, 2015, from UW Health Sciences and UW Medicine: http://www.washington.edu/news/2013/05/23/depression-raises-diabetics-risk-of-severe-low-blood-sugar-episodes/

MedResources Inc. (1996-2015). *Study: Depression and diabetes combination can be deadly.* Retrieved March 8, 2015, from Canada.com: http://bodyandhealth.canada.com/channel_section_details.asp?text_id=3814&channel_id=11&relation_id=30085

Melinda Smith, M. a. (2015). *How to Reduce, Prevent, and Cope with Stress.* Retrieved March 9, 2015, from Stress Management: http://www.helpguide.org/articles/stress/stress-management.htm

Melinda Smith, M. R. (2015). *The Effects of Stress Overload and What You Can Do About It.* Retrieved March 9, 2015, from Stress Symptoms, Signs, and Causes: http://www.helpguide.org/articles/stress/stress-symptoms-causes-and-effects.htm

Melone, L. (2014, June 8). *14 Bad Habits That Drain Your Energy.* Retrieved March 8, 2015, from ABC News - Health-Wellness - Health.com: http://abcnews.go.com/Health/Wellness/14-bad-habits-drain-energy/story?id=24032270#14

Mind Tools Ltd. (1996-2015). *The Holmes and Rahe Stress Scale.* Retrieved March 9, 2015, from Understanding the Impact of Long-term Stress: http://www.mindtools.com/pages/article/newTCS_82.htm

Nelson, J. (2005-2015). *Stress and Diabetes.* Retrieved March 8, 2015, from WebMd Feature - Health Feature: http://www.medicinenet.com/script/main/art.asp?articlekey=47115

Remedy Health Media, LLC. (2010, June 29). *Top Ten Stressful Life Events as Predictors of Mental and Physical Illness.* Retrieved March 8, 2015, from Anxiety - Health Guide: http://www.healthcentral.com/anxiety/c/157571/115211/life-predictors/

Reuters. (2014, May 27). *Stressful relationships may raise risk of death.* Retrieved March 8, 2015, from Fox News Health - Longevity: http://www.foxnews.com/health/2014/05/27/stressful-relationships-may-raise-risk-death/?intcmp=obnetwork

Shawn Talbott, P. F. (2007). *The Cortisol Connection: Why Stress Makes You Fat and Ruins Your Health – And What You Can Do About It.* Alameda: Hunter House.

Surwit RS, S. M. (1992). *Stress and diabetes mellitus.* Retrieved March 8, 2015, from US National Library of Medicine - National Institutes of Health: http://www.ncbi.nlm.nih.gov/pubmed/1425110

University of Maryland Medical Center. (2013). *Stress.* Retrieved March 8, 2015, from Health Information: http://umm.edu/health/medical/reports/articles/stress

Wales, J. (1995, February 12). *Does psychological stress cause diabetes?* Retrieved March 8, 2015, from US National Library of Medicine - National Institutes of Health: http://www.ncbi.nlm.nih.gov/pubmed/7743755

WebMd. (2008). *Serotonin: 9 Questions and Answers.* Retrieved March 8, 2015, from Depression Health Center: http://www.webmd.com/depression/features/serotonin?page=4

WebMd Inc. (2004). *Stress and Diabetes.* Retrieved March 8, 2015, from Diabetes Health Center: http://www.webmd.com/diabetes/features/stress-diabetes

CHAPTER 11

Agency for Healthcare Research and Quality. (2011). *Research comparing diabetes medications helps patients and clinicians choose the right one.* Retrieved March 8, 2015, from http://archive.ahrq.gov/news/newsletters/research-activities/feb11/0211RA1.html

Alonzo Krangle LLP. (2015). *Victoza Lawsuit | Side Effects: Thyroid Cancer, Pancreatitis, Renal Failure Or Kidney Failure, Death.* Retrieved March 8, 2015, from http://fightforvictims.com/defective-drugs/victoza-lawsuit

American Diabetes Association (ADA). (1995-2015). *Herbs, Supplements and Alternative Medicines.* Retrieved March 8, 2015, from Living With Diabetes > Treatment and Care > Medication > Other Treatments: http://www.diabetes.org/living-with-diabetes/treatment-and-care/medication/other-treatments/herbs-supplements-and-alternative-medicines/

American Diabetes Association (ADA). (1995-2015). *Medication.* Retrieved March 8, 2015, from Living With Diabetes > Treatment and Care > Medication: http://www.diabetes.org/living-with-diabetes/treatment-and-care/medication/

American Diabetes Association (ADA). (2015). *Insulin Pumps.* Retrieved March 8, 2015, from Living With Diabetes > Treatment and Care > Medication > Insulin & Other Injectables: http://www.diabetes.org/living-with-diabetes/treatment-and-care/medication/insulin/insulin-pumps.html

American Diabetes Association (ADA). (n.d.). *Diabetes Myths.* Retrieved March 8, 2015, from Diabetes Basics: http://www.diabetes.org/diabetes-basics/myths/

American Heart Association. (2014). *Potassium and High Blood Pressure.* Retrieved March 8, 2015, from Conditions.

Arpesella, P. (2012). *Diabetes Misinformation on TV.* Retrieved March 8, 2015, from Medical Information - How About This?: http://www.peterarpesella.com/blog/diabetes-misinformation-on-tv/

Brown-Riggs, C. (2012, November 26). *Diabetes Myths and Misinformation.* Retrieved March 8, 2015, from Eating Soulfully Blog: http://www.eatingsoulfully.com/blog/?p=1334

Campbell, L. (2013, July 26). *Increased Disability with Diabetes - Will This Affect Disability Insurance Claims?* Retrieved March 8, 2015, from News Articles: http://www.lawyersandsettlements.com/articles/Diabetes-Medication-Side-Effects/diabetes-disability-insurance-claims-18931.html#.VP0MYfnF-Ah

CBS News. (2015). *Diabetes: 10 Deadliest Myths.* Retrieved March 8, 2015, from http://www.cbsnews.com/pictures/diabetes-10-deadliest-myths/

ConsumerReports.org. (2009, July). *10 diabetes myths.* Retrieved March 8, 2015, from http://www.consumerreports.org/cro/2013/01/10-diabetes-myths/index.htm

Dahl, M. (2013, August 16). *Iowa woman tries 'tapeworm diet', prompts doctor warning* . Retrieved March 13, 2015, from Today Health: http://www.today.com/health/iowa-woman-tries-tapeworm-diet-prompts-doctor-warning-6C10935746

Diabetes Medication Lawsuits. (2013). Retrieved March 8, 2015, from Potential Lawsuit >> Diabetes Medication Side Effects Lawsuits: http://www.lawyersandsettlements.com/lawsuit/Diabetes-Medication-Side-Effects.html?opt=b&utm_expid=3607522-2.QRdCdW42SWGLZa0nRc6K3w.1&utm_referrer=http%3A%2F%2Fwww.google.com%2Furl%3Fsa%3Dt%26rct%3Dj%26q%3D%26esrc%3Ds%26source%3Dweb%26cd%3D1%26ved%3D0CE8Q

Diet.st 20. (2015, March 11). *20 Crazy Ways People Used To Diet.* Retrieved March 13, 2015, from http://www.diet.st/20-crazy-ways-people-used-to-diet/6/

Diet.st 20. (2015, March 11). *Tapeworm Diet.* Retrieved March 13, 2015, from 20 Crazy Ways People Used To Diet: http://www.diet.st/20-crazy-ways-people-used-to-diet/9/

FDA Medwatch Report. (2013, July 23). *Beware of Illegally Sold Diabetes Treatments.* Retrieved March 8, 2015, from U.S. Food and Drug Administration - For Consumers: http://www.fda.gov/ForConsumers/ConsumerUpdates/ucm361487.htm

Gary Coody, R. (2013, February 15). *FDA Cracks Down on Flu Product Scammers.* Retrieved March 8, 2015, from FDA Voice: http://blogs.fda.gov/fdavoice/index.php/2013/02/fda-cracks-down-on-flu-product-scammers-2/

Huff, E. (2011, May 19). *Prevent illness by increasing your intake of potassium.* Retrieved March 8, 2015, from Natural News: http://www.naturalnews.com/032456_potassium_disease_prevention.html

Imber, S. (2013, February 26). *Avoid The Top 3 "Natural" Products That Threaten Your Heart.* Retrieved March 8, 2015, from The Partnership for Safe Medicines.org: http://www.safemedicines.org/2013/02/be-heart-smart-516.html

Imber, S. (2013, August 8). *FDA Warns Consumers To Beware Bogus Diabetes Treatments.* Retrieved March 8, 2015, from The Partnership for Safe Medicines.org: http://www.safemedicines.org/2013/08/fda-warns-consumers-to-beware-bogus-diabetes-treatments-545.html

Jenny Ruhl. (2014 (e)). *Other Dangerous Drugs for People with Diabetes.* Retrieved March 8, 2015, from Blood Sugar 101: http://www.phlaunt.com/diabetes/14046942.php

Joslin Diabetes Center. (2015). *Four Myths About Diabetes.* Retrieved March 8, 2015, from http://www.joslin.org/info/4_Myths_About_Diabetes.html

Joslin Diabetes Center. (2015). *Oral Diabetes Medications Summary Chart.* Retrieved March 8, 2015, from Managing Diabetes: http://www.joslin.org/info/oral_diabetes_medications_summary_chart.html

Justice Matters Action Center. (2014 (e)). *What Class Action Lawsuits Mean to You.* Retrieved March 8, 2015, from National Partnership for Women and Families: http://www.justicemattersactioncenter.org/class-action-lawsuits/

Lihn AS, P. S. (2005, February). *Adiponectin: action, regulation and association to insulin sensitivity.* Retrieved March 8, 2015, from US National Library of Medicine National Institutes of Health: http://www.ncbi.nlm.nih.gov/pubmed/15655035

Main, D. (2013, December 5). *Sharks Do Get Cancer: Tumor Found in Great White.* Retrieved March 13, 2015, from Sharks: http://news.discovery.com/animals/sharks/sharks-do-get-cancer-tumor-found-in-great-white-131205.htm

Manju Chandran, M. S. (2003, May 7). *Adiponectin: More Than Just Another Fat Cell Hormone?* Retrieved March 8, 2015, from American Diabetes Association (ADA) Diabetes Care: http://care.diabetesjournals.org/content/26/8/2442.full

Mayo Clinic Staff. (2013, May 30). *Sodium: How to tame your salt habit.* Retrieved March 8, 2015, from Healthy Lifestyle - Nutrition and healthy eating: http://www.mayoclinic.org/healthy-living/nutrition-and-healthy-eating/in-depth/sodium/art-20045479

Mayo Clinic Staff. (2014, September 20). *Diabetes treatment: Medications for type 2 diabetes.* Retrieved March 8, 2015, from Disease and Conditions - Type 2 Diabetes: http://www.mayoclinic.org/diseases-conditions/type-2-diabetes/in-depth/diabetes-treatment/art-20051004

Mayo Clinic Staff. (2014, August 12). *Reye's Syndrome.* Retrieved March 13, 2015, from Diseases and Conditions: http://www.mayoclinic.org/diseases-conditions/reyes-syndrome/basics/definition/con-20020083

Medicinenet.com. (1996-2015). *Diabetes Treatment.* Retrieved March 10, 2015, from http://www.medicinenet.com/diabetes_treatment/article.htm#medications_for_type_2_diabetes

MedWatch The FDA Safety Information and Adverse Event Reporting Program. (2010, October 8). *Meridia (sibutramine): Market Withdrawal Due to Risk of Serious Cardiovascular Events.* Retrieved March 8, 2015, from FDA - Safety: http://www.fda.gov/Safety/MedWatch/SafetyInformation/SafetyAlertsforHumanMedicalProducts/ucm228830.htm

Moore, E. A. (2014, October 10). *New diabetes breakthrough 'bigger than the discovery of insulin.* Retrieved March 8, 2015, from Fox News Health: http://www.foxnews.com/health/2014/10/10/new-diabetes-breakthrough-bigger-than-discovery-insulin/?intcmp=obmod_ffo&tintcmp=obnetwork

Nancy Klobassa Davidson, R. a. (2011, August 4). *Top 10 diabetes myths.* Retrieved March 8, 2015, from Living with diabetes blog: http://www.mayoclinic.org/diseases-conditions/diabetes/expert-blog/diabetes-myths/bgp-20056514

National Cancer Institute. (n.d.). *Artificial Sweeteners and Cancer.* Retrieved March 8, 2015, from 2009: http://www.cancer.gov/cancertopics/causes-prevention/risk-factors/diet/artificial-sweeteners-fact-sheet

Payne, J. W. (2010, November 11). *6 Common Myths and Misconceptions About Diabetes.* Retrieved March 8, 2015, from http://health.usnews.com/health-news/family-health/diabetes/articles/2010/11/11/6-common-myths-and-misconceptions-about-diabetes-2

Ponder, D. S. (2012). *Dr. Ponder: Best Intentions Can Lead To Misinformation About Diabetes.* Retrieved March 8, 2015, from http://m.oaoa.com/people/health/dr_ponder_on_diabetes/article_f897b04a-7590-52ed-8a8d-123d37719d10.html?mode=jqm

Richards, C. (2011, July 18). *Misinformation.* Retrieved March 8, 2015, from Country Girl Diabetic Blogspot: http://countrygirldiabetic.blogspot.com/2011/07/misinformation.html

SCOPPE, C. R. (2013, August 14). *Scoppe: Lonnie Randolph case triggers avalanche of misinformation.* Retrieved March 8, 2015, from The State - Opinion: http://www.thestate.com/2013/08/14/2917690_scoppe-lonnie-randolph-case-triggers.html?rh=1

Steven D. Ehrlich, N. (2011). *Potassium.* Retrieved March 8, 2015, from Health Information: http://umm.edu/health/medical/altmed/supplement/potassium

The Washington Times. (2004, August 16). *Edwards' malpractice suits leave bitter taste.* Retrieved March 8, 2015, from http://www.washingtontimes.com/news/2004/aug/16/20040816-011234-1949r/?page=all

Thomson Healthcare. (2015). *Glyburide And Metformin (Oral Route).* Retrieved March 8, 2015, from Drugs and Supplements - Precautions: http://www.mayoclinic.org/drugs-supplements/glyburide-and-metformin-oral-route/precautions/drg-20061991

U.S. Food and Drug Administration. (2013, March 14). *Incretin Mimetic Drugs for Type 2 Diabetes: Early Communication - Reports of Possible Increased Risk of Pancreatitis and Pre-cancerous Findings of the Pancreas.* Retrieved March 8, 2015, from FDA - Safety: http://www.fda.gov/Safety/MedWatch/SafetyInformation/SafetyAlertsforHumanMedicalProducts/ucm343805.htm

University of Gothenburg. (2011, November 2). *Obesity hormone adiponectin increases the risk of osteoporosis in the elderly, study finds.* Retrieved March 8, 2015, from Science Daily - Featured Research: http://www.sciencedaily.com/releases/2011/11/111101171036.htm

WebMd. (2005-2015). *Drugs & Medications Search.* Retrieved March 8, 2015, from Drugs and Medications Center: http://www.webmd.com/drugs/condition-594-Type+2+Diabetes+Mellitus.aspx

WebMd. (2005-2015). *Potassium and Your Heart.* Retrieved March 8, 2015, from Heart Disease Health Center: http://www.webmd.com/heart-disease/potassium-and-your-heart?page=2

WebMd. (2005-2015). *Vitamins and Supplements Lifestyle Guide.* Retrieved March 8, 2015, from http://www.webmd.com/vitamins-and-supplements/lifestyle-guide-11/supplement-guide-potassium

WebMd. (2013). *Why is potassium important?* Retrieved March 8, 2015, from A-Z Guides: http://www.webmd.com/a-to-z-guides/potassium-content-of-fruits-vegetables-and-other-foods-topic-overview

WiseGeek. (2003-2015). *What Are the Effects of High Potassium Levels?* Retrieved March 8, 2015, from http://www.wisegeekhealth.com/what-are-the-effects-of-high-potassium-levels.htm

CHAPTER 12

Ablow, D. K. (2013, October 22). *President Obama wants you and your kids to be his co-victims.* Retrieved March 9, 2015, from Fox News Opinion: http://www.foxnews.com/opinion/2013/10/22/president-obama-wants-and-your-kids-to-be-his-co-victims/?intcmp=HPBucket

Ballotpedia. (2015). *Barack Obama.* Retrieved March 15, 2015, from Ballotpedia: http://ballotpedia.org/Barack_Obama

Beaumont-Thomas, B. (2014, March 25). *Gérard Depardieu launches 'Proud to be Russian' line of watches.* Retrieved March 15, 2015, from Gérard Depardieu: http://www.theguardian.com/film/2014/mar/25/gerard-depardieu-cvstos-watches-proud-to-be-russian

Berger, J. (2014, January 20). *Parallel universe': Woman spends 6 weeks trying to disenroll from ObamaCare.* Retrieved March 9, 2015, from Fox News Politics: http://www.foxnews.com/politics/2014/01/20/parallel-universe-woman-spends-6-weeks-trying-to-disenroll-from-obamacare/?intcmp=latestnews

Berwick, D. D. (2012, August). *Affordable Care Act Overview.* Retrieved March 15, 2015, from "The Triple Aim: Health, Care, and Cost: Public Health and the Health Care Transition: https://www.apha.org/~/media/files/pdf/topics/aca/aca_overview_aug2012.ashx

Blake, A. (2014, November 13). *Nancy Pelosi says she doesn't know who Jonathan Gruber is. She touted his work in 2009.* Retrieved March 9, 2015, from The Washington Post Blogs: http://www.washingtonpost.com/blogs/the-fix/wp/2014/11/13/nancy-pelosi-says-she-doesnt-know-who-jonathan-gruber-is-she-touted-his-work-in-2009/

Brown, (. S. (2013, December 3). *Stunning hypocrisy from Democrats in wake of ObamaCare's broken promises.* Retrieved March 9, 2015, from Fox News - Opinion: http://www.foxnews.com/opinion/2013/12/03/stunning-hypocrisy-from-democrats-in-wake-obamacare-broken-promises/?intcmp=trending

Bureau of Labor Statistics. (2015, February). *The Employment Situation.* Retrieved March 10, 2015, from http://www.bls.gov/news.release/pdf/empsit.pdf

Christopher, T. (2013, October 23). *CNN's Carol Costello: Obama's People Can Be 'Nasty,' Willing to 'Threaten Your Job'.* Retrieved March 9, 2015, from Mediaite: http://www.mediaite.com/tv/cnns-carol-costello-obamas-people-can-be-nasty-willing-to-threaten-your-job/

Christopher, T. (2013, November 8). *Fox News Cancer Patient Bill Elliott Doesn't Have to Die.* Retrieved March 9, 2015, from Mediaite: http://www.mediaite.com/tv/fox-news-cancer-patient-bill-elliott-doesnt-have-to-die/

Conover, C. (2014, April 1). *How Well Is Obamacare Covering The Uninsured? A Glass Half Empty Moment.* Retrieved March 9, 2015, from Forbes - Opinion: http://www.forbes.com/sites/theapothecary/2014/04/01/how-well-is-obamacare-covering-the-uninsured-a-glass-half-empty-moment/

Consumer Reports. (2013, October). *Guide to health care reform.* Retrieved March 9, 2015, from http://www.consumerreports.org/cro/health/insurance/health-care-countdown/index.htm?EXTKEY=AFOXDIG01

C-SPAN Video. (2014, December 9). *Hearing Jonathan Gruber Marilyn-Tavenner Health Care Enrollment.* Retrieved March 15, 2015, from Health Care Law Enrollment: http://www.c-span.org/video/?323115-1/hearing-jonathan-gruber-marilyn-tavenner-health-care-enrollment

Davis, M. J. (2013, August 23). *Misconceptions about the ACA and COBRA.* Retrieved March 9, 2015, from Employee Benefits Adviser: http://eba.benefitnews.com/news/Misconceptions-about-aca-cobra-2735536-1.html?ET=ebabenefitnews:e8059:2102959a:&tst=email&utm_source=editorial&utm_medium=email&utm_campaign=EBA_inBrief_082913

Dayen, D. (2014, November 21). *http://www.thefiscaltimes.com/Columns/2014/11/21/Why-Gruber-gate-So-Devastating-Democrats.* Retrieved March 9, 2015, from The Fiscal Times - Opinion: http://www.thefiscaltimes.com/Columns/2014/11/21/Why-Gruber-gate-So-Devastating-Democrats

EDELMAN, A. (2013, October 2). *Jimmy Kimmel proves that many Americans don't understand there's no difference between Obamacare and the Affordable Care Act.* Retrieved March 9, 2015, from New York Daily News: http://www.nydailynews.com/news/politics/jimmy-kimmel-proves-americans-don-understand-no-difference-obamacare-affordable-care-act-article-1.1474442

Ehley, B. (2014, November 21). *Obamacare Deductibles, Already High, Climb in 2015.* Retrieved March 15, 2015, from Policy + Politics: http://www.thefiscaltimes.com/2014/11/21/Obamacare-Deductibles-Already-High-Climb-2015

Elizabeth Davis, R. (2014). *Copay Vs Coinsurance—What's the Difference & Which Is Riskier?* Retrieved March 9, 2015, from About Health - Health Insurance: http://healthinsurance.about.com/od/faqs/f/Whats-The-Difference-Between-Copay-And-Coinsurance.htm

Elizabeth Davis, R. (2015). *Out-of-Pocket Maximum—How It Works and Why to Beware.* Retrieved March 9, 2015, from Health Insurance - Health Insurance Basics: http://healthinsurance.about.com/od/healthinsurancebasics/a/Out-of-pocket-Maximum-how-It-Works-And-Why-To-Beware.htm

Feyman, Y. (2013, October 2). *Three things you don't know about ObamaCare (but should).* Retrieved March 9, 2015, from Fox News Opinion: http://www.foxnews.com/opinion/2013/10/02/what-dont-know-about-obamacare-but-should/?intcmp=obinsite

Foxnews.com. (2013, December 8). *Just a PR problem? ObamaCare architect claims 'big PR campaign' needed.* Retrieved March 9, 2015, from Politics: http://www.foxnews.com/politics/2013/12/08/what-holding-back-obamacare-architect-says-big-pr-campaign/

Gottlieb, S. (2013, December 9). *No, You Can't Keep Your Drugs Either Under Obamacare.* Retrieved March 9, 2015, from Forbes - Pharma & Healthcare: http://www.forbes.com/sites/scottgottlieb/2013/12/09/no-you-cant-keep-your-drugs-either-under-obamacare/

Governor Tommy Thompson, (.-W. a. (1997, March 6). *The Good News About Welfare Reform: Wisconsin's Success Story.* Retrieved March 9, 2015, from Welfare and Welfare Spending: http://www.heritage.org/research/lecture/hl593nbsp-the-good-news-about-welfare-reform

Hagar, R. (2013, December 5). *Harry Reid denies CNN report that he's only top congressional leader to exempt some staff from health exchanges.* Retrieved March 9, 2015, from Inside Nevada Politics: http://blogs.rgj.com/politics/2013/12/05/harry-reid-denies-cnn-report-that-hes-only-congressional-leader-to-exempt-some-staff-from-health-exchanges/

Hall, W. (2013, November 8). *Cancer Patient's Plan Canceled: 'I Will Pay $95 Fine And Let Nature Take Its Course'.* Retrieved March 9, 2015, from http://www.breitbart.com/big-government/2013/11/08/cancer-patient-plan-canceled-i-will-pay-95-fine-and-let-nature-take-its-course/

Health Insurance Marketplace. (2014 (e)). *A one-page guide to the Health Insurance Marketplace.* Retrieved March 9, 2015, from A quick guide to the marketplace: https://www.healthcare.gov/quick-guide/

Healthcare.gov. (2014 (e)). *What Marketplace health plans cover.* Retrieved March 9, 2015, from What Plans Cover: https://www.healthcare.gov/coverage/what-marketplace-plans-cover/

Hoskins, M. (2013, March 11). *Why Less Costly Diabetes Supplies Might Not Be Good News.* Retrieved March 9, 2015, from Diabetes Mine: http://www.healthline.com/diabetesmine/why-less-costly-diabetes-supplies-might-not-be-good-news

Howard, P. (2013, September 27). *How to cut through the spin about ObamaCare premiums.* Retrieved March 9, 2015, from Fox News Opinion: http://www.foxnews.com/opinion/2013/09/27/beyond-spin-on-obamacare-premiums/

Howley, P. (2013, October 25). *Michelle Obama's Princeton classmate is executive at company that built Obamacare website.* Retrieved March 9, 2015, from The Daily Caller - US: http://dailycaller.com/2013/10/25/michelle-obamas-princeton-classmate-is-executive-at-company-that-built-obamacare-website/

iHealthcare Updates. (2014). *List of Obamacare Premium Rates Across the US.* Retrieved March 9, 2015, from Healthcare Reform: http://www.ihealthcareupdates.com/obamacare-premium-rates/?utm_source=OutBrain&utm_medium=cpc_brain_HCR&utm_campaign=Out+Brain+Campaing+US+HealthcareReform

Kaczynski, A. (2014, June 2). *7 Times Barack Obama Promised To Reform The VA.* Retrieved March 15, 2015, from Buzzfeed News: http://www.buzzfeed.com/andrewkaczynski/7-times-barack-obama-promised-to-reform-the-va#.eo4BrJBwx

Kaiser Family Foundation. (2012, December 26). *Health Coverage Under the*

Affordable Care Act. Retrieved March 9, 2015, from Journal of the American Medical Association - Visualizing Health Policy: http://jama.jamanetwork.com/article.aspx?articleid=1487506

Kathleen Sebelius won't intervene in girl's lung transplant case. (2013, June 4). Retrieved March 9, 2015, from CBS News - CBS/AP: http://www.cbsnews.com/news/kathleen-sebelius-wont-intervene-in-girls-lung-transplant-case/

Killough, A. (2013, October 2). *Reid gets fiery over question about shutdown's effect on clinical trials for kids.* Retrieved March 9, 2015, from CNN - Political Ticker: http://politicalticker.blogs.cnn.com/2013/10/02/reid-gets-fiery-over-question-about-shutdowns-effect-on-clinical-trials-for-kids/

Kip Sullivan, J. (2014, May 9). *Why Obamacare can't lower costs.* Retrieved March 15, 2015, from Truthdig: http://www.pnhp.org/news/2014/may/why-obamacare-cant-lower-costs

Kohn, S. (2013, September 13). *Five reasons Americans already love ObamaCare – plus one reason why they're gonna love it even more, soon.* Retrieved March 9, 2015, from Fox News Opinion: http://www.foxnews.com/opinion/2013/09/30/five-reasons-americans-already-love-obamacare-plus-one-reason-why-theyre-gonna/?intcmp=trending

Lytle, T. (2013, June 6). *Why Do People Oppose Obamacare? The Answer May Surprise You.* Retrieved March 9, 2015, from CNN Survey: http://blog.aarp.org/2013/06/11/why-do-people-oppose-obamacare-the-answer-may-surprise-you/?cmp=BAC-OUTBRAIN-BLOG_15425878_Why-Do-People-Oppose-Obamacare-The-Answe

Madison K, S. H. (2013, July 10). *Smoking, obesity, health insurance, and health incentives in the Affordable Care Act.* Retrieved March 9, 2015, from US National Library of Medicine National Institutes of Health: http://www.ncbi.nlm.nih.gov/pubmed/23765171

Manhattan Institute for Policy Research, Inc. (2014). *The Obamacare Impact - How The Health Law Affects The Affordability Of Your Health Care.* Retrieved March 9, 2015, from http://www.manhattan-institute.org/knowyourrates/

McClanahan, C. (2012, July 9). *Cliffs Notes Version of the Affordable Care Act.* Retrieved March 9, 2015, from Forbes - Advisor Network: http://www.forbes.com/sites/carolynmcclanahan/2012/07/09/cliffs-notes-version-of-the-affordable-care-act/

Metcal, N. (2013, October 11). *Heard of this little-known benefit of the new health law?* Retrieved March 9, 2015, from Fox Business: http://www.foxbusiness.com/personal-finance/2013/10/11/heard-this-little-known-benefit-new-health-law/?intcmp=obinsite

Michael Bihari, M. (2014). *Out-of-Pocket Maximums*. Retrieved March 9, 2015, from Definitions of Health Insurance Terms: http://healthinsurance.about.com/od/healthinsurancetermso/g/OOP_maximums_definition.htm

Morrissey, E. (2014, May 1). *Obama's Biggest Lie: The ACA Will Lower Health Care Spending - See more at: http://www.thefiscaltimes.com/Columns/2014/05/01/Obama-s-Biggest-Lie-ACA-Will-Lower-Health-Care-Spending#sthash.l7upbQTE.dpuf*. Retrieved March 15, 2015, from Opinion: http://www.thefiscaltimes.com/Columns/2014/05/01/Obama-s-Biggest-Lie-ACA-Will-Lower-Health-Care-Spending

Nussbaum, A. (2013, September 28). *Obamacare Exchanges to Start as Questions Persist: Q&A*. Retrieved March 9, 2015, from Bloomberg Business: http://www.bloomberg.com/news/articles/2013-09-28/obamacare-exchanges-to-start-as-questions-persist-q-a

Obamacare Facts. (2013 (e)). *How ObamaCare Affects Health Insurance Premium Rates*. Retrieved March 9, 2015, from ObamaCare Insurance Premiums: http://obamacarefacts.com/obamacare-health-insurance-premiums/

Obamacare Facts. (2013 (e)). *Learn About Your State's Health Insurance Exchange Marketplace*. Retrieved March 9, 2015, from State Health Insurance Exchange: State Run Exchanges: http://obamacarefacts.com/state-health-insurance-exchange/

Obamacare Facts. (2013 (e)). *New Benefits, Rights and Protections in the Affordable Care Act*. Retrieved March 9, 2015, from Benefits Of ObamaCare: Advantage of ObamaCare: http://obamacarefacts.com/benefitsofobamacare/

Physicians for a National Health Program. (2015). *What is Single Payer?* Retrieved March 9, 2015, from http://www.pnhp.org/facts/what-is-single-payer

Poe, S. (2013, September 24). *Obamacare's Pink Slip Prescription: Hospitals Cut Staff, Services*. Retrieved March 9, 2015, from Free Enterprise: http://archive.freeenterprise.com/health-care/obamacares-pink-slip-prescription-hospitals-cut-staff-services?utm_medium=rss&utm_campaign=sitewide_feed&utm_source=0&utm_source=Taboola&utm_medium=Article_RSS_Feed&utm_campaign=OngoingPaid

ProCon.org. (2015). *Is the Patient Protection and Affordable Care Act (Obamacare) Good for America?* Retrieved March 9, 2015, from Obamacare/Health Care Laws - Pros and Cons: http://healthcarereform.procon.

Przybyla, H. (2013, September 25). *Americans Reject Effort to End Obamacare Amid Ad Barrage*. Retrieved March 9, 2015, from Bloomberg Business: http://www.bloomberg.com/news/articles/2013-09-26/americans-reject-republican-bid-to-end-obamacare-amid-ad-barrage

Reuters. (2013, November 14). *Diabetes battle 'being lost' as cases hit record*

382 million. Retrieved March 9, 2015, from Fox News Health: http://www.foxnews.com/health/2013/11/14/diabetes-battle-being-lost-as-cases-hit-record-382-million/?intcmp=obnetwork

Root, W. A. (2013, October 21). *Why ObamaCare is a fantastic success*. Retrieved March 9, 2015, from Fox News Opinion: http://www.foxnews.com/opinion/2013/10/21/why-obamacare-is-fantastic-success/?intcmp=obnetwork

ROWINGS, L. (2013, October 25). *Boiling down the ACA*. Retrieved March 9, 2015, from Employee Benefits Adviser: http://eba.benefitnews.com/news/boiling-down-aca-2737126-1.html#Login

Roy, A. (2013, October 14). *Obamacare's Website Is Crashing Because It Doesn't Want You To Know How Costly Its Plans Are*. Retrieved March 9, 2015, from Forbes - Pharma & Healthcare: http://www.forbes.com/sites/theapothecary/2013/10/14/obamacares-website-is-crashing-because-it-doesnt-want-you-to-know-health-plans-true-costs/

Roy, A. (2015, February 5). *The Impressive New Obamacare Replace Plan From Republicans Burr, Hatch, And Upton*. Retrieved March 30, 2015, from http://www.forbes.com/sites/theapothecary/2015/02/05/the-impressive-new-obamacare-replace-plan-from-republicans-burr-hatch-and-upton/

Sheppard, N. (2013, October 18). *Dr. Carson Tells Roland Martin Why ObamaCare's The Worst Thing Since Slavery*. Retrieved March 9, 2015, from Newsbusters.org: http://newsbusters.org/blogs/noel-sheppard/2013/10/18/dr-carson-tells-roland-martin-why-obamacare-s-worst-thing-slavery

Starnes, T. (2013, September 27). *President Obama lied to us -- he told America some real whoppers about ObamaCare*. Retrieved March 9, 2015, from Fox News Opinion: http://www.foxnews.com/opinion/2013/09/27/president-obama-lied-to-us-told-america-some-real-whoppers-about-obamacare/?intcmp=trending

Tapper, J. (2012, August 19). *Stephanie Cutter: I Didn't Know 'Facts' of Joe Soptic's Wife's Sickness, Even Though He'd Told Story on Obama Campaign Conference Call*. Retrieved March 9, 2015, from ABC News - Political Punch: http://abcnews.go.com/blogs/politics/2012/08/stephanie-cutter-i-didnt-know-facts-of-joe-soptics-wifes-sickness-even-though-hed-told-story-on-obama-campaign-conference-call/

The Henry J. Kaiser Foundation. (2013). *State Marketplace Profiles: California*. Retrieved March 9, 2015, from Health Reform: http://kff.org/health-reform/state-profile/state-exchange-profiles-california/

The Henry J. Kaiser Foundation. (2013, July 17). *The YouToons Get Ready for Obamacare: Health Insurance Changes Coming Your Way Under the Affordable Care Act*. Retrieved March 9, 2015, from Health Reform: http://kff.org/health-reform/video/youtoons-obamacare-video/

The Henry J. Kaiser Foundation. (2015). *Health Insurance Marketplace Calculator.* Retrieved March 9, 2015, from Health Reform: http://kff.org/interactive/subsidy-calculator/#state=sc&zip=29002&income-type=dollars&income=45000&employer-coverage=0&people=4&talternate-plan-family=individual&adult-count=2&adults%5B0%5D%5Bage%5D=21&adults%5B0%5D%5Btobacco%5D=0&adults%5B1%5D%5Bage%5D=21

The Heritage Foundation. (2013, October 21). *After Repeal of Obamacare: Moving to Patient-Centered, Market-Based Health Care.* Retrieved March 9, 2015, from Health Care: http://www.heritage.org/research/reports/2013/10/after-repeal-of-obamacare-moving-to-patient-centered-market-based-health-care

Thornton, P. (2013, October 2). *Jimmy Kimmel's Obamacare stunt: How infallible is public opinion?* Retrieved March 9, 2015, from LA Times: http://www.latimes.com/opinion/opinion-la/la-ol-jimmy-kimmel-obamacare-government-shutdown-20131002-story.html

Tobak, S. (2013, November 14). *Lies, Damn Lies and ObamaCare.* Retrieved March 9, 2015, from Fox Business - Critical Thinking: http://www.foxbusiness.com/business-leaders/2013/11/14/lies-damn-lies-and-obamacare/?intcmp=fbfeatures

Tuttle, I. (2014, November 14). *Gruber Who?* Retrieved March 9, 2015, from http://www.nationalreview.com/article/392669/gruber-who-ian-tuttle

Volsky, I. (2013, December 10). *No, Obamacare Won't Cover Every Drug — Just Like Every Other Insurance Policy.* Retrieved March 9, 2015, from Think Progress - Health: http://thinkprogress.org/health/2013/12/10/3042741/drugs-obamacare-coverage/

Warren, M. (2013, July 22). *Former ABC News Reader Charles Gibson Touts Obamacare in New Cartoon.* Retrieved March 9, 2015, from The Weekly Standard - The Blog: http://www.weeklystandard.com/blogs/former-abc-news-reader-charles-gibson-touts-obamacare-new-cartoon_740223.html

Wayne, A. (2013, August 19). *ACA success hinges on combating 'misinformation'.* Retrieved March 9, 2015, from Employee Benefits Adviser: http://eba.benefitnews.com/news/aca-success-hinges-combating-misinformation-bloomberg-2735472-1.html

Wayne, A. (2013, September 5). *'Obamacare' insurance costs affordable, Kaiser survey finds.* Retrieved March 9, 2015, from Employee Benefits Adviser: http://eba.benefitnews.com/news/obamacare-insurance-costs-affordable-kaiser-survey-finds-bloomberg-2735895-1.html?ET=ebabenefitnews:e8114:2102959a:&st=email&utm_source=editorial&utm_medium=email&utm_campaign=EBA_inBrief_090513

WebMd. (2005-2015). *Health Care Reform: Health Insurance & Affordable Care Act.* Retrieved March 9, 2015, from Heatlh Care Reform: http://www.webmd.com/health-insurance/default.htm?ecd=wgt_taboola_aca_ad19

Weigel, D. (2014, November 11). *Meet the Mild-Mannered Investment Adviser Who's Humiliating the Administration Over Obamacare.* Retrieved March 15, 2015, from Bloomberg Politics: http://www.bloomberg.com/politics/articles/2014-11-11/meet-the-mildmannered-investment-advisor-whos-humiliating-the-administration-over-obamacare

Wieczner, J. (2013, November 12). *10 things Obamacare won't tell you.* Retrieved March 9, 2015, from Market Watch: http://www.marketwatch.com/story/10-things-health-exchanges-wont-tell-you-2013-09-27/print?guid=A3C21C28-27BC-11E3-944C-00212803FAD6

WIECZNER, J. (2013, October 1). *The 50 states of Obamacare.* Retrieved March 9, 2015, from Market Watch: http://www.marketwatch.com/story/the-50-states-of-obamacare-2013-09-27

Wikipedia. (2015). *Medicare (United States).* Retrieved March 9, 2015, from http://en.wikipedia.org/wiki/Medicare_(United_States)

Williams, J. (2013, October 10). *My ObamaCare surprise.* Retrieved March 9, 2015, from Fox News Opinion: http://www.foxnews.com/opinion/2013/10/10/my-obamacare-surprise/?intcmp=HPBucket

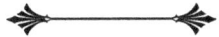

www.ingramcontent.com/pod-product-compliance
Lightning Source LLC
Chambersburg PA
CBHW070846290526
45795CB00001B/9